NUTRITION
IN
OBESITY AND DIABETES

NUTRITION
IN
OBESITY AND DIABETES

Authors

Rebecca Kuriyan Raj MSc MPhil PhD
Associate Professor
St John's Medical College and Research Institute
Head, Nutrition and Lifestyle Clinic, St John's Medical College Hospital
St John's National Academy of Health Sciences
Bengaluru, Karnataka, India

Anura V Kurpad MD PhD FAMS FIUNS
Professor
St John's Medical College
Head, Division of Nutrition, St John's Research Institute
St John's National Academy of Health Sciences
Bengaluru, Karnataka, India

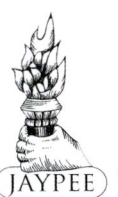

JAYPEE | The Health Sciences Publisher

New Delhi | London | Philadelphia | Panama

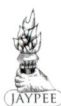 **Jaypee Brothers Medical Publishers (P) Ltd**

Headquarters
Jaypee Brothers Medical Publishers (P) Ltd
4838/24, Ansari Road, Daryaganj
New Delhi 110 002, India
Phone: +91-11-43574357
Fax: +91-11-43574314
Email: jaypee@jaypeebrothers.com

Overseas Offices

J.P. Medical Ltd
83 Victoria Street, London
SW1H 0HW (UK)
Phone: +44 20 3170 8910
Fax: +44 (0)20 3008 6180
Email: info@jpmedpub.com

Jaypee-Highlights Medical Publishers Inc
City of Knowledge, Bld. 237, Clayton
Panama City, Panama
Phone: +1 507-301-0496
Fax: +1 507-301-0499
Email: cservice@jphmedical.com

Jaypee Medical Inc
The Bourse
111 South Independence Mall East
Suite 835, Philadelphia, PA 19106, USA
Phone: +1 267-519-9789
Email: jpmed.us@gmail.com

Jaypee Brothers Medical Publishers (P) Ltd
17/1-B Babar Road, Block-B, Shaymali
Mohammadpur, Dhaka-1207
Bangladesh
Mobile: +08801912003485
Email: jaypeedhaka@gmail.com

Jaypee Brothers Medical Publishers (P) Ltd
Bhotahity, Kathmandu, Nepal
Phone: +977-9741283608
Email: kathmandu@jaypeebrothers.com

Website: www.jaypeebrothers.com
Website: www.jaypeedigital.com

© 2015, Jaypee Brothers Medical Publishers

The views and opinions expressed in this book are solely those of the original contributor(s)/author(s) and do not necessarily represent those of editor(s) of the book.

All rights reserved. No part of this publication may be reproduced, stored or transmitted in any form or by any means, electronic, mechanical, photocopying, recording or otherwise, without the prior permission in writing of the publishers.

All brand names and product names used in this book are trade names, service marks, trademarks or registered trademarks of their respective owners. The publisher is not associated with any product or vendor mentioned in this book.

Medical knowledge and practice change constantly. This book is designed to provide accurate, authoritative information about the subject matter in question. However, readers are advised to check the most current information available on procedures included and check information from the manufacturer of each product to be administered, to verify the recommended dose, formula, method and duration of administration, adverse effects and contraindications. It is the responsibility of the practitioner to take all appropriate safety precautions. Neither the publisher nor the author(s)/editor(s) assume any liability for any injury and/or damage to persons or property arising from or related to use of material in this book.

This book is sold on the understanding that the publisher is not engaged in providing professional medical services. If such advice or services are required, the services of a competent medical professional should be sought.

Every effort has been made where necessary to contact holders of copyright to obtain permission to reproduce copyright material. If any have been inadvertently overlooked, the publisher will be pleased to make the necessary arrangements at the first opportunity.

Inquiries for bulk sales may be solicited at: jaypee@jaypeebrothers.com

Nutrition in Obesity and Diabetes / Rebecca Kuriyan Raj and Anura V Kurpad

First Edition: **2015**

ISBN: 978-93-5152-421-2

Printed at: Samrat Offset Pvt. Ltd.

Dedications

We dedicate this book to our families for their constant guidance, strength, understanding, and love

Contents

Preface ix
Acknowledgments xi

Chapter 1
Energy Requirements 1

Chapter 2
Nutritional Assessment and Body Composition 12

Chapter 3
Role of Nutrition and Lifestyle in Obesity and Diabetes 34

Chapter 4
Goals of Nutritional Management in Obesity and Diabetes 51

Chapter 5
Nutritional Management in the Obese 54

Chapter 6
Nutrition in Type 1 Diabetic Children 91

Chapter 7
Type 2 Diabetes Mellitus 106

Chapter 8
Gestational Diabetes Mellitus 116

Chapter 9
Nutrition in Complications of Diabetes 125

Chapter 10
Complementary and Alternative Medicine Therapy for Obesity and Diabetes 136

Appendix 1:	Nutritive Value of Common Indian Cooked Foods	151
Appendix 2:	Carbohydrate Counting	190
Appendix 3:	Seven Day Menu with Recipes and Nutritive Value	198
Appendix 4:	Sample Exchange List	217
Appendix 5:	Energy Cost of Common Activities	222
Appendix 6:	Case Studies	227

Index   237

Preface

Nutrition in Obesity and Diabetes is targeted towards health professionals dealing with overweight and diabetic individuals in their daily practice. In view of the increasing prevalence of overweight and diabetes in South East Asia and India in particular, our vision has been to provide the reader with the scientific evidence required while planning prevention strategies or treatment guidelines for overweight, obese, and diabetic individuals. It provides health professionals with an updated, extensive reference source, compiled by experts. This book is an essential purchase for professionals working in nutrition, medicine, endocrinology, health sciences, and related areas. It was our aim to have a practical orientation, with emphasis on evidence based nutrition practice in obesity and diabetes.

Each chapter has a brief abstract, introduction, and conclusion. Chapters 1 and 2 cover the basic principles of estimating energy requirements of an individual and assessment of nutritional status and body composition. Readers will find these sections very useful as nutritional assessment and estimating energy requirement are the fundamental steps before planning a dietary schedule. Chapter 3 discusses the existing evidence of the role of nutrition and lifestyle factors in the etiology of obesity and diabetes. The nutritional goals in the management of obesity and diabetes are emphasized in chapter 4. Chapter 5 discusses the different treatment options for obesity and includes sections by experts on physical activity and behavioral modifications. The nutritional management of different types of diabetes and complications of diabetes are described in chapters 6–9. Complementary and alternative medicine therapies are becoming more popular and chapter 10 reviews the evidence on some of the complementary and alternative therapies used for patients with obesity and diabetes.

We are particularly pleased with providing readers with a ready reckoner appendix section. This is the main distinct and invaluable highlight of this book. This section provides tables with macro- and micronutrient content of more than 350 food items which can be used to plan individualized diets, exhaustive list of energy cost of activities which can be used to calculate energy expenditure of an individual and to plan exercise schedules. Healthy recipe options with nutritive values and menu plans with Indian, Continental, and Pan Asian options have also been included. The information in the tables and the appendix in general, will be of great use while planning diets and counseling individuals on their daily food intake. Case studies have been included to demonstrate on how to apply the theory into practice. We are very hopeful that this book will be of great utility to students, nutritionists, and all health professionals.

Rebecca Kuriyan Raj
Anura V Kurpad

Acknowledgments

The task of writing this book would not have been possible without support from so many. The authors would particularly like to thank Ms Deepa P Lokesh for all her contributions towards the textbook, especially with the ready reckoner appendices. We appreciate the efforts of Ms Farheen Dhinda and Ms Annie R Matilda in the planning and organization of the ready reckoner appendices. The authors would like to express their gratitude to Dr Sunita Simon Kurpad and Dr Sumathi Swaminathan for their contribution to the sections in Treatment of Obesity. The photographs were taken by Mr MS Shaju, Mr J Jayakumar, and Dr Dhinagaran and the authors would like to express their gratitude to them.

CHAPTER 1

Energy Requirements

> **Abstract**
>
> The goal of this chapter is to introduce the reader to the principles of energy requirement, basal metabolic rate, total energy expenditure, physical activity level and components of energy expenditure. It reviews the different methods of measuring energy expenditure such as direct calorimetry, indirect calorimetry, heart rate monitoring, doubly labeled water, and their physiological correlates. Since the estimation of energy requirement is one of the key steps in planning a dietary schedule for an obese or diabetic patient, this chapter also discusses how to arrive at estimates of energy requirements in an individual.

Introduction

The human body requires energy for maintaining body temperature, metabolic activities, physical work, and growth. Recommendations for dietary energy intake from food must satisfy these requirements for the attainment and maintenance of optimal health, physiological function, and well-being (WHO, 2004).[1] Energy intakes of individuals vary on a daily basis and it is possible for an individual to have a grossly inadequate food intake, lose weight, and become underweight or have high energy intakes leading to obesity. The methods used to assess energy intake are weighed or observed diet records, dietary recalls and food frequency questionnaires. Measurements of total energy expenditure (TEE) by doubly labelled water (DLW) has shown that reported energy intakes are underestimated[2,3] and the underreporting varies from 10% to 45% depending on age, gender, and body composition of the individuals.[4]

Currently, it is recommended that the requirements of energy should be assessed in terms of energy expenditure rather than energy intake. The energy requirements can be specified in terms of measures of energy expenditure plus the additional energy needs for growth, pregnancy, and lactation. Body weight is an important indicator of whether the energy intake is adequate, inadequate, or excess, and this is reflected over time by changes in body weight. In order to achieve energy balance, the dietary energy intake (input) must be equal to TEE (output). An individual is assumed to be in a steady state, when energy balance is maintained over a prolonged period (WHO, 2004).[1] While humans can adapt to small changes in energy intake through various physiological and behavioral responses related to energy expenditure, large changes (high or low) in energy intakes could cause biological and behavioral compromises, such as reduced growth velocity, loss of muscle mass, increased deposition of body fat, increased risk of disease, forced rest periods, and physical or social limitations in performing certain activities and tasks.

Key Terms

- **Energy requirement:** Energy requirement is the amount of food energy needed to balance energy expenditure in order to maintain body size, body composition, and a level of necessary and desirable physical activity consistent with long-term good health. This includes the energy needed for the optimal growth and development of children, for the deposition of tissues during pregnancy, and for the secretion of milk during lactation consistent with the good health of mother and child.
- **Basal metabolic rate (BMR):** The minimal rate of energy expenditure compatible with life. It is measured in the supine position under standard conditions of rest, fasting, immobility, thermoneutrality, and mental relaxation. Depending on its use, the rate is usually expressed per minute, per hour or per 24 hours.
- **Total energy expenditure:** The energy spent, on average, in a 24-hour period by an individual or a group of individuals. By definition, it reflects the average amount of energy spent in a typical day, but it is not the exact amount of energy spent each and every day.
- **Physical activity level (PAL):** Total energy expenditure for 24 hours expressed as a multiple of BMR, and calculated as TEE/BMR for 24 hours. In adult men and non-pregnant, non-lactating women, BMR times PAL is equal to TEE or the daily energy requirement.
- **Joule:** It is a unit of energy, defined as the energy required to move 1 kg of mass by 1 m by a force of 1 Newton acting on it.
- **Kilocalorie (kcal):** Kilocalorie is a commonly used unit of energy, defined as the heat required to raise the temperature of 1 kg of water by 1°C from 14.5°C to 15.5°C.

    1 kcal = 4.184 KJ (Kilo Joule)
    1 KJ = 0.239 kcal
    1,000 kcal = 4,184 KJ = 4.184 MJ
    1 MJ = 239 kcal

Components of Energy Expenditure

Total energy expenditure is composed of three main components: (1) basal energy expenditure, (2) thermic effect of food (TEF), and (3) energy expenditure of activity (activity thermogenesis). The components of energy expenditure are highly variable and the total effect of these variances determines the variability in daily energy expenditure between individuals. The main components of TEE are depicted in figure 1.

Basal Metabolic Rate

The BMR is the minimum amount of energy needed to carry on the basic functions of life. A person's BMR reflects the amount of energy used during a 24-hour period, at physical and mental rest in a thermo-neutral environment that prevents the activation of heat generating processes such as shivering. The BMR is measured under standard conditions of being awake in the supine position, 10–12 hours of fasting, 8 hours of physical rest, and being in a state of mental relaxation in an ambient environmental temperature. The BMR remains relatively constant on a daily basis. Depending on age and lifestyle, BMR represents 45–70% of daily TEE.

Due to the restrictive conditions of the BMR, it is often more practical to measure the resting metabolic rate (RMR). The RMR is measured under the same conditions as the BMR, but a 3–4 hour fasting period is adequate and is the energy expended by an individual for activities, necessary for normal body functions and homeostasis (respiration, circulation, synthesis of organic compounds, pumping of ions across the membranes, and maintenance of body temperature). Since it is practically difficult to measure BMR, the RMR

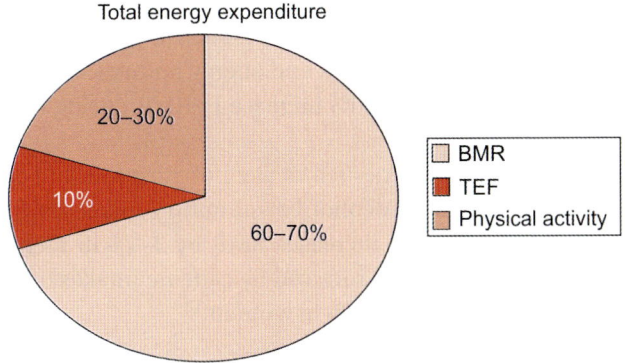

TEF, thermic effect of food; BMR, basal metabolic rate.

Figure 1 Main components of total energy expenditure.

which is about 10–20% higher is used more often.[5] There are many factors that affect the RMR. They are:

- *Age*: The RMR is highest during the first 2 years of life when there is rapid growth[6] and a growing child stores 12–15% of the energy value of food as new tissue. The RMR decreases by 1–2%/kg of fat free mass (FFM), with every decade after early adulthood,[7] may be related to age associated changes in lean body mass (LBM).[8] Regular exercise can maintain a higher LBM and RMR
- *Body composition*: The main predictor of RMR is the FFM, which is the metabolically active tissue in the body. The FFM contributes to about 80% of the variations in RMR.[9] Organs that have a high metabolic rates such as the liver, brain, heart, spleen, and kidneys account for about 60% of RMR[10] and thus the differences in FFM between different ethnic groups could be due to the total mass of these organs,[8] with the RMR being affected by small variation in the mass of these organs[11]
- *Body size*: Lean body mass is highly correlated with the total body size and thus, though obese children have a higher RMR than nonobese children, no differences in RMR are found when the RMR is adjusted for body composition, FFM, and fat mass[12]
- *Climate*: The RMR is 5–20% higher for people living in tropical climates than those living in temperate climates. Increased sweat gland activity caused by exercise in high temperature also increases the RMR
- *Gender*: The differences in body size and body composition are primarily the reason for the gender differences in metabolic rates, with women having 5–10% lower metabolic rates due to their increased fat mass[13]
- *Hormonal status*: Conditions such as hyperthyroidism and hypothyroidism can increase or decrease the metabolic rate. Menstrual cycle affects energy metabolism, with small increases in the metabolic rate during the luteal phase[14] and all the various changes in pregnancy causes a gradual change in BMR.[15] Gut hormones such as ghrelin and peptide YY are involved in appetite regulation and energy homeostatsis[16]
- *Temperature*: There is about 13% increase in RMR during fever for each degree higher than 37°C[17]
- *Miscellaneous factors*: Factors such as alcohol, nicotine, and caffeine can affect the metabolic rate. Alcohol consumption increases RMR by 9% in women,[18] while nicotine increases RMR by 3–4% in men and 6% in women. The increase in RMR induced by caffeine intakes of 200–350 mg is about 7–11% in men and 8–15% in women.[18]

Thermic Effect of Food

The TEF also known as diet induced thermogenesis, specific dynamic action of food is the energy expenditure associated with the consumption, digestion, and absorption of food and accounts for about 10% of TEE. The size and the macronutrient content of a meal affect the TEF.

Physical Activity Thermogenesis

The most variable component of TEE is the energy expenditure for physical activity. It is of two types—(1) exercise and (2) non-exercise activity thermogenesis (NEAT). For individuals who do not take part in any sporting activity, the exercise related activity is zero, while it is about 10% for individuals who exercise regularly. The PAL is the ratio of the TEE to BMR (TEE/BMR).

Measurement of Energy Expenditure

There are many methods available to measure human energy expenditure. They include:
- Direct calorimetry
- Indirect calorimetry
- Heart rate monitoring
- Doubly labelled water
- Physiological correlates.

Direct Calorimetry

Direct calorimetry involves the measurement of an individual in a whole body calorimeter, which is equipped to measure the amount of heat produced by the individual inside the chamber. There are three principal types of direct calorimeter: (1) isothermal, (2) heat sink, and (3) convection systems. These approaches have on occasion been used in combination. This method of measuring energy expenditure is not representative of a free living condition as the physical activity is restricted.

Indirect Calorimetry

Indirect calorimetry estimates heat production indirectly by measuring oxygen consumption (VO_2), the CO_2 production and the respiratory quotient (RQ), which is the ratio of the VCO_2 to VO_2. The RQ reflects substrate utilization and reflect the fuel mixture being metabolized.

Carbohydrate = 1.0
Fat = 0.71
Protein = 0.84
Mixed meal = 0.85

The RMR is obtained from the oxygen consumption using the Wier's equation.[19] A mouthpiece, mask, or a ventilated hood is generally used to

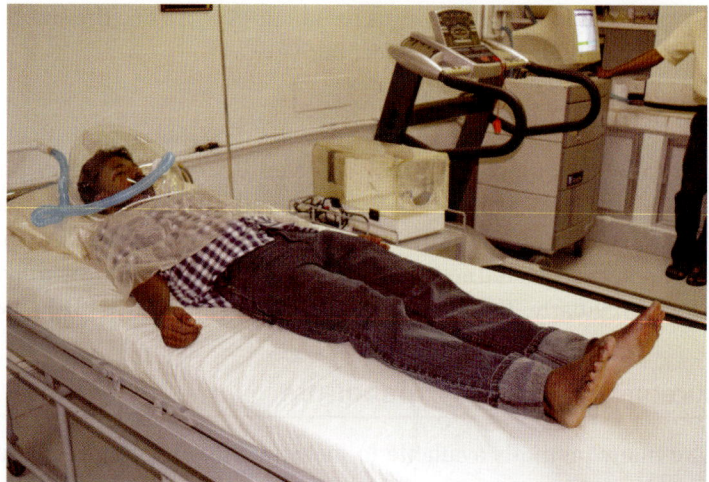

Figure 2 A volunteer undergoing indirect calorimeter using a ventilated hood.

collect the expired carbon dioxide. The indirect calorimetry can be measured using total collection system (rigid total collection system, flexible total collection system), open-circuit indirect calorimeter system (ventilated open-circuit system, expiratory collection open circuit systems), and closed circuit system. Figure 2 depicts a volunteer undergoing indirect calorimeter using a ventilated hood.

Heart Rate Monitoring

The heart rate monitoring method is based on the linear relationship between heart rate and energy expenditure;[20] however, the relationship needs to be calibrated for every individual as there are variations due to age, gender, body size, and nutritional status.[21] The factors that could affect the energy expenditure to heart rate relationship are ambient temperature, hydration status, food intake, emotional state, and smoking. Heart rate monitors are portable, nonrestraining, and can be measured for several days. The heart rate monitoring method provides a reasonably accurate estimate of TEE on a group of individuals rather than on individuals, where it is likely to be subjected to errors.

Doubly Labelled Water

The measurement of TEE by the DLW technique provides a means of validating other methods and measures TEE in free living conditions. DLW is a mixture of stable isotope labelled waters (^2H_2O and $H_2^{18}O$). TBW is measured by isotope dilution as part of the DLW procedure, therefore, an estimate of body composition can be made at the same time as TEE using the DLW technique.

Two stable isotopic forms of water ($H_2^{18}O$ and ^2H_2O) are administered to the individual and their ^{18}O and ^2H_2O disappearance rates from the body are measured for 7–21 days, which is equivalent for these isotopes. The sample used is urine, saliva, or blood. The method is based on the principle that carbon dioxide production can be estimated from the difference in the elimination rates of body hydrogen and oxygen. The water flux is reflected by the disappearance rate of ^2H_2O, while the water flux plus the VCO_2 is reflected by $H_2^{18}O$, due to the rapid equilibrium of body water and bicarbonate pools by carbonic anhydrase. VCO_2 is calculated by the difference between the two disappearance rates, and then assuming a RQ, energy expenditure is calculated. In conditions of energy balance, the RQ is calculated from the composition of the diet using the food quotient (FQ). The accuracy of the DLW method is about 5% and the main advantage is that it is noninvasive, and can be measured in a free living state, while the disadvantages are the high costs of the isotope and the mass spectrometric equipment needed for the analysis.

Physiological Correlates

Activity Recall and Time and Motion Studies

Habitual activity and information on NEAT can be obtained using questionnaires, interviews, and time and motion studies. Although the errors in the data are highly possible due to inaccurate recall and improper data recording, the approaches can be used to assess trends in certain activities such as occupational activities.

Measuring Activity Related Energy Expenditure

Uniaxial monitors are portable devices which measure the degree and intensity of movements in a vertical plane. These monitors have found to be acceptable for estimates of activity related energy expenditure in groups, but have limitations in individuals. A triaxial monitor employs three uniaxial monitors to measure multidirectional movement and has shown to correlate well with energy expenditure from DLW technique.[22]

Estimating Energy Requirements for Indian Adults

The FAO/WHO/UNU expert consultation in 1985 (FAO/WHO/UNU, 1985)[23] used the BMR factors (factorial method) for estimating the energy requirements and this method was adopted by the Indian Council of Medical Research (ICMR) expert group in 1989 to arrive at energy requirements

TABLE 1: Prediction equations for BMR (kcal/day)[26]

Category	Age (years)	FAO/WHO/UNU 1985	ICMR expert group 2010
Males	18–30	15.1 × Bwt + 692.2	14.5 × Bwt + 645
	30–60	11.5 × Bwt + 873	10.9 × Bwt + 833
	>60	11.7 × Bwt + 587.7	12.6 × Bwt + 463
Females	18–30	14.8 × Bwt + 486.6	14.0 × Bwt + 471
	30–60	8.1 × Bwt + 845.6	8.3 × Bwt + 788
	>60	9.1 × Bwt + 658.5	10.0 × Bwt + 565

BMR, basal metabolic rate; FAO, Food and Agricultural Association; UNU, United Nations University; ICMR, Indian Council of Medical Research; Bwt, body weight in kg.

estimates for Indian man and woman. This method is based on the time allotted to activities that are performed habitually and the energy cost of those activities and it combines two or more factors such as the sum of energy spent while sleeping, resting, or in household or leisure activities. The time allotted to each activity and its energy cost is used to calculate the energy spent. The TEE is measured as product of predicted BMR and PAL. Equations to predict BMR using body weight of an individual are available.[23] Since the BMR of Indians is about 5% lower[24] than the BMR reported in developed countries, the ICMR developed a set of equations for computing BMR of Indian adults.[25] Table 1 provides the list of equations for predicting BMR, proposed by FAO/WHO/UNU and those for Indians.[26]

Physical Activity Level

The PAL is a major determinant of TEE and can be measured or estimated from the TEE and BMR.

$$PAL = \frac{TEE}{BMR}$$

The PAL values for Indian reference adult man and woman for different categories of work are 1.53 for sedentary work, 1.8 for moderate work, and 2.3 for heavy work.[26] The PAL of an individual can also be obtained from the different physical activity ratio (PAR) values of activities performed in a day.

The PAR is the ratio of energy cost of an individual activity per minute to the cost of the BMR per minute

$$PAR = \frac{\text{Energy cost of an activity per minute}}{\text{Energy cost of basal metabolism per minute}}$$

The metabolic equivalent of task (MET), is a physiological measure of expressing the energy cost of physical activities and is defined as the ratio of metabolic rate (and, therefore, the rate of energy consumption) during a specific physical activity to a reference metabolic rate, set by convention to 3.5 mL of oxygen/min/kg.[27] The MET values of activities range from 0.9 (sleeping) to 18 (running at 17.5 km/h). The Compendium of Physical Activities, published in 1993, 2000, and updated in 2011[27-29] is used mainly in epidemiologic studies to standardize the assignment of MET intensities in physical activity questionnaires and has been used widely to assign intensity units to physical activity questionnaires. MET is a measure of intensity and rate, and thus "MET-minute" can be used to quantify the total amount of physical activity in a way comparable across different persons and types of activities.

Example of Calculating Physical Activity Level of an Individual Spending (Box 1)

A detailed list with PAR values for various activities has been provided in Appendix 5. The energy requirements of Indians at different ages are summarized in table 2.

Box 1	Example of calculating Physical Activity Level of an individual spending
8 hours of sleep (PAR = 1; 8 × 1 = 8 PAR-hours)	
9 hours at work (PAR = 1.7; 9 × 1.7 = 15.3 PAR-hours)	
4 hours of domestic work (PAR = 2; 4 × 2 = 8 PAR hours)	
3 hours of leisure = (PAR = 1.4; 3 × 1.4 = 4.2 PAR hours)	
Total PAR hours = 35.5 hours	
$PAL = \dfrac{Total\ PAR\ hours}{Total\ time} = \dfrac{35.5}{24} = 1.5$	
PAR, physical activity ratio; PAL, physical activity level.	

TABLE 2: Energy requirements of Indians at different ages[26]

Age group	Category	Body weight (kg)	Requirement (kcal/day)	Requirement (kcal/kg/day)
Men	Sedentary	60	2,320	39
	Moderate	60	2,730	46
	Heavy	60	3,490	58
Women	Sedentary	55	1.900	35
	Moderate	55	2.230	41
	Heavy	55	2.850	52
	Pregnant	55 + GWG	+350	
	Lactating	55 + WG	+600	
			+520	

Continued

Continued

Age group	Category	Body weight (kg)	Requirement (kcal/day)	Requirement (kcal/kg/day)
Infants	0–6 months	5.4	500	92
	6–12 months	8.4	670	80
Children	1–3 years	12.9	1,060	82
	4–6 years	18.1	1,350	75
	7–9 years	25.1	1,690	67
Boys	10–12 years	34.3	2,190	64
Girls	10-12 years	35.0	2,010	57
Boys	13–15 years	47.6	2,750	58
Girls	13–15 years	46.6	2,330	50
Boys	16–17 years	55.4	3,020	55
Girls	16–17 years	52.1	2,440	47

GWG, gestational weight gain; WG, gestational weight gain remaining after delivery.

In order to promote weight loss, regardless of the type of diet, it is important to reduce the energy intake to achieve weight loss and once weight loss is achieved, the lower energy intake has to be sustained to prevent weight gain. Calorie restriction of 500–600 kcal/day results in weight loss of 0.5 kg/week and 10% weight loss in 6 months.[30] The amount of energy required for each overweight/obese patient varies and should be planned individually with the help of a dietician.

References

1. Joint FAO/WHO/UNU. Human Energy Requirements. Report of a Joint FAO/WHO/UNU Expert Consultation, Rome, 17-24 Oct 2001. Rome, FAO/WHO/UNU 2004.
2. Schoeller DA. How accurate is self-reported dietary energy intake? Nutr Rev. 1990;48(10):373-9.
3. Goldberg GR, Black AE, Jebb SA, Cole TJ, Murgatroyd PR, Coward WA, et al. Critical evaluation of energy intake data using fundamental principles of energy physiology: 1. Derivation of cut-off limits to identify under-recording. Eur J Clin Nutr. 1991;45(12):569-81.
4. Johnson RK, Soultanakis RP, Matthews DE. Literacy and body fatness are associated with underreporting of energy intake in US low-income women using the multiple-pass 24-hour recall: a doubly labeled water study. J Am Diet Assoc. 1998;98(10):1136-40.
5. Institute of Medicine of the National Academies, Food and Nutrition Board. Dietary reference intakes for energy, carbohydrate, fiber, fat, fatty acids, cholesterol, protein and amino acids. Washington DC: The National Academies Press; 2005.
6. Butte NF, Hopkinson JM, Wong WW, Smith EO, Ellis KJ. Body composition during the first 2 years of life: an updated reference. Pediatr Res. 2000;47(5):578-85.
7. van Pelt RE, Dinneno FA, Seals DR, Jones PP. Age-related decline in RMR in physically active men: relation to exercise volume and energy intake. Am J Physiol Endocrinol Metab. 2001;281(3):E633-9.

8. Gallagher D, Albu J, He Q, Heshka S, Boxt L, Krasnow N, et al. Small organs with a high metabolic rate explain lower resting energy expenditure in African American than in white adults. Am J Clin Nutr. 2006;83(5):1062-7.
9. Bosy-Westphal A, Reinecke U, Schlörke T, Illner K, Kutzner D, Heller M, et al. Effect of organ and tissue masses on resting energy expenditure in underweight, normal weight and obese adults. Int J Obes Relat Metab Disord. 2004;28(1):72-9.
10. Gallagher D, Belmonte D, Deurenberg P, Wang Z, Krasnow N, Pi-Sunyer FX, et al. Organ-tissue mass measurement allows modeling of REE and metabolically active tissue mass. Am J Physiol. 1998; 275(2 Pt 1):E249-58.
11. Javed F, He Q, Davidson LE, Thornton JC, Albu J, Boxt L, et al. Brain and high metabolic rate organ mass: contributions to resting energy expenditure beyond fat-free mass. Am J Clin Nutr. 2010;91(4):907-12.
12. Byrne NM, Weinsier RL, Hunter GR, Desmond R, Patterson MA, Darnell BE, et al. Influence of distribution of lean body mass on resting metabolic rate after weight loss and weight regain: comparison of responses in white and black women. Am J Clin Nutr. 2003;77(6):1368-73.
13. Poehlman ET. Regulation of energy expenditure in aging humans. J Am Geriatr Soc. 1993;41(5):552-9.
14. Ferraro R, Lillioja S, Fontvieille AM, Rising R, Bogardus C, Ravussin E. Lower sedentary metabolic rate in women compared with men. J Clin Invest. 1992;90(3):780-4.
15. Butte NF, Wong WW, Treuth MS, Ellis KJ, O'Brian Smith E. Energy requirements during pregnancy based on total energy expenditure and energy deposition. Am J Clin Nutr. 2004;79(6):1078-87.
16. Larson-Meyer DE, Ravussin E, Heilbronn L, DeJonge L. Ghrelin and peptide YY in postpartum lactating and nonlactating women. Am J Clin Nutr. 2010;91(2):366-72.
17. Hardy JD, DuBois EF. Regulation of heat loss from the human body. Proc Natl Acad Sci U S A. 1937;23(12):624-31.
18. Compher C, Frankenfield D, Keim N, Roth-Yousey L, Evidence Analysis Working Group. Best practice methods to apply to measurement of resting metabolic rate in adults: a systematic review. J Am Diet Assoc. 2006;106(6):881-903.
19. Weir JB. New methods for calculating metabolic rate with special reference to protein metabolism.1949. Nutrition. 1990;6(3):213-21.
20. Levine JA. Measurement of energy expenditure. Public Health Nutr. 2005;8(7A):1123-32.
21. Research Methods in Nutritional Anthropology. Edited by Gretel H Pelto, Pertti J Petto. Ellen Messer. United Nations University Press; 1989.
22. Plasqui G, Westerterp KR. Physical activity assessment with accelerometers: an evaluation against doubly labelled water. Obesity (Silver Spring). 2007;15(10):2371-9.
23. Joint FAO/WHO/UNU: Energy and Protein requirements. Report of Joint FAO/WHO/UNU Expert Consultants, WHO Tech Rep Series 724, 1985.
24. Shetty PS, Soares MJ, Sheela ML. Basal metabolic rates of South Indian males. Report of FAO, Rome, 1986.
25. Indian Council of Medical Research: Nutrient Requirements and recommended dietary allowances for Indians. A report of the expert group of the Indian Council of Medical Research, ICMR, New Delhi, 1989.
26. Indian Council of Medical Research: Nutrient requirements and recommended dietary allowances for Indians. A report of the expert group of the Indian Council of Medical Research, ICMR, New Delhi, 2010.
27. Ainsworth BE, Haskell WL, Herrmann SD, Meckes N, Bassett Jr DR, Tudor-Locke C, et al. 2011 Compendium of Physical Activities: a second update of codes and MET values. Med Sci Sports Exerc. 2011;43(8):1575-81.
28. Ainsworth BE, Haskell WL, Leon AS, Jacobs DR Jr, Montoye HJ, Sallis JF, et al. Compendium of physical activities: classification of energy costs of human physical activities. Med Sci Sports Exerc. 1993;25(1):71-80.
29. Ainsworth BE, Haskell WL, Whitt MC, Irwin ML, Swartz AM, Strath SJ, et al. Compendium of physical activities: an update of activity codes and MET intensities. Med Sci Sports Exerc. 2000;32(9 Suppl): S498-504.
30. Klein S. Medical management of obesity. Surg Clin North Am. 2001;81:1025-38.

CHAPTER 2

Nutritional Assessment and Body Composition

> **Abstract**
>
> This chapter focuses on nutritional assessment and describes the crucial steps in nutritional assessment such as anthropometry, biochemistry, and clinical and dietary assessment. An accurate assessment of body composition is necessary to identify an individual's health risk associated with an excessively low or high body fat and this chapter provides a comprehensive overview of the different methods for measuring body composition. Equations to estimate percentage body fat using various compartment models (2, 3, 4) are provided in the chapter. The advantages and limitations of the different methods of body composition such as hydrodensitometry, air displacement plethysmography, hydrometry, and dual energy X-ray absorptiometry are discussed.

Nutritional Assessment of the Overweight/Obese Individual

Maintaining optimal nutritional status at any age is important and can contribute to preventing chronic diseases, frequent episodes of illness, shorter and less expensive hospital stays, fewer complications, and a higher survival rate. The nutritional assessment of an individual/patient requires a combination of the history, physical examination, anthropometrics, and laboratory assessment. Nutritional assessment can provide information on the individual before the start of nutritional intervention and can also help to identify individuals needing detailed screening. The assessment of the patient is critical for three purposes:
1. Identification of modifiable lifestyle behaviors (dietary, physical activity, and behavioral practices).
2. Assessment of current and future risks for medical comorbidities.

Nutritional Assessment and Body Composition

3. Assessment of the patient's and family's readiness to make lifestyle changes.

The assessment process includes:
- Review of patient's background data
- Accurate data collection and recording
    - Anthropometric
    - Biochemical
    - Clinical
    - Dietary
- Assessment of physical activity level
- Assessment of individual/patient's motivation and readiness to participate in treatment plan.

Review of Patient's Background Data

This data will provide an insight into the medical history and other factors that may directly or indirectly affect the patient's nutrition needs and health status.

Medical history: It helps to identify health problems and family history that may influence the patient's nutritional status. It is important to assess the presence of underlying diseases such as coronary heart disease, atherosclerotic disease, hypertension, sleep apnea, hypothyroidism, gynecological abnormalities, osteoarthritis, and gall stones.

Drug history: It reviews medications (drugs, nutrient supplements, herbal/ayurvedic drugs that may affect nutritional status).

Socioeconomic history: Details on environmental, personal, religious, social, and economic factors that can influence food availability, food needs, food intake, and nutrient needs.

Accurate Data Collection and Recording

This data can be summarized as: (i) anthropometry, (ii) biochemical, (iii) clinical, and (iv) dietary.

Anthropometric Data

Anthropometric measurements are noninvasive and measure the human body size and proportion. Body weight and height are measures of body size, while ratio of body weight to height represents body proportion. It helps in assessing the nutritional status, identifying individuals at risk, monitoring the efficacy of a nutrition intervention, and in providing information about the body's stores of fat and muscle.

- *Height*—The height is measured to the nearest 0.1 cm using an accurate stadiometer
- *Weight*—Weight is a sensitive indicator of nutritional status. The body weight is measured to the nearest 0.1 kg using a calibrated digital weighing scale. The patient, wearing light clothing is made to stand on the platform of the weighing scale with the body weight evenly distributed. It is important to calibrate the weighing scale on a regular basis using standard weights (WHO, 1995).[1]

The body mass index (BMI), which relates height and weight, can be mathematically calculated as:

$$\frac{\text{Weight in kg}}{\text{height (meters)}^2}$$

The BMI is used to classify individuals as obese, overweight, normal, and underweight. It is popularly used in studies to identify individuals at risk. The World Health Organization (WHO, 1998) classification of BMI is as follows (Table 1).[2]

Studies have shown that for a given BMI, Indians have more body fat than other ethnic groups, both within and outside Asia.[3,4] This is important, because measures of overall obesity and the location of body fat are strongly associated with insulin sensitivity in Indians. Due to the evidence of the relative increase in adiposity in Indians, it has been suggested that the BMI cut-off for noncommunicable diseases should be reduced for Indians and Asians to about 23 kg/m² or even lower (WHO/IASO/IOTF, 2000).[5] The recent WHO Expert Committee while acknowledging this, stopped short of actually suggesting a new BMI cut-off for Indians, instead preferring to refer to a "public health action point" at a BMI of 23 kg/m² (WHO, 2004).[6] This approach will help to define the burden of risk of chronic disease in a population, since reducing BMI cut-off values for overweight and obesity would immediately increase their prevalence rates and, therefore, increase public and clinical awareness, but it is not clear whether it would be ideal for the long-term prevention of death in terms of individuals.

TABLE 1: Classification of body mass index[2]

	Obesity class	BMI (kg/m²)
Underweight		<18.5
Normal		18.5–24.9
Overweight		25.0–29.9
Obesity	I	30.0–34.9
	II	35.0–39.9
Extreme obesity	III	≥40.0

BMI, body mass index.

In children, cut off based on distribution of anthropometric measurements (weight and BMI) are used to define obesity. The Center for Disease Control and Prevention (CDC) 2000 growth reference charts were developed on American children.[7] BMI categories based on pooled six international data sets were developed in 2000, on children aged 2–18 years and these reference curves have been referred to as the International Obesity Task Force (IOTF) standards.[8] These charts assume that the most appropriate cut-off points for overweight and obesity in children are those corresponding to the BMI of 25 kg/m^2 and 30 kg/m^2, respectively, in the BMI distribution for adults, that are recognized internationally as defining overweight and obesity. The IOTF standards have been widely used to classify overweight and obesity in children. IOTF charts, however, provide only overweight and obesity categories and not a full array of percentile levels and are thus not useful for monitoring the BMI progress of individual children. The WHO developed growth standards on children (WHO, 2006)[9,10] and these standards provide an effective tool for detecting both under nutrition and obesity, thus addressing the double burden of malnutrition. For Indian children, age and gender specific BMI cut offs, based on a reference population of urban Indian affluent children have been recently developed by Khadilkar et al.,[11] such that the cut-offs are linked to the adult accepted BMI of 23 kg/m^2 and 28 kg/m^2 for overweight and obesity for Asians. These cut offs can be used to identify overweight and obesity.

Waist circumference: Waist circumference has received recent attention as an indicator of fat and health risks in children and adults (Table 2). The interest in waist circumference stems from research linking accumulated visceral adipose tissue to increased health risks and metabolic disorders in children and adults. Waist circumference is a good indicator of intra-abdominal fat and is normally measured with a nonstretchable tape by trained staff (exerting the same standard pressure on the tape) at the midpoint of the lowest rib cage and the iliac crest, to the nearest 0.1 cm, in a standing position during end-tidal expiration (WHO, 1995).[1]

Misra et al. in 2006,[12] evaluated several waist circumference cut-off points in relation to BMI cut-off points and cardiovascular diseases in Asian Indians residing in north India and proposed action level for adult Asian Indians: action level 1: men, greater than or equal to 78 cm, women, greater than

TABLE 2: The indicators of risk based on waist circumference[2]

Gender	Waist circumference
Men	≥102 cm
Women	≥88 cm

or equal to 72 cm; and action level 2: men, greater than or equal to 90 cm, women, greater than or equal to 80 cm. Kuriyan et al. recently developed waist percentile curves for children aged 3–16 years from urban south India.[13] For a start, until larger dataset from different regions in the country are available, these curves can be used to assess abdominal obesity in Indian children.

Waist-hip ratio: The waist-hip ratio is used as an indirect measure of lower and upper body fat distribution (Table 3). Waist-to-hip ratio is a way of measuring where body fat is stored. "Android" or excess upper body fat is seen more typically in men, while gynoid or excess lower body fat is seen more in women. A high waist-to-hip ratio indicates an increased risk of obesity-related health problems. Waist-to-hip ratio is calculated by dividing the measured waist circumference by the measured hip circumference.

$$\frac{W}{H} = \text{waist-to-hip ratio (WHR)}$$

The accuracy of WHR in assessing visceral fat decreases with increasing levels of fatness.

Body fat estimation: The assessment of the body fat and body composition of the patients will provide an insight into the distribution of fat and lean tissue in the body. Increased body fat has been associated with increased risk for chronic diseases. The various methods of body composition have been discussed in the latter part of the chapter.

Biochemical or Laboratory Data Assessment

Based on the patient's existing signs and symptoms, tests are carried out to identify associated comorbidities. There is no single biochemical test that is indicated for all patients with obesity. Some of the common tests performed to rule out certain conditions are presented in table 4.

Clinical Data

The patient's medical, social, and family history for current and potential obesity related symptoms and diseases need to be reviewed. This includes recording of signs and symptoms of the disease, diagnosis, treatment

TABLE 3: The indicators of risk based on waist-hip ratio[2]

The Indicators of risk	
Gender	WHR circumference
Men	≥1.0
Women	≥0.85

WHR, waist:hip ratio.

TABLE 4: Tests to rule out obesity related comorbidity

Test performed	Condition to rule out
• Fasting blood glucose • Postprandial blood glucose • Glycosylated hemoglobin • Fasted insulin levels	• Diabetes
Fasting blood lipid profile	• Hyperlipidemia
Recording of two or more properly measured blood pressure readings	• Hypertension
Serum thyroid stimulating hormone	• Hypothyroidism
• Serum triglycerides • High density lipoprotein cholesterol • Blood pressure • Fasting glucose	• Metabolic syndrome
Cortisol levels	• Cushing's syndrome
• Total testosterone • Prolactin • Thyroid stimulating hormone	• Polycystic ovarian syndrome

information, medical problems relating to food intake (dysphagia), gastrointestinal problems, and blood pressure. Obesity could affect many organs of the body and thus it is important to clinically evaluate for type 2 diabetes, hypertension, gall bladder disease, and metabolic syndrome. Additionally, in an obese individual, the psychosocial complications may be as significant as the health concerns, since these individuals often experience discrimination, difficulties in work place, and personal life leading to low self-esteem, social withdrawal, depression, and other mental health problems. Thus, a comprehensive clinical assessment of an overweight/obese individual needs to be carried out.

Dietary Data

An accurate diet history is an important component of the nutritional assessment process. The diet history provides valuable information about the patient's past and current food intake patterns. The data recorded must capture what the patient usually eats and drinks. The nutritionist collecting the data must be skilled as patients, especially obese patients, tend to omit important information or underestimate the amounts of food intake. Details captured should include quantity eaten, number of meals eaten, snacking habits, meal preparation methods, and social and family history. The nutritionist should avoid reacting to information provided by the patient and remember that both verbal and nonverbal communication can influence the patient.

Points to remember while performing a dietary assessment include:
- Self-introduction
- Explain the benefits of the assessment to the patient
- Avoid being judgmental
- Use standard measurements to help in getting an idea of the amount of food intake
- Always make plans for follow up.

There are many methods for obtaining a dietary history. The various methods of dietary assessment with their advantages and disadvantages are given in table 5.

Additional data that can be recorded include data on the patient's general health, food habits, and eating habits
- Monthly family consumption of oil, ghee, coconut, and salt
- History of cigarette smoking and alcohol consumption
- Method of meal planning and preparation
- Food purchasing ability
- Usual meal pattern
- Snack consumption
- Place where meals are eaten regularly
- Food preferences/allergies
- Previous dietary restriction
- Use of supplements (vitamin, herbal, nutritional, or mineral)
- Weight changes
- Bowel habits
- Duration of television viewing, frequency of consumption of meals while watching television
- Frequency of eating meals together with family
- Sleep pattern.

Assessment of Physical Activity

Physical activity is an important component of health and well being. Individuals who are physically active have health benefits of lower risk of coronary heart disease, type 2 diabetes, hypertension, hyperlipidemia, osteoporosis, cancer, and depression rates. There are many methods by which the physical activity can be measured—questionnaire, direct observation, electronic monitoring such as pedometers, accelerometers, and heart rate monitors. Appropriate assessment of physical activity patterns requires accurate and reliable instruments. Physical activity questionnaire is a checklist of frequency, intensity, and duration of specific activities within

TABLE 5: Dietary assessment methods

Method	Details	Advantages	Disadvantages
24-hour recall	Information on food intake in the previous 24 hours	Quick and easy Patient need not be literate	• Over-/underestimation is possible • Memory dependent • Not representative of patient's usual intake • Requires a skilled interviewer
Food frequency questionnaire	List of foods or food groups from which the patient selects the frequency with which they are consumed	• Beneficial when used with 24-hour recall • Provides details on food consumption over a period of time with key nutrients • Does not influence the usual diet.	• Needs the patient to be literate, unless interviewed • Details is lacking on meal patterns
Food records/diary	Provides 3–7 days record of actual food intake	• Eliminates errors of recall • Provides an accurate record of food eaten and time of consumption	• Needs the patient to be literate • The patients could alter the food intake during the recording period • Requires recording period of at least 3 days (must include a weekend)

a defined time period (past 24 hours, 1 week, or 1 month). A single page, simple and easy to use physical activity questionnaire has been developed in urban middle class Indians.[14] This questionnaire can be applied to Indian populations to provide valuable insights to physical activity patterns. While the questionnaire is primarily designed for epidemiological use, it can provide insights into physical activity patterns of an individual.

Assessment of Patient's Motivation

Effective treatment for obesity is based on skillful and empathetic communication between the nutritionist/doctor and patients. It is important to evaluate the patient's readiness to make necessary lifestyle changes to lose weight. Suggesting change when patients are not ready, often, leads to frustration and may hamper future efforts. The nutritionist/physician must first assess the patients' readiness for behavior change, and then help them to overcome the barriers to change. The benefits and difficulties of weight management should be discussed with the patient before treatment goals are developed. The patient's readiness and motivation is assessed by evaluating reasons for weight reduction, history of successful and unsuccessful weight loss attempts, family, friends and work support for weight loss, patient's understanding of obesity and its risks, attitude towards physical activity, time available for weight loss, appropriateness of expectations to help establish the likelihood of lifestyle change, psychiatric status, and financial and other barriers.

After the comprehensive assessment of the patient, a nutritional care plan with goals is made catering to individual patient needs.

Body Composition

The measurement of body composition provides an objective means of nutritional assessment and is of interest to nutritionists, medical personnel, and sports scientists. An accurate assessment of body composition is necessary to identify an individual's health risk associated with an excessively low or high relative body fat (% BF). The age adjusted suggested body fat recommendations for adults are provided in table 6.[15]

Periodic body composition measurements can be used to assess the effectiveness of exercise and dietary interventions or monitor changes in body composition associated with growth and maturation or disease states. Body composition has been linked to numerous health conditions, such as cardiovascular disease, diabetes, some types of cancers, osteoporosis, and osteoarthritis. Thus, there is a clinical need to measure not only % BF, but fat distribution, muscle mass, and bone mass.

TABLE 6: Age adjusted suggested body fat recommendation for adults[15]

Age (years)	Low fat (BMI <18.5)	Healthy range (BMI 18.5–24.9)	Overweight (BMI 25–29.9)	Obese (BMI ≥30)
Women				
20–39 years	≤25	25.1–34.9%	35–39.9%	≥40
40–59 years	≤25	25.1–34.9%	35–40.9%	≥41
60–79 years	≤25	25.1–35.9%	36–40.9%	≥41
Men				
20–39 years	≤13	13.1–22.9%	23–27.9%	≥28
40–59 years	≤13	13.1–23.9%	24–28.9%	≥29
60–79 years	≤14	14.1–23.9%	24–28.9%	≥29

BMI, body mass index.

Regardless of the reason for assessing body composition, it is important to understand the various techniques that are available for assessing body composition. The various techniques used for body composition are based on two compartment (2C), three compartment (3C), four compartment (4C), or multi-compartment model. The models of body composition have been briefly described below.

Two-compartment Model

The most common approach in body composition assessment is to utilize the 2C model, dividing body weight into fat mass (FM) and fat-free mass (FFM). The FM, which is defined as chemically extractable fat, is assumed to have a density of 0.9007 g/cm^3 and be anhydrous, whereas the FFM is assumed to have a density of 1.1000 g/cm^3 with a water content of 73.72%.[16] Most of the error associated with these 2C models lies not in the technical accuracy of the measurements, but in the validity of the assumptions, which are based on analyses of just three male cadavers.[17] The most frequently used 2C models are hyrodensitometry, air displacement plethysmography, and hydrometry.

Three-compartment Model

In order to reduce the limitations of 2C model, the 3C model was developed. In the 3C model, the FFM is divided into total body water (TBW) and the remaining solids [protein and minerals, fat free dry mass (FFDM)]. This is based on measurements of both, body density (Db) and TBW, while assuming a constant mineral-to-protein ratio of 0.35.[18] The 3C model, thus, controls for inter-individual variation in FFM hydration. The 3C model shows better results over the 2C model, while measuring healthy adults and older children, but have to be used with caution in patients with depleted body protein or bone mineral mass, as the estimated values for density would not be accurate.[16]

Four-compartment Model

A 4C model (FM, water, and bone mineral, residual) of body composition analysis is theoretically more valid than the 3C model, because it controls for biological variability in both bone mineral and TBW. The density of protein and mineral is assumed to be 1.34 kg/L and 3.075 kg/L.[16] The dual-energy X-ray absorptiometry (DEXA) is used to measure the amount of mineral (bone mass) (Fig. 1).

This model involves independent assessment of Db, body water, and bone and can account for deviations in the quality of fat-free mass, in part, because the 4C model measures the individual constituents of the fat-free mass (aqueous and bone) rather than assuming a constant density of 1.100 g/cm^3 and hydration of 73.2%. Although this approach is preferred, it is impractical for most laboratories because of the cost and necessary equipment needed to measure TBW and bone mineralization.

Multicompartment Models

Atomic models of body composition require the direct analysis of the chemical composition of the body. The total body content of elements (calcium, sodium, chloride, phosphorus, nitrogen, hydrogen, oxygen, and carbon) can be measured using neutron activation analysis (NAA). The 6C model, divides the body into water + nitrogen + calcium + potassium + sodium + chloride.[19] While these multicompartment models provide accurate measures of body

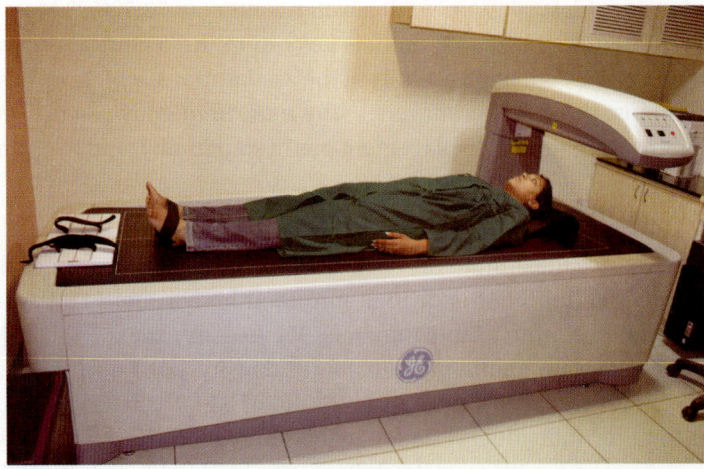

Figure 1 Measurement of body composition using dual-energy X-ray absorptiometry.

TABLE 7: Equations for estimating percent body fat

Model	Assumption	Equations	Other methods needed	References
2C	BW = FM + FFM	% BF = [(4.95/Db − 4.50)] × 100		Siri 1956[20]
		% BF = [(4.57/Db − 4.142)] × 100		Brozek et al. 1963[17]
3C	BW = FM + TBW + (mineral and protein combined)	% BF = [(2.118//Db) − 0.78 W − 1.354] × 100	D_2O dilution	Siri 1961[21]
		% BF = [(6.386//Db) + 3.961M − 6.090] × 100	DEXA	Lohman 1986[22]
4C	BW = FM + TBW + BM + Protein	% BF = [(2.747//Db) − 0.714 W + 1.146 B − 2.0503] × 100	D_2O dilution and DEXA	Selinger 1977[23]
		% BF = [(2.513//Db) − 0.739 W + 0.947 B − 1.790] × 100		Heymsfield 1996[24]
		% BF = [(2.747//Db) − 0.718 W + 1.148 B − 2.050] × 100		Baumgartner 1991[25]
6C	BW = TBW + TBN + TBCa + TBK + TBNa + TBCl	FM (kg) = BW − (TBW + 6.525 TBN + 2.709 TBCa + 2.76 TBK + TBNa + 1.43 TBCl)		Wang et al. 1998[26]

% BF, relative body fat; Db, body density from underwater weighing/air displacement plethysmography; FM, fat mass; BW, body weight; FFM, fat free mass; BM, bone mass; W, total body water/body weight; M, total body mineral/body weight; B, total body bone mineral/body weight; TBN, total body nitrogen; TBCa, total body calcium; TBK, total body potassium; TBNa, total body sodium; TBCl, total body chloride.

composition, for evaluating other methods, the lack of facilities, the high expense, and the exposure to radiation limits the use. The various equations for estimating % BF are provided in table 7.

The various body composition techniques can be divided into laboratory methods and field methods and have been briefly described below.

Laboratory Method

Laboratory techniques are frequently used as reference methods in clinical and research settings for the evaluation of field methods. The common laboratory methods for body composition assessment include hydrodensitometry (HD), air displacement plethysmography, isotope dilution, and DEXA.

Hydrodensitometry (Underwater Weighing)

Underwater weighing (UWW) or HD involves the estimations of Db. FM has lower density as compared to the FFM. The HD measures the water displaced by the body, when it is fully submerged and from this, provides an estimate of total body volume (BV). HD in combination with residual lung volume measurements can provide accurate measure of BV, from which Db can be estimated. Estimates of % BF from Db can be obtained using HD along with 2C model, which assumes the human body to be the sum of the FM and FFM. The HD method uses Archimedes principle, which states that when a body is submerged in water, there is a buoyant counter force equal to the weight of the water which is displaced. Because bone and muscle are denser than water, a person with a higher percentage of FFM will weigh more in the water and have a lower percent body fat. Fat, on the other hand, will float. Therefore, a large amount of FM will make the body lighter in the water and have a higher percent body fat. The individual's underwater weight is used to calculate the weight loss. In order to arrive at an accurate estimate of Db using HD, the BV should be corrected for the amount of air in the lungs and gastrointestinal tract at the time of measurement. Residual lung volume is the amount of air remaining in the lungs after a maximal expiration and is measured by oxygen dilution and nitrogen washout techniques. The volume of gas in the gastrointestinal tract is assumed to be about 100 mL.

Validity of hydrodensitometry: The HD method is considered to be a valid method for measuring BV and Db, with values of chemically determined Db agreeing with 0.6% of Db measured by HD.[27] When % BF estimates from HD were compared to estimates of % BF from 4C models, the difference was 0.6% BF, with a confidence interval level of 0.1–1.2% BF.[28] More recent studies have found average errors ranging from –2.8% BF to 1.8% BF.[18,29]

Errors and limitations: Sources of error for HD besides the assumptions include subject factor, technician skill, and equipment. The HD method has disadvantages such as causing discomfort and anxiety to the subject and the testing being time consuming.

Air Displacement Plethysmography

Body density has been conventionally measured by UWW, but now a commercial apparatus (BOD POD) provides a simpler alternative for the measurement of wide ranges of ages and population subgroups. The BOD POD is a relatively new device for measuring BV and uses air displacement, instead of water displacement, to estimate BV. The BOD POD is a large, egg-shaped fiberglass chamber, with two internal chambers separated by a moving diaphragm. The diaphragm oscillates back and forth to create small

Nutritional Assessment and Body Composition

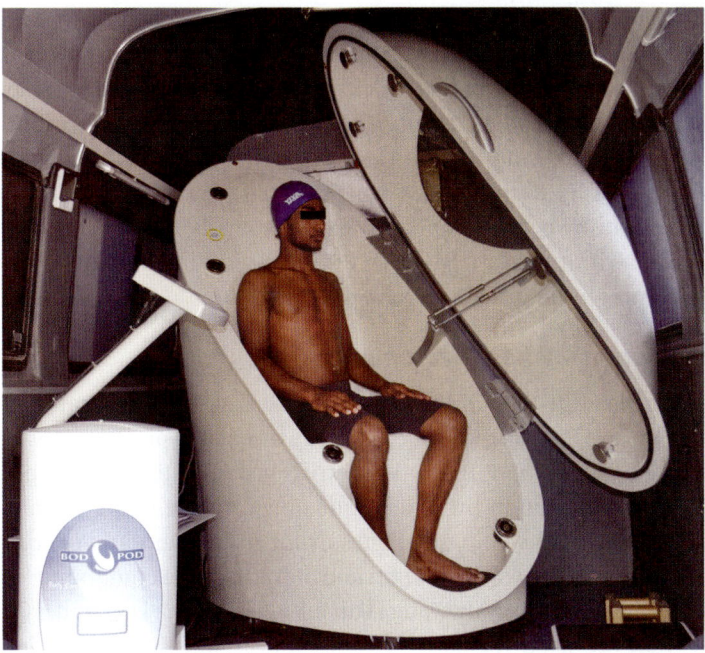

Figure 2 Measurement of body composition using air displacement plethysmography.

volume changes in the two chambers that are exactly equal in magnitude but opposite in sign. These volume shifts result in complementary pressure fluctuations in the two chambers. The principle of the instrument is based on air displacement plethysmography and uses the relationship between pressure and volume (Boyle's law) to derive BV for a subject seated aside the chamber (Fig. 2). BV is equal to the volume of air in an empty chamber minus the volume of air remaining in the chamber after the subject has been placed into it. Measurement time takes roughly 5-8 minutes per individual. The advantages of the BOD POD are it is easy to use, quick, and can be used in special population such as children, obese and elderly.

Validity of air displacement plethysmography: Many studies have reported small differences in Db (≤ 0.002 g/cc), measured by the BOD POD and HD,[29,30] while others[31,32] have reported slightly higher differences (0.003–0.007 g/cc). When % BF estimates of ADP was compared to those obtained using HD or DEXA, the average difference ranged from −4.0% to 1.9% with standard error of estimate (SEE) ranging from 2.2% to 3.7% BF.[33] When evaluated against 4C models, the predictive accuracy of the BOD POD and HW was found to be similar.[30,32] When the 4C model was used to validate the BOD POD in South Indian adult men and women, the SEE was 1.3 kg FM.[34]

Errors and limitation: The factors that may affect the accuracy of the BOD POD include hydration status and it is imperative to breathe normal and sit still, as any slight movement or change in breathing pattern may affect the results. The BOD POD assumes that isothermal effects (clothing, hair, thoracic gas volume, and body surface area) that alter the BV estimates are controlled. In order to minimize the isothermal effects of clothing and hair, the clothing attire needed for the measurement is tight fitting swimsuit/shorts and a swimming cap. The BOD POD instrument, though easy to use, is expensive and only few facilities have the machine.

Isotope Dilution Method (Hydrometry)

Water comprises 40-60% of the human body weight and because water is present mainly in the fat-free tissue, TBW can be used to provide an estimate of FFM and, consequently, % BF. Hydrometry is based on the dilution principle. According to the dilution principle, the concentration of a compound in a solvent depends on the volume of the solvent and the amount of compound added to it. Thus, if the concentration and amount of the compound (isotope) are known, the solvent (body water) can be calculated.[35] D_2O and ^{18}O are the isotopes that are used regularly. Two samples (saliva, urine or blood) are collected; one before administration of the dose, to determine the natural background levels, and the second provides a measure of the concentration of the tracer, taken after a sufficient amount of time for the tracer to equilibrate with all water spaces. The isotopic enrichment can be measured from either isotope ratio mass spectrometry or infrared spectrophotometry.

Validity of hydrometry: The precision and accuracy of this method for measuring TBW varies from 1% to 2%.[36,37] The FFM is estimated from TBW based on the assumption that, the hydration factor of FFM is about 73%, and the biological variability in the water content of FFM could lead to errors in % BF. The percentage of water in the FFM to range from 70% to 76% in most species and thus the assumption of 73% could cause an error.[38] It is important to use population specific hydration factor of FFM. The hydration factor of FFM was found to be 0.74 in South Indian adults.[34] Studies have reported small differences (<1% BF) for the TBW method as compared to 4C model of estimates of % BF.[18,39]

Errors and limitation: The technical errors in estimating TBW from isotope dilution could exist from variations in (a) the physiological fluid measured (saliva, urine, blood, or respiratory water), (b) equilibration time of the isotope, (c) water changes during equilibration, (d) correction for isotopic dilution space, and (e) the method for measuring the isotopic enrichment following equilibration. The cost of the isotopes and the technical expertise needed in analyzing the results, make this method not widely used.

Dual Energy X-ray Absorptiometry

Dual energy X-ray absorptiometry uses two X-ray energies to measure body fat, muscle, and total body bone mineral (TBBM). The DEXA is quick, radiation exposure is low, and needs little technical skill and preparation by the subject. DEXA provides a very precise and accurate measurement of TBBM. The DEXA works on the principle that the attenuation of X-rays with high and low photon energies is measureable and depends on the thickness, density, and chemical composition of the underlying tissue. The differences in the density and chemical composition of fat, lean tissue, and bone causes variations in the attenuation of X-ray through the tissues.

During a DEXA measurement, the subject lies supine on a padded table, and an X-ray beam passes in a posterior-to-anterior direction through the bone and soft tissue upward to a detector. The radiation exposure is low. DEXA requires minimal cooperation from the participant, is quick, and is less affected by and less prone to the errors associated with the underlying assumptions inherent in HD. The greatest advantage of DEXA over the other laboratory methods is the ability to assess regional as well as total body composition and analyze separate compartments of the body (fat, soft tissue, and bone).

Validity of dual energy X-ray absorptiometry: The variability in results reported in DEXA validation studies have been sometimes attributed to the different models and software versions. DEXA estimates of % BF were within from 1% to 3% of multicomponent model estimates.[38] The DEXA estimates of body FM when compared to 4C model in South Indian men and women, showed a mean error of -0.5 kg.[34]

Errors and limitations: While the accuracy and precision of DEXA for measuring TBBM and BMD is accepted, the method has its limitations for assessing the composition of bone-free soft tissue. The DEXA method assumes that the amount of fat over bone is the same as the amount of fat over bone free tissue, when, in fact, it varies and this is a major drawback in using DEXA to estimate % BF.

Field Method

While laboratory methods are generally more precise, they are also more time-consuming, inconvenient, and costly than field methods. Thus, field methods are a more attractive means of assessing % BF for the clinical and field research. Each of the methods has strengths and limitations. The common field methods used are bioelectrical impedance analysis (BIA) and skinfold measurements.

Bioelectrical Impedance Analysis

Bioelectrical impedance analysis is the technique used to predict body composition based, on the electrical conductive properties of the body. This method involves measuring the impedance (Z) to the flow of a low-level electrical current (800 microamperes), at a fixed frequency (50 kHz). The TBW is estimated from the impedance measurement as the electrolytes in the body water are good conductors of electrical current. BIA is based on the principle that lean tissue, which contains large amounts of water and electrolytes, is a good electrical conductor, and fat, which is anhydrous, is a poor conductor. FFM is predicted from TBW using the hydration factor of 73%. Several BIA prediction equations for TBW have been developed and the prediction SEE ranged from 0.9 kg to 1.8 kg TBW.[40] The BIA device can be single frequency, when it operates at a frequency of 50 kHz or multifrequency, which uses a wide range of frequencies.

Certain guidelines have to be followed for a BIA analysis and the subjects should be instructed to:
- Abstain from eating and drinking 4 hour prior to the test
- Avoid exercising within 12 hours of the test
- Avoid alcohol consumption within 48 hours of the test
- Completely empty the bladder prior to testing
- Avoid diuretics prior to testing unless instructed by the attending physician.

The BIA measurement is a relatively simple procedure. The subject lies supine on a nonconducting surface with arms and legs abducted at an angle of 30–45° from the trunk (Fig. 3). Source electrodes are placed on the dorsal surfaces of the right hand and foot proximal to the metacarpal-phalangeal and metatarsal-phalangeal joints, respectively. Voltage-sensing electrodes are placed at the midpoint between the distal prominences of the radius and ulna of the right wrist, and between the medial and lateral malleoli of the right ankle. A current of 800 microamperes at 50 kHz is passed between the outer two electrodes.[41] BIA does not require a high degree of technician skill. With proper standardization of methods, instrumentation, and subject preparation, the BIA can provide quick, easy, and relatively inexpensively estimates of FFM and TBW in healthy populations. It is useful in obese individuals, where the skinfold measurement is limited. It is, however, crucial that, prior to BIA testing, strict guidelines for standardizing hydration levels are followed. It is not recommended to use the FFM and % BF values directly from the BIA analyzer, unless it is clear, as to which equations have been used, what the accuracy and validity of the equations are and whether these equations are population specific.

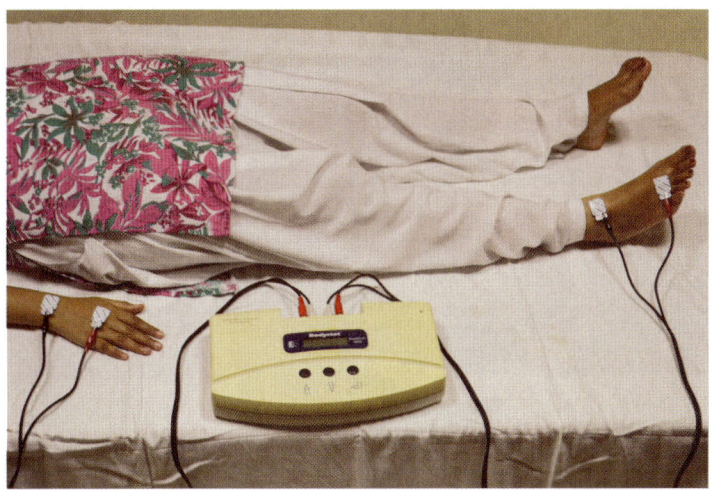

Figure 3 Measurement of body fat using bioelectrical impedance analysis.

The precision and accuracy of the BIA method is affected by the type of instrument, subject factor, and technician skill. Most of the equations are population specific and are applicable only to individuals from that specific group. If the BIA equation is not appropriately chosen based on age, gender, level of physical activity, level of body fat, and ethnicity, the results of the study will not be reliable. The validity of BIA to measure body fat was compared with D_2O dilution in Indian men, and BIA was found to overestimate body fat by 1.2 kg.[42] Estimates of body fat using BIA underestimated percent body fat by 5.5% when compared to the 4C method.[34] Thus, there is a need to develop population specific equations for estimating body fat in Indians.

Skinfold Measurements

The skinfold technique is an indirect measure of subcutaneous adipose tissue, by estimating Db to derive % BF. The skinfold technique involves pinching the skin with the thumb and forefinger, pulling it away from the body slightly, and placing the calipers on the fold (Fig. 4). It measures the thickness of two layers of skin and the underlying subcutaneous fat. The equipment used is a skinfold caliper, which is designed specifically for simple accurate measurement of subcutaneous tissue. The commonly used calipers are Holtain, Lange, and Harpenden which measure to the nearest 0.2 mm and vary in cost from $200 to $400. Measurements are made at sites such as biceps, triceps, subscapular, and suprailiac and the measurements need adequate practice. These measurements are used in formulas, which are age

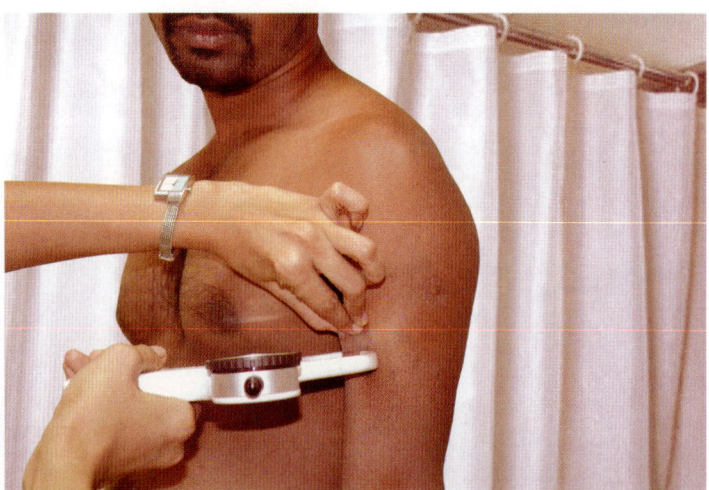

Figure 4 Measurement of body fat using skinfold thickness.

and gender specific, to arrive at values of Db. Most equations use three or four skinfold measurements to predict Db. Body fat is obtained from Db using a population specific conversion formula.[21] The prediction equations are developed either using linear (population specific) or quadratic (generalized) regression models. The equations of Durnin and Womersley[43] for estimating Db and % fat from skinfold thickness based on large numbers of subjects have been found to be some of the most widely applicable estimation equations. The % BF from skinfold method (where Db was from Durnin and Womersly equation and % BF from Db using Siri's equation) was found to accurately estimate % BF and FFM in Indian male and female subjects, when HD was used as reference.[44] However, when body FM estimates from skinfold techniques were compared to the 4C method, the average estimates of fat mass by skinfold method was 8% lower than 4C method.[34]

Some of the potential sources of error in the skinfold technique include variation in subcutaneous to total fat, variation in skinfold thickness to subcutaneous fat, and technical error in the SKF measurement. The skinfold method precisely measures Db; however, it requires a considerable amount of technical skill, being meticulous with site location and measurement, and is restricted to populations from whom the prediction equation was derived. Although an excellent field method to use on lean participants, it is difficult to obtain reliable and accurate readings on older participants with loose connective tissue or obese individuals with large folds.

Conclusion

There is no single method which is "best"; rather, the nutritionist/doctor or researcher must weigh the practical considerations of their assessment needs with the limitations of the methods. For example, combining data from several laboratory methods, such as TBW from isotope dilution, bone mineral content from DXA, and Db from HD into a multicomponent model would produce a precise but expensive and time-consuming body composition assessment. The expense and time involved with combining several laboratory methods may be essential for validation studies that require a high degree of accuracy and precision. On the other hand, for large epidemiological studies involving several thousand, subjects, anthropometry with skinfold technique may be ideal. The laboratory methods are more precise than the field methods; however, they are also more expensive, more time intensive, and require a higher degree of technical training and skill. Numerous factors need to be considered prior to selecting a method for body composition assessment. They include cost, ease of operation, technician skill requires, subject cooperation and comfort, whether or not the assessment will be conducted on multiple occasions to assess changes in body composition parameters.

Regardless of which instrument is chosen to assess body composition, it is very important to follow the standard guidelines and protocols associated with each method to limit measurement error. Additionally, the conversion formulas and prediction equations selected for use must be restricted to the populations from which they were derived to remain valid.

References

1. World Health Organization. Physical status: the use and interpretation of anthropometry: a report of a WHO expert committee. Geneva: WHO; 1995.
2. World Health Organization Report 1998. Obesity, prevention and managing the global epidemic. Report of a WHO consultation on obesity. Geneva: World Health Organization.
3. Dudeja V, Misra A, Pandey RM, Devina G, Kumar G, Vikram NK. BMI does not accurately predict overweight in Asian Indians in northern India. Br J Nutr. 2001;86(1):105-12.
4. Deurenberg-Yap M, Chew SK, Deurenberg P. Elevated body fat percentage and cardiovascular risks at low body mass index levels among Singaporean Chinese, Malays and Indians. Obes Rev. 2002;3(3): 209-15.
5. WHO/IASO/IOTF. The Asia-Pacific perspective: Redefining obesity and its treatment. Health Communications Australia: Melbourne; 2000.
6. who Expert Consultation. Appropriate body mass index for Asian populations and its implication for policy and implementation strategies. Lancet. 2004;363:157-63.
7. Kuczmarski RJ, Ogden CL, Grummer-Strawn LM, Flegal KM, Guo SS, Wei R, et al. CDC growth charts: United States. Adv Data. 2000;(314):1-27.
8. Cole TJ, Bellizzi MC, Flegal KM, Dietz WH. Establishing a standard definition for child overweight and obesity worldwide: international survey. BMJ. 2000;320(7244):1240-3.
9. WHO Multicentre Growth Reference Study Group. WHO Child Growth Standards. Acta Pædiatrica. 2006; Suppl 450:76-85.

10. WHO Multicentre Growth Reference Study Group. WHO Child Growth Standards: Length/height-for-age, weight-for-age, weight-for-length, weight-for-height and body mass index-for-age: Methods and development. Geneva: World Health Organization; 2006. p. 312.
11. Khadilkar VV, Khadilkar AV, Borade AB, Chiplonkar SA. Body mass index cut-offs for screening for childhood overweight and obesity in Indian children. Indian Pediatr. 2011;49(1):29-34.
12. Misra A, Vikram NK, Gupta R, Pandey RM, Wasir JS, Gupta VP. Waist circumference cutoff points and action levels for Asian Indians for identification of abdominal obesity. Int J Obes (Lond). 2006;30(1):106-11.
13. Kuriyan R, Thomas T, Lokesh DP, Sheth NR, Mahendra A, Joy R, et al. Waist circumference and waist for height percentiles in urban South Indian children aged 3-16 years. Indian Pediatr. 2011;48(10):765-71.
14. Bharathi AV, Sandhya N, Vaz M. The development & characteristics of a physical activity questionnaire for epidemiological studies in urban middle class Indians. Indian J Med Res. 2000;111:95-102.
15. Gallagher D, Heymsfield SB, Heo M, Jebb SA, Murgatroyd PR, Sakamoto Y. Healthy percentage body fat ranges: an approach for developing guidelines based on body mass index. Am J Clin Nutr. 2000;72(3):694-701.
16. Ellis JK. Human body composition: in vivo methods. Physiological Reviews. 2000;8(2).
17. Brozek J, Grande F, Anderson JT, Keys A. Densitometric analysis of body composition: Revision of some quantitative assumptions. Ann N Y Acad Sci. 1963;110:113-40.
18. Withers RT, LaForgia J, Pillans RK, Shipp NJ, Chatterton BE, Schultz CG, et al. Comparisons of two-, three-, and four-compartment models of body composition analysis in men and women. J App Physiol (1985). 1998;85(1):238-45.
19. Heyward VH and Wagner DR. Applied Body Composition Assessment, 2nd Edition. USA: Human Kinetics; 2004.
20. Siri WE. The gross composition of the body. In: Lawrence JH, Tobias CA (eds). Advances in Biological and Medical Physics. New York, NY: Academic Press, Inc.; 1956. pp. 239-80.
21. Siri WE. Body composition from fluid spaces and density: Analysis of methods. In: Brozek J, Henschel A (Eds). Techniques for measuring body composition. Washington DC: National Academy of Sciences; 1961. pp. 223-44.
22. Lohman TG. Applicability of body composition techniques and constants for children and youth. In: Pandolf KB (Ed). Exercise and Sports Science Reviews, Vol. 14. New York, NY: Macmillan; 1986. pp. 325-57.
23. Selinger A. The body as a three component system. Unpublished doctoral dissertation. University of Illinois, Urbana; 1977.
24. Heymsfield SB, Wang ZM, Withers RT. Multicomponent molecular level models of body composition analysis. In: Roche AF, Heymsfield SB, Lohman TG (Eds). Human body composition. Champaign IL: Human Kinetics; 1996. pp. 129-48.
25. Baumgartner RN, Heymsfield SB, Lichtman S, Wang J, Pierson RN Jr. Body composition in elderly people: effect of criterion estimates on predictive equations. Am J Clin Nutr. 1991;53(6):1345-53.
26. Wang ZM, Deurenberg P, Guo SS, Pietrobelli A, Wang J, Pierson RN Jr, et al. Six-compartment body composition model: inter-method comparisons of total body fat measurement. Int J Obes Relat Metab Disord. 1998;22(4):329-37.
27. Heymsfield SB, Wang J, Lichtman S, Kamen Y, Kehayias J, Pierson RN Jr. Body composition in elderly subjects: a critical appraisal of clinical methodology. Am J Clin Nutr. 1989;50(5 Suppl):1167-75.
28. Fogelholm M, van Marken Lichtenbelt W. Comparison of body composition methods: a literature analysis. Eur J Clin Nutr. 1997;51(8):495-503.
29. Yee AJ, Fuerst T, Salamone L, Visser M, Dockrell M, Van Loan M, et al. Calibration and validation of an air-displacement plethysmography method for estimating percentage body fat in an elderly population: a comparison among compartmental models. Am J Clin Nutr. 2001;74(5):637-42.
30. Fields DA, Wilson GD, Gladden LB, Hunter GR, Pascoe DD, Goran MI. Comparison of the BOD POD with the four-compartment model in adult females. Med Sci Sports Exerc. 2001;33(9):1605-10.

31. Wagner DR, Heyward VH, Gibson AL. Validation of air displacement plethysmography for assessing body composition. Med Sci Sports Exerc. 2000;32(7):1339-44.
32. Millard-Stafford ML, Collins MA, Evans EM, Snow TK, Cureton KJ, Rosskopf LB. Use of air displacement plethysmography for estimating body fat in a four-component model. Med Sci Sports Exerc. 2001;33(8):1311-7.
33. Fields DA, Goran MI, McCrory MA. Body-composition assessment via air-displacement plethysmography in adults and children: a review. Am J Clin Nutr. 2002;75(3):453-67.
34. Kuriyan R, Tinku Thomas, Sangeetha Ashok, Jayakumar J, Anura V Kurpad. A 4 compartment model based validation of air displacement plethysmography, dual energy X-ray absorptiometry, skinfold technique and bio-electrical impedance for measuring body fat in Indian adults. Indian Journal of Medical Research Indian J Med Res. 2014;139(5):700-7.
35. Edelman IS, Olney JM, James AH, Brooks L, Moore FD. Body Composition: Studies in the Human Being by the Dilution Principle. Science. 1952;115(2991):447-54.
36. Schoeller DA, Kushner RF, Taylor P, Dietz WH, Bandini L. Measurement of total body waster: isotope dilution techniques. In: Roche AF (Ed). Report of the sixth Ross conference on medical research. Columbus OH: Ross Laboratories; 1985. pp. 24-9.
37. Scholeller DA. Hydrometry. In: Roche AF, Heymsfield SB, Lohman TG (Eds). Human body composition. Champaign, IL: Human Kinetics; 1996. pp. 25-43.
38. Lohman TG, Harris M, Teixeira PJ, Weiss L. Assessing body composition and changes in body composition. Another look at dual-energy X-ray absorptiometry. Ann N Y Acad Sci. 2000;904:45-54.
39. Fuller NJ, Sawyer MB, Elia M. Comparative evaluation of body composition methods and predictions, and calculation of density and hydration fraction of fat-free mass, in obese women. Int J Obes Relat Metab Disord. 1994;18(7):503-12.
40. Houtkooper LB, Going SB, Sproul J, Blew RM, Lohman TG. Comparison of methods for assessing body-composition changes over 1 y in postmenopausal women. Am J Clin Nutr. 2000;72(2):401-6.
41. National Institute of Health (NIH) Technology Assessment Conference Statement. (December 12-14, 1994). Bioelectrical Impedance Analysis in Body Composition Measurement. [online] Available from: http://consensus.nih.gov/1994/1994BioelectricImpedanceBodyta015PDF.pdf. [Accessed July 2014].
42. Bhat DS, Yajnik CS, Sayyad MG, Raut KN, Lubree HG, Rege SS, et al. Body fat measurement in Indian men: comparison of three methods based on a two-compartment model. Int J Obes (Lond). 2005;29(7):842-8.
43. Durnin JV, Womersley J. Body fat assessed from total body density and its estimation from skinfold thickness: measurements on 481 men and women aged from 16 to 72 years. Br J Nutr. 1974;32(1):77-97.
44. Kuriyan R, Petracchi C, Ferro-Luzzi A, Shetty PS, Kurpad AV. Validation of expedient methods for measuring body composition in Indian adults. Indian J Med Res. 1998;107:37-45.

CHAPTER 3

Role of Nutrition and Lifestyle in Obesity and Diabetes

Abstract

Nutrition and lifestyle play an important role in the etiology of chronic diseases like diabetes and obesity. This chapter summarizes the evidence available for the nutritional factors related to excessive weight gain and diabetes. The role of dietary factors such as increased intake of high energy foods, carbohydrates, protein, fat, alcohol, and eating behaviors, and home and school environments in the development of diabetes and obesity are discussed. This chapter also reviews the factors that play a role throughout the life cycle in obesity and diabetes mellitus.

Introduction

Nutrition and diet play an important role in the etiology of chronic diseases. Nutrition related noncommunicable chronic diseases are becoming more common in the low- and middle-income countries. Rapid changes in diet and lifestyles caused by urbanization and economic development have significantly impacted the health and nutritional status of developing countries and countries in transition. Increased consumption of energy-rich diets, high in fat, saturated fat, and low in unrefined carbohydrates, coupled with decrease in energy expenditure have become increasingly common. Epidemiological research suggests that a relationship exists between chronic noninfectious disease and diets that include excessive amount of energy, fat, and refined sugars but are low in complex carbohydrates. Increasing evidence also suggests that chronic disease risks begins in fetal life and continues into old age.[1] Thus prevention through interventions of diet and physical activity can be a supportive strategy in retarding the progression of existing chronic diseases and decreasing mortality and the disease burden from such diseases.

Factors Related to Excessive Weight Gain and Obesity

Optimal nutrition plays an important role in the prevention of obesity. Although the causes of obesity are multifactorial, social and environmental factors that either increase energy intake or decrease physical activity will create additional load on the normal mechanism of appetite control and metabolic regulation. Table 1 summarizes the evidence of factors that might promote or protect against weight gain and obesity.

Dietary Factors

Factors linked to overweight and obesity include nutrients (high intake of energy, fat, low intake of fiber, type of carbohydrate), eating behaviors (excessive snacking/eating frequency, binge-eating patterns, eating out), and environmental (obesogenic or obesity promoting).

TABLE 1: Strength of evidence on factors that might promote or protect against weight gain and obesity[1]

Evidence	Decreased risk	No relationship	Increased risk
Convincing	• Regular physical activity • High dietary intake of nonstarch polysaccharide dietary fiber		• Sedentary lifestyles • High intake of energy-dense micronutrient-poor foods
Probable	• Home and school environments that support healthy food choices for children • Breastfeeding		• Heavy marketing of energy-dense foods • High intake of sugar-sweetened soft drinks and fruit juices • Adverse socioeconomic conditions (in developed countries, especially for women)
Possible	Low glycemic index foods	Protein content of the diet	• Large portion sizes • High proportion of food prepared outside the home (developed countries)
Insufficient	Increased eating frequency		Alcohol

Nutrients

Nutrition transition includes both quantitative and qualitative changes in the diet, with shift towards higher intake of energy, fat, refined sugars, saturated fat and reduced intake of fruits, vegetables, complex carbohydrates, and dietary fiber,[2] coupled with reduced physical activity, both at work and leisure time activities. India is in the phase of a rapid demographic transition with rapid urbanization and huge shifts in populations from rural to urban areas. Traditional diets rich in complex carbohydrates are being replaced by diets high in sugar, fat, and animal products.

Increased intake of high energy foods: Food rich in energy are often high in fat, highly processed, low in dietary fiber, and micronutrients and the increased consumption of these foods have shown to promote weight gain. Evidence from long-term randomized trials and epidemiological studies linking fat intake to weight gain or obesity is weak and inconsistent.[3-5] Short-term studies of ad libitum total intakes, with manipulations of fat and carbohydrate proportions have observed an increase in the total energy intake and body weight on higher percent fat diets and the reverse on lower percent fat diets, suggesting that the physiological and behavioral consequence of high-fat diet is a slow weight gain through the "passive overeating" of total energy.[6,7] Satiety, palatability, and energy density are some of the mechanism suggested to be responsible for the passive overeating of total energy through high-fat diets. Trials of ad libitum high-fat versus low-fat diets suggested that a 10% reduction in fat content results in about 3 kg reduction in body weight.[8] Results from a large longitudinal study of women observed that overall, percent of calories from fat had only a weak association with weight gain, while percentage of calories from animal, saturated, and trans fat has stronger associations. Overweight women with either overweight parents or with normal weight parents appeared to be more susceptible to weight gain due to dietary fat composition, suggesting that the association may not be genetic. Trans fat intake was shown to be more predictive than total fat of changes in waist circumference[9] but more research is needed to determine the mechanism.

Intake of carbohydrate and dietary fiber [non-starch polysaccharide (NSP)]: Inverse relation between sugar intake (as a percent of energy) and body mass index (BMI) have been observed[10] and this may be due to confounding factors such as selective underreporting of high sugar foods and drinks by overweight individuals.[11] Lower energy intake and greater weight loss was observed on high-starch diet, while high-fat and high-sucrose diets had similar amounts of energy intakes.[12] The evidence for the role of high intake of sugar-sweetened drinks in promoting weight gain is strong and a high intake of sugar drinks was found to predict the development of obesity in a longitudinal study of 12-year-old children.[13] Although more research is needed, adequate evidence is available to discourage consumption of sugary drinks as part of a healthy lifestyle.

High intake of dietary fiber promotes weight loss and studies involving ad libitum eating[14] observed mean weight loss of 1.9 kg over 3.8 months, with no difference between fiber type or source of fiber either as in food or as supplements. The intrinsic effects, such as energy density and palatability of NSP, hormonal effect (gastric emptying, postprandial glycemia) and colonic effects (effects on satiety and fermentation to short chain fatty acids), have been suggested as some of the potential mechanism for the effects of NSP on energy.[15,16] Glycemic index (GI) of foods could have a possible effect on body weight,[17,18] but there is a need for longitudinal studies to confirm these findings.

Protein intake: Higher intakes of protein may be beneficial for weight control in some individuals.[19,20] Consumption of high-protein diets (18% of total energy) during weight maintenance period, resulted in a 50% lower body weight regain, only consisting of fat-free mass, and was related to increased satiety and decreased energy efficiency.[21] However, more research is needed to establish the benefits of high-protein on weight control at a population level.

Alcohol: The association between BMI and reported alcohol intake shows conflicting results with some studies showing positive association and others no association.[22,23] Light-to-moderate alcohol intake, especially wine intake, may protect against weight gain, whereas consumption of spirits has been positively associated with weight gain. The results of a recent review do not conclusively confirm that alcohol consumption has an effect on weight gain with positive findings between alcohol intake and weight gain being observed only with higher levels of drinking.[24] Further research should be directed towards assessing the specific roles of different types of alcoholic beverages and also consider the effect of consumption patterns.

Eating Behaviors

Eating behaviors that have been studied for their role in weight gain and obesity include: frequency of food consumption, skipping of main meals (breakfast), and frequency of meals eaten away from home (eating out). The existing limited evidence suggests that increased meal frequency may not play a significant role in weight loss/gain after accounting for under-reporting, restrained eating, and exercise. Increased meal frequency accompanied with energy restriction could decrease hunger, nitrogen loss, improve lipid oxidation, and improve insulin, total and low-density lipoprotein (LDL) cholesterol and insulin.[25] However, more well-designed studies involving various meal frequencies are needed. Bigger portion sizes have been suggested as a possible causative factor for unhealthy weight gain.[26] The increased frequency of eating out may play a role in weight gain, since those who eat out more were observed to have higher BMI than those who ate more at home,[27] although these findings have been mainly observed in US. Skipping breakfast has been associated with higher BMI and obesity[28,29] and the reason suggested is that having breakfast was associated with better dietary macronutrient composition and healthy habits such as physical activity and avoidance of alcohol. Late dinner has been associated with obesity[28,29] and the mechanism has been suggested to be the accumulation of energy in the form of glycogen after eating a carbohydrate-rich late dinner.[30] Increased consumption of bakery items, nonvegetarian foods, eating while watching television, snacking between meals, family meals and skipping breakfast were found to be positively related to waist circumference in a cross sectional study of South Indian children aged between 6 and 16 years.[31]

Additionally in developing countries, the overfeeding of stunted population should be avoided and it is crucial to assess stature in combination with weight in feeding programs to prevent providing excess energy to children of low weight-for-age but normal weight-for-height. Appropriate education and encouragement should be provided to mothers and food decision makers to retain traditional foods such as fruit, vegetables, and reduce the intake of refined foods.

Home and School Environments

An "obesogenic" environment is "the sum of the influences that the surroundings, opportunities or conditions of life have on promoting obesity in individuals and populations".[32] A supportive home and school environment plays a role in obesity in children. Parents as "role models" with their knowledge, attitude, and behavior related to healthy diet and physical activity are determinants of children's eating behaviors.[33] Fruit and vegetable consumption in children were related to their availability, accessibility, and variety at home.[34] Using foods as reward or restricting their availability was associated with increased preference for those foods, while higher parental control of a child's food intake was related to lower ability of the child to self-regulate energy intake.[33] Food marketing also is thought to play a role in weight gain/obesity. The foods most commonly advertised on television are high energy foods and drinks, with the targeted audience often being children.[35] It is possible that the heavy advertising of fast foods and energy dense foods and drinks could increase the consumption of these foods.

Some of the factors that contribute to the role of school environment in weight gain are school food policies, types of food served at school, promotion

TABLE 2: General strategies for obesity prevention[1]

Infants and young children
• Promotion of exclusive breastfeeding for 6 months • Avoid/restrict the use of added sugars • Avoiding "force feeding" of the child • Ensure adequate intake of appropriate micronutrients to promote optimal linear growth of the child
Children and adolescents
• Promote an active lifestyle • Limit the duration of television viewing • Ensure adequate intake of fruits and vegetables • Restrict the intake of sugar sweetened beverages • Restrict the intake of energy dense, high-fat, and salt foods • Encourage children to eat family meals • Encourage parents to be "role models" • Modifying environment to create a healthy home and school environment which increases physical activity, decreases sedentary time and reduces obesogenic environment

of healthy options in food brought from home, and education on food and nutrition. These factors along with physical activity environment could affect the prevalence of obesity but more conclusive evidence is needed. Some of the strategies that can be employed to prevent obesity are provided in table 2.

Physical Activity and Physical Fitness

Physical activity and physical fitness (which relates to the ability to perform physical activity) are important modifiers of mortality and morbidity related to overweight and obesity. Regular physical activity prevents unhealthy weight gain while sedentary lifestyles (sedentary occupations, increased television viewing) promotes it. Individuals engaging in regular moderate physical activity have decreased risk of weight gain, overweight, and obesity.[36] At least 30 minutes of moderate-intensity physical activity on most days of the week is recommended to reduce overall mortality and cardiovascular diseases, while higher amounts of about 45–60 minutes of physical activity is needed on most days/every day to prevent unhealthy weight gain.[37] Reduction of sedentary behaviors have focused primarily on reducing television viewing in children. Decreased sleep duration has shown to be associated with increased risk of obesity in children and young adults.[38,39] Sleep duration was found to be one of the main determinants of increased waist circumference in South Indian children aged between 6 and 16 years.[31]

Low cardiovascular fitness is a common comorbidity of obesity and fitness is influenced strongly by physical activity and genetic factors.[40] Thus besides the role of physical activity on body weight, it also has an independent effect in the prevention of overweight and obesity. Education campaign about the health benefits of physical activity to improve cardiorespiratory fitness, in combination with changes in health care policy to make environments more conducive to physical activity needs to be initiated.

Factors Related to Diabetes

Lifestyle modification is the cornerstone for the prevention and treatment of type 2 diabetes.[41] Figure 1 summarizes the evidence on lifestyle factors and the risk of developing type 2 diabetes.

Weight Gain, Obesity, Abdominal Obesity

The onset of diabetes is strongly related to obesity and thus weight loss or weight maintenance is important to prevent type 2 diabetes. The association between excessive weight gain, central adiposity, and the development of type 2 diabetes is strong and waist circumference or waist-to-hip ratio (WHR) (surrogate for abdominal or visceral adiposity) have shown to be determinants of subsequent risk of type 2 diabetes[42] and insulin resistance.[43] Insulin sensitivity has shown to improve with weight loss[44] and weight loss reduces the risk of progression from impaired glucose tolerance (IGT) to

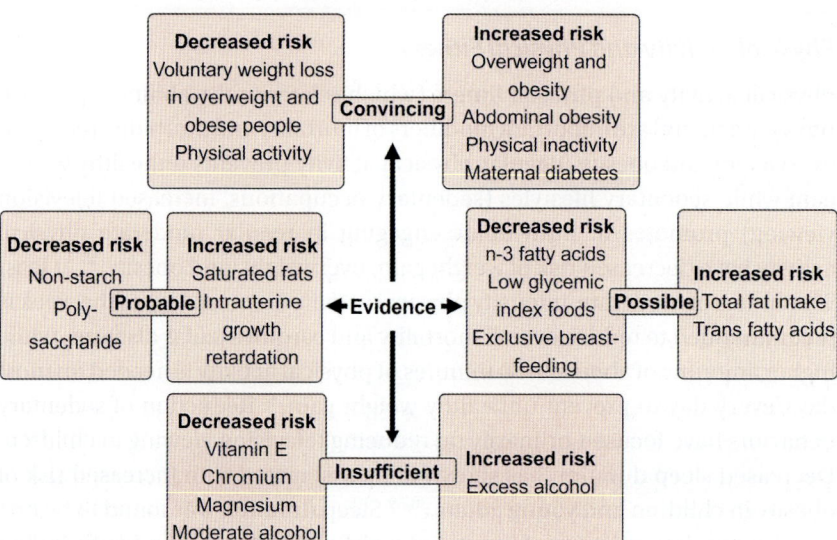

Figure 1 Summary of strength of evidence on lifestyle factors and risk of developing type 2 diabetes.[1]

> **Box 1** **Strategies for diabetes prevention**
> - Prevention/treatment of overweight and obesity, particularly in high risk groups
> - Maintaining an optimum BMI and avoiding weight gain (>5 kg) in adult life
> - Voluntary weight reduction in overweight or obese individuals with impaired glucose tolerance
> - Performing an endurance activity at moderate or greater level of intensity (e.g., brisk walking) for 1 hour or more per day on most days per week
> - Reducing the saturated fat intake to below 10% of total energy
> - Ensuring adequate intakes of NSP through regular consumption of wholegrain cereals, legumes, fruits, and vegetables. A minimum daily intake of 20 g is recommended

type 2 diabetes.[45,46] The Diabetes Prevention Program (DPP) demonstrated that modest weight loss through dietary changes and increased physical activity reduced the risk of developing diabetes in participants by 58%.[46] The benefit of physical activity includes not only better glycemic control by preventing weight gain but also improved metabolism. The progression of IGT to diabetes is high in native Asian Indians and the Indian DPP demonstrated that both lifestyle modifications and metformin significantly reduced the incidence of diabetes in Asian Indians with IGT.[47] The strategies for the prevention of diabetes are listed in box 1.

Dietary Factors

Dietary Fiber (Non-starch Polysaccharide)

The increased intakes of refined carbohydrates, low in dietary fiber have been suggested to promote the development of diabetes. NSP was shown to have a protective effect independent of age, BMI, smoking, and physical activity in women.[48,49] Blood glucose and insulin levels were reduced in people with type 2 diabetes and IGT who consumed high amounts of NSP (dietary fiber).[50] Additionally, higher intake of wholegrain cereals, vegetables, and fruits (all rich in NSP) were found to be associated with a reduced risk of progression of IGT to type 2 diabetes.[45,46] Diets low in cereal fiber increased the risk of type 2 diabetes, particularly in women with a sedentary lifestyle and a family history of diabetes,[51] reinforcing the importance of the quality of carbohydrates consumed in preventing type 2 diabetes. The information on the type of NSP having beneficial effects is conflicting with some studies suggesting that soluble forms of NSP exert benefit,[50,52] while others suggest that it is the cereal-derived insoluble forms that are protective.[48]

Glycemic Index

Foods low in glycemic index (GI) are associated with a reduced glycemic response after ingestion and overall improvement in glycosylated hemoglobin (HbA1c) in people with diabetes.[53,54] A large population-based cohort study in China found that a diet high in carbohydrates with a high GI was associated with a higher risk of type 2 diabetes mellitus, especially in individuals with increased WHR and BMI.[55] Recently, clear positive association was observed between GI and incidence of type 2 diabetes.[56] However, it should be noted that food with low GI may not always have overall health benefits, since a high-fat or energy dense food will also have low GI.

Fat Intake

High fat intake in the diet predicted development of IGT in healthy subjects and progression from IGT to type 2 diabetes.[57] Increased fasting insulin levels and lowered insulin sensitivity were associated with high total fat intake.[58] On the contrary, some studies have found no association between diabetes risk and total fat intake.[59] The long-term effects of specific types of dietary fatty acids on insulin resistance and risk of type 2 diabetes is inconclusive with the epidemiologic data being sparse. Increased intake of saturated fat is associated with a higher risk of IGT, and higher fasting glucose and insulin levels[60,61] and higher proportions of saturated fatty acids in serum lipid or muscle phospholipid have been associated with higher fasting insulin, lower insulin sensitivity, and a higher risk of type 2 diabetes.[62] Replacement of saturated fatty acids by unsaturated fatty acids leads to improved glucose tolerance[63] and enhanced insulin sensitivity.[64] Long-chain polyunsaturated fatty acids do not, however, appear to confer additional benefit over monounsaturated fatty acids in intervention studies. The epidemiological data with regards to monounsaturated fatty acids are inconsistent with some studies even indicating that high intake of monounsaturated fatty acids may be detrimental in terms of increasing diabetes risk and these reported findings may be due to the effects of saturated fatty acids in these food sources,[61] since in a typical "Western" diet the monounsaturated fatty acids may not be only from vegetable oils but also from saturated fat in sources such as meat and milk products.

Altering the quality of dietary fat appears to have little effect, when the total fat intake is high greater than 37% of total energy,[64] especially since observational studies have demonstrated that a high intake of total fat to predict development of IGT and the progression of IGT to type 2 diabetes.[61] Reduced risk of type 2 diabetes was associated with increased consumption of unsaturated fatty acids and polyunsaturated fatty acids from vegetable sources and lower fasting and 2-hour glucose concentrations.[65] Increased insulin sensitivity was seen with higher proportions of long chain polyunsaturated fatty acids in skeletal muscle phospholipids.[59,66] These finding indicate a probable causal link between saturated fatty acids and type 2 diabetes and a possible causal association between total fat intake and type 2 diabetes. Studies on the effect of trans fatty acid on risk of type 2 diabetes is limited with studies showing a positive association,[67] while another had no effect.[68]

Micronutrients

Convincing evidence is still lacking for the role of vitamin E, chromium, and magnesium in preventing type 2 diabetes.

Alcohol Intake

Moderate alcohol has been associated with a reduced incidence of type 2 diabetes in some studies. The Nurses' Health Study observed reduced incidence of diabetes in women who consumed alcohol compared with those who did not[69] and male physicians consuming greater than 2-4 drinks/week had a lower incidence of type 2 diabetes in the subsequent 12 years compared with non-drinkers.[70] Another study,[71] after adjusting for other diabetes risk factors observed that men consuming more than 21 drinks per week had a significant increase in the incidence of diabetes, while this association was not seen in women. More recently, moderate alcohol consumption was associated with a lower risk of type 2 diabetes only among women and the relation was stronger for overweight than normal-weight women.[72] In view of the present inconsistencies in results, clear recommendations regarding the role of alcohol in preventing type 2 diabetes is not available.

Physical Activity and Fitness

The risk of developing type 2 diabetes is reduced by increased physical activity, irrespective of the level of adiposity. Exercise with an intensity of 80–90% of age predicted maximum heart rate for at least 20 minutes, at least five times per week could improve insulin sensitivity.[44] Lifestyle interventions which included 150 minutes/week of physical activity and diet-induced weight loss of 5-7% reduced the risk of progression from IGT to type 2 diabetes by 58% (DPP Research Group 2002). The recommendations for people with IGT are to include at least 150 minutes/week of moderate to vigorous physical activity and a healthful diet.[73]

Factors Playing A Role Throughout the Life Cycle in Obesity and Type 2 Diabetes

Maternal Factors and Early Fetal Life

Early life environment can determine the risk of later obesity. Indications of intergenerational factors in obesity have been observed and factors include parental obesity, maternal gestational diabetes, and maternal birth weight. Maternal birth size was found to be a significant predictor of a child's birth size after controlling factors such as gestational age, sex of the child, socioeconomic status, and maternal age, height, and prepregnant weight.[74] Children born from mothers who had gestational diabetes tend to be large and heavy at birth with increased risk for obesity in childhood and are at high risk of developing type 2 diabetes at an early age. Lower insulin secretion has been observed in these individuals as compared to age matched children of nondiabetic pregnancies.[75]

Intrauterine growth retardation (IUGR) is associated with an increased risk of coronary heart disease, stroke, diabetes, and raised blood pressure.[1,76] The "Barker hypothesis", proposes that the risk for chronic diseases, such as type 2 diabetes and cardiovascular diseases, originate through adaptations of the fetus when it is undernourished, causing permanent changes in the structure and function of the body.[77,78] High risk of diabetes was observed with low birth weight, followed by subsequent adult obesity.[79]

Rapid postnatal catch-up growth, caused by postnatal overnutrition following the restricted fetal growth may be pathogenetic for the cause of obesity and type 2 diabetes.[80] The association between poor fetal growth and subsequent development of type 2 diabetes/metabolic syndrome results from the effects of poor intrauterine nutrition, producing permanent changes in glucose-insulin metabolism such as reduced capacity for insulin secretion and insulin resistance.[81]

Existing literature suggests that optimal birth weight and length distribution affects not only immediate health outcomes but also has long-term effects such as risk of chronic disease in later life.[82] India is experiencing a rapidly increasing epidemic of type 2 diabetes with the incidence being higher among urban populations. Thus, a life-course model of evolution of insulin resistance and type 2 diabetes incorporating fetal, postnatal, and adult components needs to be applied.

Prevention of type 2 diabetes must begin *in utero* and continue throughout the life course.

Growth and Feeding During Infancy

The extent of growth during infancy could contribute to development of chronic diseases in later life. Diabetes has shown to be associated with short stature.[83]

Breastfeeding is protective against weight gain in childhood[84] and this is important since childhood obesity tracks into adulthood. A 20% reduction in the risk of becoming overweight was observed in children aged between 9 and 14 years who were mainly breastfed in the first 6 months of life, after adjusting for measured confounders.[85] The length of exclusive breastfeeding was associated with a lower risk of developing obesity[85,86] although the effects are seen later in childhood.[84] A systematic review to quantify the strength of the associations between breastfeeding and risk of type 2 diabetes in later life concluded that breastfeeding in infancy was associated with a reduced risk of type 2 diabetes and lower insulin concentrations in later life.[87]

Childhood and Adolescence

Childhood obesity has shown to track into adulthood in some studies,[88,89] while a prospective cohort study in UK, found little tracking from childhood overweight to adulthood obesity, while using percent body fat for age as an index.[90] Overweight and obesity once established is likely to persist into adolescence and about 60% of the overweight children were found to have at least one additional risk factor for cardiovascular disease, such as raised blood pressure, hyperlipidemia, or hyperinsulinemia, and more than 20% have two or more risk factors.[84] The phenomenon of "thin-fat babies" exists in Indian babies which is characterized by low birth weight, poor muscle, but higher fat mass. Indian children also have increased central adiposity in childhood.[91,92] Young girls who grow inadequately become stunted women and are more likely to give birth to low-birth-weight babies, who are then likely to continue the cycle by being stunted in adulthood.[93]

The development of healthy/unhealthy habits during adolescence that tend to persist throughout the life, such as increased television viewing, lack of exercise, diets rich in fat, cholesterol and salt, and low in vegetables and fruits, are associated with increased weight gain, IGT and high lipid levels in children and adolescent.[83] Most of these factors persist throughout the life cycle.

Adulthood

Adulthood period is important since it is the period during when most chronic diseases are expressed, and it is the critical time for the reducing the risk factors and increasing effective treatment.[94] Obesity, physical inactivity, high cholesterol, high blood pressure, and increased alcohol consumption are known to be associated with type 2 diabetes and cardiovascular disease.

Low birth weight, followed by subsequent adult obesity, has been shown to increase the risk for IGT and diabetes.[79]

Elderly

Many chronic diseases exist in older people as a result of interactions between multiple disease processes as well as more general losses in physiological functions. Elderly patients are likely to gain from risk factor modification and interventions aimed at supporting elderly patients and promoting healthier environments, which could lead to decreased risk and increased independence in older age.

Conclusion

Recent evidences have demonstrated that type 2 diabetes is preventable by the implementation of lifestyle measures such as weight control and exercise. Thus primary prevention should be top priority and preventive interventions early in the life course can have lifelong benefits. Interventions in order to be effective must extend beyond individual risk factors and continue throughout the life course.

References

1. Diet, nutrition and the prevention of chronic diseases: report of a joint WHO/FAO expert consultation, Geneva, 28 January–1 February 2002. (WHO Technical Report Series; 916).
2. Drewnowski A, Popkin BM. The nutrition transition: new trends in the global diet. Nutr Rev. 1997;55(2):31-43.
3. Carmichael HE, Swinburn BA, Wilson MR. Lower fat intake as a predictor of initial and sustained weight loss in obese subjects consuming an otherwise ad libitum diet. J Am Diet Assoc. 1998;98(1):35-9.
4. Westerterp-Plantenga MS, Wijckmans-Duijsens NE, Venne, Verboeket-Van de WP, de Graaf K, van het Hof, KH, Weststrate, JA. Energy intake and body weight effects of six months reduced or full fat diets, as a function of dietary restraint. Int J Obes Relat Metab Disord. 1998;22(1):14-22.
5. Pirozzo S, Summerbell C, Cameron C, Glasziou P. Should we recommend low-fat diets for obesity? Obes Rev. 2003;4(2):83-90.
6. Kendall A, Levitsky DA, Strupp BJ, Lissner L. Weight loss on a low-fat diet consequence of the imprecision of the control of food intake in humans. Am J Clin Nutr. 1991;53(5):1124-9.
7. Thomas CD, Peters JC, Reed GW, Abumrad NN, Sun M, Hill JO. Nutrient balance and energy expenditure during ad libitum feeding of high-fat and high-carbohydrate diets in humans. Am J Clin Nutr. 1992;55(5):934-42.
8. Astrup A ,Grunwald GK, Melanson EL, Saris WH, Hill JO. The role of low-fat diets in body weight control: a meta-analysis of ad libitum dietary intervention studies. Int J Obes Relat Metab Disord. 2000;24(12):1545-52.
9. Koh-Banerjee P, Chu NF, Spiegelman D, Rosner B, Colditz G, Willett W, et al. Prospective study of the association of changes in dietary intake, physical activity, alcohol consumption, and smoking with 9-y gain in waist circumference among 16,587 US men. Am J Clin Nutr. 2003;78(4):719-27.

10. Hill JO, Prentice AM. Sugar and body weight regulation. Am J Clin Nutr. 1995;62(1 Suppl):264S-273S; discussion 273S-274S.
11. Bellisle F, Rolland-Cachera MF. How sugar-containing drinks might increase adiposity in children. Lancet. 2001;357(9255):490-1.
12. Raben A, Macdonald I, Astrup A. Replacement of dietary fat by sucrose or starch: effects on 14 d ad libitum energy intake, energy expenditure and body weight in formerly obese and never-obese subjects. Int J Obes Relat Metab Disord. 1997;21(10):846-59.
13. Ludwig DS, Peterson KE, Gortmaker SL. Relation between consumption of sugar-sweetened drinks and childhood obesity: a prospective, observational analysis. Lancet. 2001;357(9255):505-8.
14. Howarth NC, Saltzman E, Roberts SB. Dietary fiber and weight regulation. Nutr Rev. 2001;59(5):129-39.
15. Burton-Freeman B. Dietary fiber and energy regulation. J Nutr. 2000;130(2S Suppl):272S-275S.
16. Pereira MA, Ludwig DS. Dietary fiber and body-weight regulation. Observations and mechanisms. Pediatr Clin North Am. 2001;48(4):969-80.
17. Agus MS, Swain JF, Larson CL, Eckert EA, Ludwig DS. Dietary composition and physiologic adaptations to energy restriction. Am J Clin Nutr. 2000;71(4):901-7.
18. Spieth LE, Harnish JD, Lenders CM, Raezer LB, Pereira MA, Hangen SJ, et al. A low-glycemic index diet in the treatment of pediatric obesity. Arch Pediatr Adolesc Med. 2000;154(9):947-51.
19. Latner JD, Schwartz M. The effects of a high-carbohydrate, high-protein or balanced lunch upon later food intake and hunger ratings. Appetite. 1999;33(1):119-28.
20. Long SJ, Jeffcoat AR, Millward DJ. Effect of habitual dietary-protein intake on appetite and satiety. Appetite. 2000;35(1):79-88.
21. Westerterp-Plantenga MS, Lejeune MP, Nijs I, van Ooijen M, Kovacs EM. High protein intake sustains weight maintenance after body weight loss in humans. Int J Obes Relat Metab Disord. 2004;28(1):57-64.
22. Hellerstedt WL, Jeffery RW, Murray DM. The association between alcohol intake and adiposity in the general population. Am J Epidemiol. 1990;132(4):594-611.
23. Suter PM, Hasler E, Vetter W. Effects of alcohol on energy metabolism and body weight regulation: is alcohol a risk factor for obesity? Nutr Rev. 1997;55(5):157-71.
24. Sayon-Orea C, Martinez-Gonzalez MA, Bes-Rastrollo M. Alcohol consumption and body weight: a systematic review. Nutr Rev. 2011;69(8):419-31.
25. La Bounty PM, Campbell BI, Wilson J, Galvan E, Berardi J, Kleiner SM, et al. International Society of Sports Nutrition position stand: meal frequency. J Int Soc Sports Nutr. 2011;8:4.
26. Nielsen SJ, Popkin BM. Patterns and trends in food portion sizes, 1977-1998. JAMA. 2003;289(4):450-3.
27. Binkley JK, Eales J, Jekanowski M. The relation between dietary change and rising US obesity. Int J Obes Relat Metab Disord. 2000;24(8):1032-9.
28. Ma Y, Bertone ER, Stanek EJ, Reed GW, Hebert JR, Cohen NL, et al. Association between eating patterns and obesity in a free-living US adult population. Am J Epidemiol. 2003;158(1):85-92.
29. Cho S, Dietrich M, Brown CJ, Clark CA, Block G. The effect of breakfast type on daily energy intake and body mass index: results from the Third National Health and Nutrition Examination Survey (NHANES III). J Am Coll Nutr. 2003;22(4):296-302.
30. Keim NL, Van Loan MD, Horn WF, Barbieri TF, Mayclin PL. Weight loss is greater with consumption of large morning meals and fat-free mass is preserved with large evening meals in women on a controlled reduction regimen. J Nutr. 1997;127(1):75-82.
31. Kuriyan R, Thomas T, Lokesh DP, Sheth NR, Mahendra A, Joy R, et al. Waist circumference and waist for height percentiles in urban South Indian children aged 3-16 years. Indian Pediatr. 2011;48(10):765-71.
32. Swinburn B, Egger G. Preventative strategies against weight gain and obesity. Obes Rev. 2002;3(4):289-301.
33. Campbell K, Crawford D. Family food environments as determinants of preschool aged children's eating behaviours: implications for obesity prevention policy: A review. Australian Journal of Nutrition and Dietetics. 2001;58(1):19-25.

34. Hearn MD, Baranowski T, Baranowski J, Doyle C, Smith M, Lin LS, et al. Environmental influences on dietary behavior among children: availability and accessibility of fruits and vegetables enable consumption. Journal of Health Education. 1998;29(1):26-32.
35. French SA, Story M, Jeffery RW. Environmental influences on eating and physical activity. Annu Rev Public Health. 2001;22:309-35.
36. Fogelholm M, Kukkonen-HarjulaK. Does physical activity prevent weight gain — a systematic review. Obes Rev. 2000;1(2):95-111.
37. Saris WHM. Dose-response of physical activity in the treatment of obesity-How much is enough to prevent unhealthy weight gain. Outcome of the First Mike Stock Conference. Int J Obes. 2002; 26(Suppl. 1):S108.
38. Hasler G, Buysse DJ, Klaghofer R, Gamma A, Ajdacic V, Eich D, et al. The association between short sleep duration and obesity in young adults: a 13-year prospective study. Sleep. 2004;27(4):661-6.
39. Reilly JJ, Armstrong J, Dorosty AR, Emmett PM, Ness A, Rogers I, et al. Early life risk factors for obesity in childhood: cohort study. BMJ. 2005;330(7504):1357.
40. Carnethon MR, Gulati M, Greenland P. Prevalence and cardiovascular disease correlates of low cardiorespiratory fitness in adolescents and adults. JAMA. 2005;294(23):2981-8.
41. Mann J. Stemming the tide of diabetes mellitus. Lancet. 2000;356(9240):1454-5.
42. Boyko EJ, Fujimoto WY, Leonetti DL, Newell-Morris L. Visceral adiposity and risk of type 2 diabetes: a prospective study among Japanese Americans. Diabetes Care. 2000;23(4):465-71.
43. Despre's JP. Health consequences of visceral obesity. Ann Med. 2001;33(8):534-41.
44. McAuley KA, Williams SM, Mann JI, Goulding A, Chisholm A, Wilson N, et al. Intensive lifestyle changes are necessary to improve insulin sensitivity: a randomized controlled trial. Diabetes Care. 2002;25(3):445-52.
45. Tuomilehto J, Lindström J, Eriksson JG, Valle TT, Hämäläinen H, Ilanne-Parikka P, et al. Prevention of type 2 diabetes mellitus by changes in lifestyle among subjects with impaired glucose tolerance. N Engl J Med. 2001;344(18):1343-50.
46. Knowler WC, Barrett-Connor E, Fowler SE, Hamman RF, Lachin JM, Walker EA, et al. Reduction in the incidence of type 2 diabetes with lifestyle intervention or metformin. N Engl J Med. 2002;346(6):393-403.
47. Ramachandran A, Snehalatha C, Mary S, Mukesh B, Bhaskar AD, Vijay V, et al. Indian Diabetes Prevention Programme. The Indian Diabetes Prevention Programme shows that lifestyle modification and metformin prevent type 2 diabetes in Asian Indian subjects with impaired glucose tolerance (IDPP-1). Diabetologia. 2006;49(2):289-97.
48. Salmeron J, Manson JE, Stampfer MJ, Colditz GA, Wing AL, Willett WC, et al. Dietary fiber, glycemic load, and risk of non-insulin-dependent diabetes mellitus in women. JAMA. 1997;277(6):472-7.
49. Meyer KA, Kushi LH, Jacobs DR, Slavin J, Sellers TA, Folsom AR, et al. Carbohydrates, dietary fiber, and incident type 2 diabetes in older women. Am J Clin Nutr. 2000;71(4):921-30.
50. Mann J. Dietary fibre and diabetes revisited. Eur J Clin Nutr. 2001;55(11):919-21.
51. Schulze MB, Liu S, Rimm EB, Manson JE, Willett WC, Hu FB. Glycemic index, glycemic load, and dietary fiber intake and incidence of type 2 diabetes in younger and middle-aged women. Am J Clin Nutr. 2004;80(2):348-56.
52. ChandaliaM, Garg A, Lutjohann D, von Bergmann K, Grundy SM, Brinkley LJ. Beneficial effects of high dietary fiber intake in patients with type 2 diabetes mellitus. N Engl J Med. 2000;342(19):1392-8.
53. Fontvieille AM, Rizkalla SW, Penfornis A, Acosta M, Bornet FR, Slama G. The use of low glycaemic index foods improves metabolic control of diabetic patients over five weeks. Diabet Med. 1992;9(5):444-50.
54. Wolever TMS, Jenkins DJ, Vuksan V, Jenkins AL, Buckley GC, Wong GS, et al. Beneficial effect of a low glycaemic index diet in type 2 diabetes. Diabet Med. 1992;9(5):451-8.
55. Villegas R, Liu S, Gao YT, Yang G, Li H, Zheng W, Shu XO. Prospective study of dietary carbohydrates, glycemic index, glycemic load, and incidence of type 2 diabetes mellitus in middle-aged Chinese women. Arch Intern Med. 2007;167(21):2310-6.
56. Greenwood DC, Threapleton DE, Evans CE, Cleghorn CL, Nykjaer C, Woodhead C, et al. Glycemic index, glycemic load, carbohydrates, and type 2 diabetes: systematic review and dose-response meta-analysis of prospective studies. Diabetes Care. 2013;36(12):4166-71.

57. Marshall JA, Hoag S, Shetterly S, Hamman RF. Dietary fat predicts conversion from impaired glucose tolerance to NIDDM. The San Luis Valley Diabetes Study. Diabetes Care. 1994;17(1):50-6.
58. Marshall JA, Bessesen DH, Hamman RF. High saturated fat and low starch and fibre are associated with hyperinsulinemia in a non-diabetic population: the San Luis Valley Diabetes Study. Diabetologia. 1997;40(4):430-8.
59. Meyer KA, Kushi LH, Jacobs DR, Folsom AR. Dietary fat and incidence of type 2 diabetes in older Iowa women. Diabetes Care. 2001;24(9):1528-35.
60. Parker DR, Weiss ST, Troisi R, Cassano PA, Vokonas PS, Landsberg L. Relationship of dietary saturated fatty acids and body habitus to serum insulin concentrations: the Normative Aging Study. Am J Clin Nutr. 1993;58(2):129-36.
61. Feskens EJM, Virtanen SM, Rasanen L, Tuomilehto J, Stengard J, Pekkanen J, et al. Dietary factors determining diabetes and impaired glucose tolerance. A 20-year follow-up of the Finnish and Dutch cohorts of the Seven Countries Study. Diabetes Care. 1995;18(8):1104-12.
62. Folsom AR, Ma J, McGovern PG, Eckfeldt H. Relation between plasma phospholipid saturated fatty acids and hyperinsulinemia. Metabolism. 1996;45(2):223-8.
63. Uusitupa M, Schwab U, Makimattila S, Karhapaa P, Sarkkinen E, Maliranta H, et al. Effects of two high-fat diets with different fatty acid compositions on glucose and lipid metabolism in healthy young women. Am J Clin Nutr. 1994;59(6):1310-6.
64. Vessby B, Uusitupa M, Hermansen K, Riccardi G, Rivellese AA, Tapsell LC, et al. Substituting dietary saturated for monounsaturated fat impairs insulin sensitivity in healthy men and women: the KANWU Study. Diabetologia. 2001;44(3):312-9.
65. Mooy JM, Grootenhuis PA, de Vries H, Valkenburg HA, Bouter LM, Kostense PJ, et al. Prevalence and determinants of glucose intolerance in a Dutch Caucasian population. The Hoorn Study. Diabetes Care. 1995;18(9):1270-3.
66. Salmeron J, Hu FB, Manson JE, Stampfer MJ, Colditz GA, Rimm EB, et al. Dietary fat intake and risk of type 2 diabetes in women. Am J Clin Nutr. 2001;73(6):1019-26.
67. Christiansen E, Schnider S, Palmvig B, Tauber-Lassen E, Pedersen O. Intake of a diet high in trans monounsaturated fatty acids or saturated fatty acids. Effects on postprandial insulinemia and glycemia in obese patients with NIDDM. Diabetes Care. 1997;20(5):881-7.
68. Louheranta AM, Turpeinen AK, Vidgren HM, Schwab US, Uusitupa MI. A high-trans fatty acid diet and insulin sensitivity in young healthy women. Metabolism. 1999;48(7):870-5.
69. Rimm EB, Chan J, Stampfer MJ, Colditz GA, Willett WC. Prospective study of cigarette smoking, alcohol use, and the risk of diabetes in men. BMJ. 1995;310(6979):555-9.
70. Ajani UA, Hennekens CH, Spelsberg A, Manson JE. Alcohol consumption and risk of type 2 diabetes mellitus among US male physicians. Arch Intern Med. 2000;160(7):1025-30.
71. Kao WH, Puddey IB, Boland LL, Watson RL, Brancati FL. Alcohol consumption and the risk of type 2 diabetes mellitus: atherosclerosis risk in communities study. Am J Epidemiol. 2001;154(8):748-57.
72. Beulens JW, van der Schouw YT, Bergmann MM, Rohrmann S, Schulze MB, Buijsse B, et al. Alcohol consumption and risk of type 2 diabetes in European men and women: influence of beverage type and body size The EPIC-InterAct study. J Intern Med. 2012;272(4):358-70.
73. Sigal RJ, Kenny GP, Wasserman DH, Castaneda-Sceppa C, White RD. Physical activity/exercise and type 2 diabetes: a consensus statement from the American Diabetes Association. Diabetes Care. 2006;29(6):1433-8.
74. Ramakrishnan U, Martorell R, Schroeder DG, Flores R. Role of intergenerational effects on linear growth. J Nutr. 1999;129(2S Suppl):544S-549S.
75. Gautier JF, Wilson C, Weyer C, Mott D, Knowler WC, Cavaghan M, et al. Low acute insulin secretory responses in adult offspring of people with early onset type 2 diabetes. Diabetes. 2001;50(8):1828-33.
76. Rich-Edwards JW, Colditz GA, Stampfer MJ, Willett WC, Gillman MW, Hennekens CH, et al. Birth weight and the risk of type II diabetes mellitus in adult women. Ann Intern Med. 1999;130(4 Pt 1):278-84.
77. Bateson P, Barker D, Clutton-Brock T, Deb D, D'Udine B, Foley RA, et al. Developmental plasticity and human health. Nature. 2004;430(6998):419-21.

78. Barker DJ. Adult consequences of fetal growth restriction. Clin Obstet Gynecol. 2006;49(2):270-83.
79. Lithell HO, McKeigue PM, Berglund L, Mohsen R, Lithell UB, Leon DA. Relation of size at birth to non-insulin dependent diabetes and insulin concentrations in men aged 50-60 years. BMJ. 1996;312(7028):406-10.
80. Barker DJ, Eriksson JG, Forsén T, Osmond C. Fetal origins of adult disease: strength of effects and biological basis. Int J Epidemiol. 2002;31(6):1235-9.
81. Hales CN Barker DJ. Type 2 (non-insulin-dependent) diabetes mellitus: the thrifty phenotype hypothesis. Diabetologia. 1992;35(7):595-601.
82. Fall CH, Stein CE, Kumaran K, Cox V, Osmond C, Barker DJ, et al. Size at birth, maternal weight, and type II diabetes in South India. Diabet Med. 1998;15(3):220-7.
83. Aboderin I, Kalache A, Ben-Shlomo Y, Lynch JW, Yajnik CS, Kuh DY, et al. Life course perspectives on coronary heart disease, stroke and diabetes: the evidence and implications for policy and research. Geneva, World Health Organization, 2002 (document WHO/NMH/NPH/02.1).
84. Dietz WH. The obesity epidemic in young children. BMJ. 2001;322(7282):313-4.
85. Gillman MW, Rifas-Shiman SL, Camargo CA, Berkey CS, Frazier AL, Rockett HR, et al. Risk of overweight among adolescents who were breastfed as infants. JAMA. 2001;285(19):2461-7.
86. von Kries R, Koletzko B, Sauerwald T, von Mutius E. Does breast-feeding protect against childhood obesity? Adv Exp Med Biol. 2000;478:29-39.
87. Owen CG, Martin RM, Whincup PH, Smith GD, Cook DG. Does breastfeeding influence risk of type 2 diabetes in later life? A quantitative analysis of published evidence. Am J Clin Nutr. 2006;84(5):1043-54.
88. Whitaker RC, Wright JA, Pepe MS, Seidel KD, Dietz WH. Predicting obesity in young adulthood from childhood and parental obesity. N Engl J Med. 1997;337(13):869-73.
89. Wang Y, Ge K, Popkin BM. Tracking of body mass index from childhood to adolescence: a 6-y follow-up study in China. Am J Clin Nutr. 2000;72(4):1018-24.
90. Wright CM, Parker L, Lamont D, Craft AW. Implications of childhood obesity for adult health: findings from thousand families cohort study. BMJ. 2001;323(7324):1280-4.
91. Yajnik C. Interactions of perturbations of intrauterine growth and growth during childhood on the risk of adult-onset disease. Proc Nutr Soc. 2000;59(2):257-65.
92. Yajnik CS. The insulin resistance epidemic in India: fetal origins, later lifestyle, or both? Nutr Rev. 2001;59(1 Pt 1):1-9.
93. United Nations Children's Fund. The state of the world's children 1998. Oxford and New York: Oxford University Press; 1998.
94. Mann JI. Diet and risk of coronary heart disease and type II diabetes. Lancet. 2002;360(9335):783-9.

CHAPTER 4

Goals of Nutritional Management in Obesity and Diabetes

Abstract

Nutritional therapy is a critical component of comprehensive health care and the health and quality of life of individuals with different illnesses can be improved with medical nutrition therapy. This chapter summarizes the goals of the nutritional management of individuals with obesity and diabetes and highlights the importance of individualized nutrition therapy, keeping in mind the food and eating habits, metabolic profile, treatment goals, socio-economic factors, cultural beliefs, and desired outcomes.

Introduction

Medical nutrition therapy (MNT) is a therapeutic approach to treating medical conditions and their associated symptoms through the use of a specifically planned diet, devised and monitored by a registered dietician or clinical nutritionist. The diet is planned based on the patient's medical and psychosocial history, physical examination, functional examination, and dietary history. MNT is a critical component of comprehensive health care. The health and quality of life of individuals with a variety of conditions and illnesses can be improved with medical nutrition therapy. MNT by the nutritionist includes nutritional assessment, planning an appropriate intervention using evidence based practice guidelines, regular monitoring, and follow up.

Goals for Nutritional Management of Obesity

The effective management of body weight includes a judicious balance of nutrient intake, physical activity, behavior modification, and a positive attitude toward achieving appropriate body weight. The main focus should be on achieving good health. While ideal body weight may not be achieved in some cases, it is important to understand that achieving a weight loss that reduces the risk of obesity-related morbidities is beneficial.

The goals of obesity treatment are to:
- Achieve and maintain healthy body weight
- Prevent further weight gain and keep body weight stable
- Provide a comprehensive lifestyle management plan (diet, physical activity and behavior modification) to promote weight loss and subsequent weight maintenance
- Provide individualized, sustainable dietary guidelines to achieve optimal weight loss
- Target realistic weight loss goals, with focus on reduction of body fat. An initial weight loss goal of 5–7% of body weight is recommended
- Promote successful weight maintenance after optimal weight loss, by self-monitoring of body weight, consumption of low energy, low fat foods, engaging in daily physical activity of 60 minutes, decreasing sedentary and screen time
- Improve comorbidities, quality of life, and reduction in mortality rate
- Reduce risk of obesity-related health risk
- In childhood obesity, the nutritional management must achieve control of weight gain and reduction in body mass index safely and effectively, and reduce the risk for the long-term complications of obesity in childhood and adulthood. A multidisciplinary team approach to therapy, involving educators, nutritionists, exercise physiologists, and counselors is likely to prove most effective.

Goals for Diabetes Mellitus

Nutrition therapy is an integral component of successful diabetes management and is one of the most challenging aspects of diabetes care. Nutrition therapy plays a role in preventing diabetes, managing existing diabetes, and preventing or retarding the rate of development of diabetes complications. A trained and skilled registered dietician/clinical nutritionist should lead the team in providing nutrition care. However, it is important that all team members, including physicians and nurses should play active roles and support the nutrition therapy.

Exercise is an important part of the diabetes management plan, since regular exercise improves blood glucose control, reduces cardiovascular risk factors, promotes weight loss, and improves well-being. The individuals with diabetes should be encouraged to be actively involved in all levels of therapy, such as self-management, treatment, and education, along with the nutritionist in order to achieve maximum benefits.

The main goals of nutritional therapy are to:
- Achieve and maintain normal blood glucose and lipid levels
- Achieve and maintain optimal body weight. Intensive lifestyle interventions (nutrition counseling, physical activity, and behavior modifications) with regular follow-up visits are recommended in order to achieve a modest weight loss in diabetic patients
- Promote and support healthy eating patterns with emphasis on reduced energy intake and portion size
- Delay and prevent macro- and microvascular complications of diabetes
- Provide individualized optimal nutrition based on cultural preferences, access to healthy foods, socioeconomic status, willingness to make the change and barriers to change
- Monitor carbohydrate intake by carbohydrate counting in order to achieve glycemic control. Although the evidence on the effect of different levels of carbohydrate in diabetic individuals is inconclusive, evidence suggests that both the quantity and type of carbohydrate in a food influences blood glucose level and total amount of carbohydrate eaten is the primary determinant of glycemic response. The carbohydrate intake from vegetables, fruits, whole grains, legumes, and dairy products should be encouraged, while intake from refined carbohydrate sources should be restricted.
- To provide practical advice to diabetic patients rather than focusing on specific foods. Unnecessary dietary restriction should be avoided and foods should be limited based only on scientific evidence
- To encourage physical activity in children and adults. Children with diabetes or prediabetes should be encouraged to participate in physical activity for at least 60 minutes a day. Adults with diabetes should be advised to perform at least 150 minutes/week of moderate-intensity aerobic physical and in the absence of contraindications, should be encouraged to perform resistance training at least twice per week.

Conclusion

Nutrition therapy for persons with obesity and diabetes should be individualized, keeping in mind the food and eating habits, metabolic profile, treatment goals, socioeconomic factors, cultural beliefs, and desired outcomes. Regular monitoring of metabolic parameters, such as blood glucose, glycated hemoglobin, lipids, blood pressure, body weight, and renal function along with quality of life is essential to assess the need for changes in therapy and to ensure successful outcomes. Ongoing nutrition self-management education and skill should be provided. It is crucial to provide evidence based, practical nutrition therapy, rather than unnecessary restriction of specific foods and nutrients.

CHAPTER 5

Nutritional Management in the Obese

Abstract

Recent advances have been made in dietary therapy, physical activity, behavioral and pharmacologic treatment, and bariatric surgical approaches for successful long-term management of obesity. Effective weight management involves a careful balance of nutrient intake, physical activity, behavior modification, and a positive attitude toward achieving appropriate body weight. This chapter discusses the different treatment options for obesity. Principles of weight reducing diet along with the different dietary strategies for the treatment of obesity have been outlined in this chapter. Additional practical tips on recommendations for healthy eating, healthy options for food, and food choices, while eating out have been provided. The importance of physical activity intervention and behavioral modifications in weight reduction has been reviewed by experts.

Introduction

Obesity at its simplest level, within the context of environmental, social and genetic factors, results from long-term positive energy balance. The rapid increase in the prevalence of obesity in the recent years is more a result of environmental and cultural influences rather than only genetic factors. Due to rapid economic growth and progressive improvements in the standard of living in developed and developing countries, excessive eating and sedentary lifestyle have replaced controlled eating, physical labor, and regular physical activity, leading to positive energy balance and overweight. Recent advances have been made in dietary, physical activity, behavioral, pharmacologic, and bariatric surgical approaches to successful long-term management of obesity. While lifestyle interventions remain the cornerstone in the treatment of obesity, long-term adherence is poor and success is modest because of significant barriers. Effective weight management involves a careful balance of nutrient intake, physical activity, behavior modification, and a positive attitude toward achieving appropriate body weight. The essential components of weight reduction, regardless of the type of diet, are decreased energy intake, increased energy output through physical activity, behavioral modification of lifestyles, and alterations in the larger environment that foster all of these measures and contribute to the energy deficit necessary to reduce weight. The overall aim should focus on "achieving good health". The same eating and exercise habits that support a healthy lifestyle, aimed at decreasing energy intake and increasing energy expenditure, often achieve appropriate body weight. Unfortunately, there is no quick and easy remedy for curing obesity, and the best way to keep off excess weight is through lifelong obesity prevention involving physical activity, balanced with a healthy diet.[1] Pharmacotherapy and bariatric surgery are useful adjuncts for improving the health outcomes of very obese patients, but need to be used only when the benefits surpass the side-effects. The guide to selection of treatment for obesity is presented in table 1.[2]

TABLE 1: Guide to selection of treatment for obesity[2]

Treatment	Body mass index category (kg/m²)				
	25–26.9	27–29.9	30–35	35–39.9	>40
Diet, physical activity, and behavior therapy					
Drug therapy			Comorbidity	Present	
Surgery				Comorbidity	Present

Key Terms

Physical activity: Any bodily movement produced by contraction of the skeletal muscle resulting in energy expenditure above the basal level. The amount of energy expended is determined by the duration, intensity, and frequency of a particular activity and is usually measured in kilocalories. This is a broad term which also includes physical fitness and exercise.[1]

Exercise: A subcategory of physical activity. It is physical activity that is planned, structured, repetitive and purposive with improvement or maintenance of physical fitness as an objective.[2]

Physical fitness: "Ability to carry out daily tasks with vigor and alertness without undue fatigue, and with ample energy to enjoy leisure-time pursuits and to meet unforeseen emergencies." Basically it is a set of attributes that people have to achieve that relates to ability to perform physical activity. It includes health-related and skill-related components. Health-related fitness includes cardio-respiratory endurance, muscular endurance and strength, body composition and flexibility. Skill-related components that refer to athletic ability include agility, balance, coordination, speed, power and reaction time.[2]

Physical inactivity: Physical inactivity refers to insufficient activity or sedentary activity. It is a "state when body movement is minimal and energy expenditure approximates the resting metabolic rate (RMR)".[3]

References
1. US Department of Health and Human Services. Physical activity and health. A report of the surgeon general. Jones and Bartlett Publishers; 1998.
2. Caspersen CJ, Powell KE, Christenson GM. Physical activity, exercise, and physical fitness: definitions and distinctions for health-related research. Public Health Rep. 1985;100(2):126-31.
3. Dietz WH. The role of lifestyle in health: the epidemiology and consequences of inactivity. Proc Nutr Soc. 1996 Nov;55(3):829-40.

Dietary Intervention

The cornerstone of weight reduction efforts is dietary intervention. A moderate weight loss can reduce the risk of type 2 diabetes in obese patients, improve blood pressure, and lipid levels.[3] The dropout rates of a dietary intervention program are often high and this is most often due to the fact that obese patients have an unrealistic view of the amount of weight that they can lose.[4] Since modest (10%) weight reduction in obese people often results in clinical improvements of several health-related parameters, it is important that health professionals and patients should not be overwhelmed by their inability to meet excessively ambitious, or unrealistic, weight loss goals. Even small amounts of weight loss can bring considerable health and social benefits.

While the dietary treatment of obesity is primarily carried out by the nutritionist/dietician, the role of the physician should not be underplayed. The role of the physician is crucial because obese patients receiving weight reduction advice from their physicians were found to embark on weight loss attempts more than those who do not receive advice.[5] Additionally, when physicians included recommendations for lifestyle changes in counseling their obese patients, the weight loss was greater.[5]

The various steps involved in the dietary treatment of an overweight/obese individual is presented in flowchart 1.

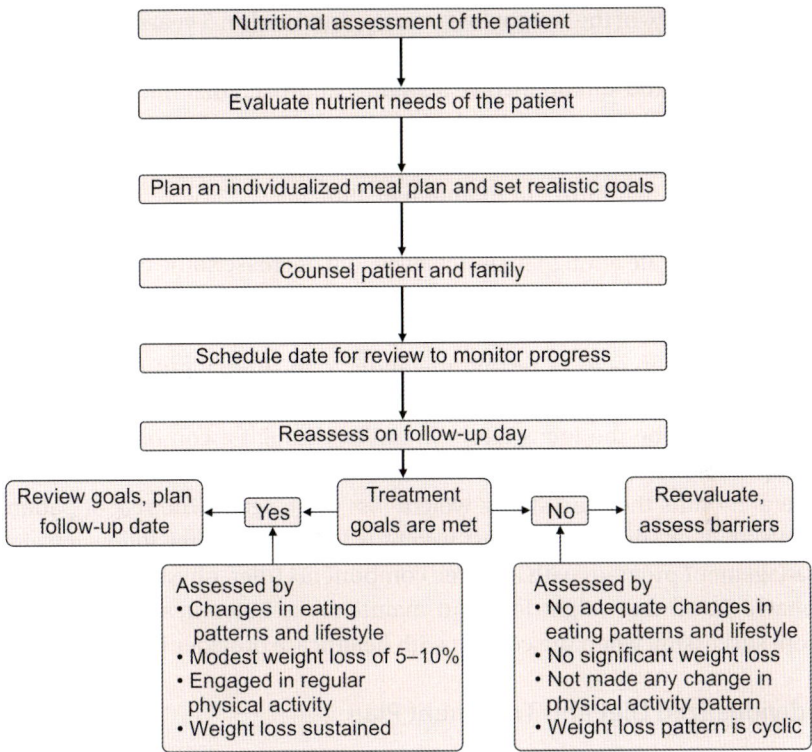

Flowchart 1 Steps in the dietary treatment of an overweight/obese individual.

Setting Reasonable Goals

Goal setting is an important part of achieving weight loss and the focus should be on an acceptable weight to achieve good health outcomes, rather than simply reaching a lower body weight. Overweight and obese patients are often hesitant to broach the topic of weight loss, but yet they wish for assistance in discussing, setting, and achieving weight loss goals. Obese patients who had discussed weight loss, with their healthcare professional were three times more likely to lose weight than those who had not.[6] Determining whether the patient's weight-related goals are realistic and attainable, and agreeing on the realistic goals facilitates maintenance of the weight loss achieved.[7] Patients are likely to go in favor of short-term drastic measures of weight loss rather than long-term "healthy" measures. Thus, it should be emphasized to the patients that the primary reason for losing weight is health, and weight control measures must be healthy. Healthy weight loss has shown to be the key for long-term weight maintenance.[7,8] Intensive very low-calorie diets (VLCD), although achieving up to 20% short-term weight loss, is not sustainable and greater than 50% of the weight loss was regained within 5 years.[9] The optimal weight reduction goal varies depending on the patient's weight and associated comorbidities and should involve a gradual approach that minimizes health risks, timed to the patient's level of readiness, motivations, and attainable short-term targets. The primary medical concern is to help the patient lose enough weight to improve or maintain health.

The target is to lose 5–10% of the baseline weight at the end of 6 months, which is moderate enough to be achieved and decrease some obesity-related risk factors, such as type 2 diabetes, hypertension, cardiovascular disease, and sleep apnea.[10] After about 6 months, the patients could have difficulty sustaining adherence, as resting metabolic rate (RMR) and energy output decreases, causing the body weight to plateau. Maintenance of the lost weight should be the focus after 6 months, through a combination of diet therapy, physical activity, and behavior modification. If successful, after several months they can start a weight loss cycle again. The risk of patients to regain all or some of their lost weight is lower when they follow a weight management program with all three components (diet, physical activity, and behavior) and the weight loss and maintenance outcomes of patients are more successful, when the contact with healthcare provider is frequent.[8]

Individualized Diet and Treatment Plan

Evidence-based reviews of successful weight control techniques increasingly emphasize the importance of individualized, multidisciplinary care, a health-outcome focus, realistic goal setting, and making permanent lifestyle changes including an increase in physical activity.[2,11] The strategies for weight reduction need to be individualized to avoid positive energy balance and promote adherence and success.[1] Since, there is no one "single formula" that works for everyone, the dietary approaches for maximizing adherence are successful to varying degrees in different patients. The weight loss strategy planned should keep in mind the previous success and failure patterns of the patients, with regards to weight loss. Patients should be encouraged to maintain daily records of their food and beverage intake, since record keeping often increases awareness of consumption and promotes dietary adherence.

General Principles of Weight Reduction Diet

Successful weight control and loss requires dietary modifications of the type, quantity, and/or frequency of food and drink consumed, to achieve and maintain a hypocaloric intake. This is followed by a maintenance phase. In order to achieve a weight loss of about 0.5 kg per week, resulting from a loss of adipose tissue, an energy deficit of 3,500 kcal per week is required. This translates to a daily energy deficit of at least 500 kcals per day.[12] The goal of the dietary treatment of obesity during energy deficit period is to decrease body fat stores, preserve the lean body mass, and to keep its loss to a minimum.[13] A very hypocaloric diet with rapid weight loss increases the loss of lean tissue, while a combination of exercise (both cardiovascular and resistance) and adequate dietary protein (0.8–1.5 g/kg of body weight) helps to minimize lean tissue loss.[14]

Calculating Daily Energy Requirements

The energy requirement of an individual is based on age, gender, physical activity and has been explained previously in chapter 2 (Nutritional Assessment and Body Composition). Ideal body weight should be aimed to maintain a body mass index (BMI) between 18 and 22.9 kg/m^2.[15] In case of patients who are to be put on a weight reducing diet, calories should be reduced by about 500 kcal/day to achieve a 0.5 kg weight loss/week.

Dietary Strategies

Dietary strategies for the treatment of obesity can be broadly divided into two types:
1. Decreased calorie content (altering quantity of diet)
   - Low-calorie diets (LCD) reduce the amounts of all macronutrients, including fat, to achieve a daily caloric intake of 1,000–1,400 kcal/day
   - Very low-calorie diets recommend a daily caloric intake of less than 1,000 kcal/day and invariably restrict fat and carbohydrate, but near normal protein intake is maintained.
2. Adjusting macronutrient balance (altering quality of diet)
   - Low-fat diets are focused primarily on limiting fat intake with no recommendations concerning caloric intake
   - Carbohydrate-restricted diets specify either a modest restriction of carbohydrate and an increase in protein intake or a severe restriction of carbohydrate intake and an increase in protein and fat intake
   - Low-glycemic-index diets mostly recommend a diet with a low glycemic load: carbohydrate intake is maintained but the type of carbohydrate consumed is changed to deliver a lower glycemic load.

Low-calorie Diets

The rationale for using a LCD of 1,000–1,200 kcals/day for women and 1,200–1,600 kcals/day for men is that there will be a deficit of approximately 500–1,000 kcals per day causing a slow progressive weight loss of about 0.5–1.0 kg/week.[2] Even with perfect adherence to the diets, the amount of weight loss will vary between individuals, due to the difference in resting energy expenditure and physical activity. While LCDs reduced body weight by about

8% over 3–12 months of treatment, with decrease in abdominal fat, there was no improvement seen in cardiorespiratory fitness (VO_2 max), unless the diet was accompanied by increased physical activity.[2] The benefits of LCD that provide portion controlled servings or liquid meal replacements have been studied. Patients on portion controlled diets, which provide a fixed amount of food with known calorie content lost significantly greater body weight when compared to those who were prescribed conventional diet of 1,000 kcal.[16] Similarly, the weight loss of patients using liquid meal replacement was more (2.5 kg more) than conventional diets[17] and it has also been suggested that long-term use of meal replacement may significantly improve the maintenance of weight loss.[18] However, randomized controlled trials (RCT) are needed to confirm these findings.

Very Low-calorie Diets

These diets are designed to produce very rapid weight loss, preserve lean body mass by providing below 800 kcals, 50–80 g of protein, and 100% of the recommended intake for vitamins and minerals per day.[19] VLCDs, often through meal replacement liquid diets, form an intensive diet therapy, to promote rapid and significant weight loss (13–23 kgs) over 3–6 month periods.[20] Randomized trials comparing the short-term and long-term results of LCD and VLCD have found no significant differences in weight loss after 1 or more years of treatment,[21,22] and this was mainly due to the greater weight gain in VLCD treated patients. The special feature of the VLCD are the low-calorie level and a relatively high percent of protein; 0.8–1.5 g/kg of ideal body weight. The amount of protein in the VLCD diets are high because, in the hypocaloric state, the efficiency of protein utilization for maintaining the body's lean cell mass is lessened and also since very heavy individuals, have more lean tissue and thus higher protein levels may help to preserve protein nutritional status. VLCD also have extremely low fat content and relatively low carbohydrate levels, making them ketogenic. It may be essential to supplement vitamins and minerals, especially potassium, calcium, iron, zinc, vitamin C, vitamin B6, copper, and possibly other nutrients. VLCDs are often used when the health risks from obesity are severe and threatening, so it is imperative to lose weight. In patients with BMI greater than 30 kg/m², the VLCDs are effective in promoting significant short-term weight loss and improving obesity-related comorbidities such as obstructive sleep apnea, poorly-controlled type 2 diabetes, and hypertriglyceridemia.[23] These diets need close metabolic supervision and should be followed only under medical supervision. The medical contraindications include recent myocardial infarction, history of cardiovascular disease, renal or hepatic disease, cancer, type 1 diabetes, and pregnancy, while the behavioral contraindications are bulimia nervosa, major depression, bipolar disorder, substance abuse,

Nutritional Management in the Obese

and acute psychiatric illness. Since dehydration could occur, patients on VLCDs should drink at least 2 liters of water/day and avoid caffeine.[8] The common minor side-effects that occur include fatigue, dizziness, muscle cramps, gastrointestinal distress (constipation and/or diarrhea), and cold intolerance. In case of very rapid weight loss, the risk of cholelithiasis (gallstones) is increased, and this can be reduced by limiting the weight loss to below 1.5 kg/week.[24] Short-term modified alternate-day fasting (ADF) is a new dietary strategy in which a patient consumes 25% of their energy needs on the fast day, and ad libitum food intake the next day. The ADF was found to help obese patients lose weight and decrease their risk of coronary artery disease.[25] However; there is a need for further research before using this approach for weight loss.

Low Fat Diet

Since fat has twice the calories as compared to carbohydrate and protein, limiting fat would result in fewer ingested calories and resultant weight loss. However, this strategy has shown mixed results. Some studies show that it is superior to simple calorie-restricted diets,[26,27] while others showed no advantage,[28,29] in the short-term. A systematic review of RCT found that a 10% decrease in fat calories is required for successful weight loss;[30] an aggressive reduction of dietary fat, rather than minimal modifications, is essential for this strategy to be effective. The low-fat diet appears more effective when coupled with exercise in the weight loss program, at least in women.[31] A low-fat diet does appear to be important for long-term weight loss maintenance.[32] Additionally, even on a low-fat diet, it is important that there should be a proper balance of fatty acids. Diets providing high intakes of both polyunsaturated fatty acid (PUFA), such as linoleic acid (LA) and α-linolenic acid (ALA), or balanced LA/ALA ratio, and long-chain n-3 PUFAs from fish/fish oils, have shown to be effective to prevent diet related noncommunicable diseases.[33-35] Thus, rather than complete dependence on one single oil, it is better to use a combination of 2–3 vegetable oils in order to endure optimal intake of all fatty acids. The recommended combination of oils to be used in Indian diets is given in table 2.

Low-carbohydrate Diets, High Protein Diets

A "low-carbohydrate" diet allows ad libitum consumption of protein and fat while limiting carbohydrate intake to 20 g/day. The proposed mechanism is that the fast-release energy of carbohydrates, compared with more slowly metabolized lipids or proteins, triggers an elevated insulin response, appetite stimulation, and weight gain. Thus, restricting carbohydrates decreases this and shifts the metabolism to lipolysis, which breaks down the body fat stores, promoting weight loss. The resultant ketosis is believed to suppress

TABLE 2: Recommended combinations of oils to be used in India (1:1 ratio)[36]

Oils containing LA + oil containing LA + ALA	Oil containing high LA + oil containing moderate or low LA
Groundnut/sesame/rice bran/cotton seed + mustard	Sunflower/safflower + palm/olive
Groundnut/sesame/rice bran/cotton seed + canola	Safflower/sunflower + groundnut/sesame/rice bran
Groundnut/sesame/rice bran/cotton seed + soya bean	
Palmolein + soya bean	
Safflower/sunflower + palmolein + mustard	

ALA, α-linoleic acid; LA, linoleic acid.

the appetite, further contributing to weight loss.[37] A low-carbohydrate diet, during the initial period of weight reduction program will cause shifts in water balance and weight. In response to reduced carbohydrate intake, glycogen stores are depleted and the resultant diuresis produces an initial steep weight loss, which however will not continue. There is less water weight to lose as the glycogen stores are rapidly depleted, and hence it is difficult to sustain the initial weight loss. Patients on very low-carbohydrate diets (e.g., less than 20 g per day) could have decreased hunger as the body produces ketones to sustain fuel utilization in the brain. The low-carbohydrate diet has been criticized because of its high saturated fat content and low fiber, vitamin, mineral content. While the low-carbohydrate diets do result in weight loss,[38] their efficacy is comparable to other diets[29,39] suggesting that total caloric intake, rather low-carbohydrate content is responsible for the weight loss. The weight loss at 6 months was more for individuals' assigned to ad libitum low-carbohydrate diets, than those assigned to low-fat, reduced-energy diets, but the difference was not significant at 12 months.[40] These results suggest that low-carbohydrate high-protein diets are effective and safe for short-term use, but additional long-term studies are needed to determine its safety and efficacy. Additionally, the low-carbohydrate diet may be inappropriate for long-term use as, globally guidelines suggest that for weight reduction and maintenance, patients should decrease the intake of saturated fat and increase the intake of fruits and vegetables.

Low-glycemic Index Diets

Glycemic index (GI) is a measure of serum glucose response to a food relative to reference food that contains equal amounts of carbohydrate. Refined carbohydrates are high-GI foods, while vegetables, fruits, and legumes have low GI. A diet rich in foods with high GI stimulates appetite, insulin oversecretion, and weight gain. Poor appetite regulation causes increased energy intake and thus increased body weight. A diet with low GI (low simple carbohydrate) was found to be more effective for weight loss rather than a low-carbohydrate diet (low glycemic load).[41] However, other studies have found no effect.[42,43] There is insufficient evidence to use GI in the long-term management of diabetes[44,45] and further studies are needed.

Thus, it can be summed that there are numerous dietary strategies for weight loss that work in the short-term. Restricting one dietary component is not effective for long-term weight loss and the main mechanism by which weight loss is attained is by decreased caloric intake. The ultimate benefit of a weight reducing diet is judged by its long-term effects on body weight and general health.

Maintenance of Weight Loss

While a reasonable weight loss of 8–10% of initial body weight is achievable at 6 months by most dietary weight-loss strategies, the big challenge of treatment for obesity is long-term weight maintenance. Since long-term changes in food habits are difficult to sustain, people who have lost weight recently are at high risk of weight regain. Weight maintenance can be achieved by following a nutritionally balanced healthy diet. The nutrient based guidelines for healthy eating is presented in table 3.[36]

TABLE 3: Recommendations for healthy eating[36]

Nutrient	Recommendations
Carbohydrate	• 50–60% of total calorie intake • Primary source should be complex carbohydrate (whole wheat, brown rice, ragi, jowar, pulses and legumes) • Food with low glycemic index such as oats, unpolished rice, whole pulses, legumes, and whole fruits are preferred • Fiber intake should be 25–40 g/day • 4–5 servings of fruits and vegetables per day • Simple sugars, such as sugar, carbonated beverages, and fruit juice, to be restricted and below 10% of total energy of diet
Fat	• Should be below 30% of diet • Saturated fat should be below 10% of diet, in patient with high low-density lipoprotein it should be < 7% of diet • Essential polyunsaturated fats to be within 5–8% of total energy • Monounsaturated fat to be 10–15% of energy • Cholesterol intake to be within 200–300 mg/day • Trans fat at <1% energy/day • In order to ensure optimal intake of fatty acids, a combination of cooking oil has to be used • Consumption of butter, ghee to be limited • The use of partially hydrogenated vegetable oils (vanaspati) to be avoided

Continued

Continued

Nutrient	Recommendations
Protein	• Requirement is about 1 g/kg body weight based on the quality of protein • Recommended non-vegetarian sources are fish, egg white, and lean chicken, while vegetarian sources are soya, whole gram (channa, rajma, green gram), and low-fat dairy foods
Salt	• Salt intake should be below 5 g/day • Addition of extra salt at the table should be avoided • Processed foods rich in salt (pickles, chutneys, namkeens, papads, bakery items, potato chips, popcorn, salty biscuits, preserved meat products, other pre-prepared and preserved foods, soups, cheese, and fast foods) should be limited • Encourage reading of food labels

Some additional points that need to be emphasized while counseling a patient on a weight reducing/maintenance diet include:
- Start the day with a healthy breakfast
- Aim to include at least five portions of fruit and vegetables each day—3 vegetables and 2 fruits
- Include either green leafy vegetables, whole gram, or a salad with every meal
- Avoid eating at the same time as doing something else (e.g., watching TV, working, or reading)
- Read food labels on the products you buy
- Boil or steam vegetables rather than frying. Use the idli vessel or a steamer for steaming the vegetables.
- Avoid fast foods and quick service counter foods as they are rich in energy and fat
- Include adequate water and fiber intake
- Portion size reduction
- Limit alcohol consumption
- Watch portion size and eat sensibly while eating out

Foods to be included in the diet of an overweight/obese patient
Dietary Fiber

Foods rich in fiber tend to be lower in total calories, saturated fat, and cholesterol. A high fiber diet is associated with increased satiety and decreased appetite, and thus can be an important adjunct to weight management plans. Increasing fruit and vegetable intake alone does not help with weight loss,[46] but consuming them along with other low energy-dense foods was shown to control hunger.[47-49] Thus, it appears that the addition of these foods to the menu does not result in weight loss independent of caloric restriction. Eating a variety of high-fiber foods is recommended as most fiber-rich foods contain a mixture of both soluble and insoluble fibers. The dietary fiber intake should be gradually increased along with the increased intake of fluids. The recommended fiber intake for adults is between 25–40 g/day.

A few tips to increase the fiber content of the diet is given below:
- Eat whole fruits instead of fruit juices and consume fruits, such as apple, guava, pear with skin, after careful washing
- Replace white rice, maida with brown rice and whole wheat flour
- Choose wheat flakes, bran, and oats for breakfast and toss in cut fruits along with milk
- Snack on fruits and vegetables rather than fried foods and sweets
- Substitute whole grams (channa, rajma, green gram, horse gram) twice a week for meat.

Dietary Calcium

An association between high calcium intake, low body weight, low fat mass, and low abdominal fat was observed,[50] which supported an earlier study which indicated that high calcium intake was significantly related to lower BMI.[51] Calcium may play a small, but significant role in people whose adipocyte status is changing, such as during weight loss, age associated weight gain and growth.[52] When the effects of a high versus low dairy calcium breakfast on satiety and subsequent food choices was evaluated, it was observed that subjects who ate high dairy calcium breakfast had significantly lower food intake over the next 24 hours.[53] A review of randomized controlled trials was conducted[54] to evaluate whether increasing intakes of calcium or vitamin D (single or combined) had an effect on weight and fat loss. Of the 15 studies evaluated, only 2 studies that supplemented calcium during calorie restriction observed fat loss. The authors concluded that while studies favored the hypothesis that calcium accelerated weight or fat loss, the studies lacked statistical power.[54]

Water

Water is necessary for metabolism and for physiological functions in the body, and is also a source of essential minerals, including calcium, magnesium, and fluoride. Fluid requirements vary depending on individuals and specific population. The normal recommendation for water is 1.5–2 L (8–10 glasses) of water every day; intake could be increased in hot climates, situations of vigorous work, and outdoor activity. Adequate water intake is important on weight reduction diets to prevent dehydration, especially if diets are ketogenic or very low in calories. Water losses accompany the

TABLE 4: Suggested foods that can be used as healthier options

Opt for these ✓	Reduce these ↓
Whole fruit	Fruit juice
Whole wheat noodles, pasta, bread, and multigrain bread	Maida noodles, maida pasta, white bread
Grilled vegetable sandwiches	Cheese burgers
Dark chocolate, rice crispy bars, whole grain, nut and fruit bars	Caramel bars
Whole nuts (baked)	Fried and salted nuts
Home-made lemonade, water, fresh lime soda with sugar syrup on the side	Aerated drinks
Milk shakes, flavored milk (preferably skim milk)	Soft drinks
Grain or fiber rich biscuits	Butter biscuits
Bhel puri, chats without fried papdi	Pani puri, masala puri, sev puri, kachori, samosa chat
Plain vegetable soup	Cream soup

loss of body glycogen and protein and thus emphasis on intake of water should be integral to every weight reducing regime.[55] Table 4 provides a list of suggested foods that can be used as healthier options.

Other Dietary Instructions/Modifications

Portion Size

Excessive portions of energy-dense foods lead to the overconsumption of energy. Since it is not just large portion sizes, but also large portion size of energy-dense foods that can increase energy intake, it may not be effective to just tell individuals to "eat less". Including large portions of foods low in energy density, such as vegetables, fruits, and clear soups, can help weight management by providing satisfying portions with little calories.[56,57] Patients should be educated on the principles of both portion size control and energy density. Food and restaurant industries, policy makers, scientists, and consumers need to work together to develop successful strategies.

Eating Right While Eating Out

Eating out has been linked to overweight and obesity as calorie intake often increases when dining out. Some of the tips that can be given to obese patients are:
- Try to avoid buffet, as the variety of choices will make you overeat on unwanted calories

- Never go hungry to a restaurant as you will snack on everything that is offered
- Choose your dish based on method of cooking (boiled, steamed, grilled, baked are better choices)
- Omit high calorie toppings such as sour cream, mayonnaise, and tartar sauce
- Avoid high calorie salad dressings and opt for simple dressing with lemon juice, vinegar, and some olive oil
- Choose water over carbonated drinks and fruit juices. If choosing fresh lime soda, ask for the sugar syrup to be got separately
- Eat smaller portions, choose healthy snacks
- Choose lean meat (fish, chicken) and plenty of vegetables
- Choose fresh fruit as dessert.

Breakfast and Eating Patterns

Eating breakfast is one way to help control weight and increase metabolism for the day.[58] Individuals, who do not eat breakfast, may tend to be hungry later in the day and thus may consume more calories in the evening than individuals who eat consistently throughout the day, resulting in increased body weight.[59] Low-meal frequency is associated with higher 24-hour insulin concentrations, when compared with high-meal frequency and thus eating multiple, small meals may suppress hunger and overall serum insulin concentrations. Insulin inhibits lipase enzyme activity and increases fat deposition. Since insulin is related to fatty acid storage, meal frequency may be one of the factors affecting body weight.[60] Finally, there is some evidence to suggest that eating late in the evening could be related to obesity, however, more controlled studies are needed to confirm these findings.

Restrict and Choose List

The use of avoid and choose lists (Table 5) can help the patient to choose the right food under each food group, without always having to count the calories and also help the patient achieve behavioral change.

Dietary Supplements

Patients on a VLCD may not meet the recommended needs of nutrients. But all individuals should check with their physician before starting a supplement as some supplements could have added herbs, enzymes, or amino acids that could interfere with medications such as anticoagulants. Additionally, since overuse of multivitamin and mineral supplements is of concern, no supplementation should be started without consulting a healthcare professional.

TABLE 5: List of foods that are restricted and allowed on a weight reducing diet

Foods	Restrict	Allowed
Cereals, bread, pasta	White bread, maida products, bakery items such as puffs, rolls	Brown bread, whole wheat chapattis, oats, bran, ragi
Vegetables	Root vegetables, vegetables prepared with cream sauce, butter, coconut, or deep fried	Fresh or frozen vegetables cooked with less oil and without coconut. Salads with low-calorie dressings like lime juice, vinaigrette, olive oil
Fruits	Banana, mango, jackfruit, avocado, canned fruits with lots of sugar syrup	All other fresh and dry fruits
Dairy Products	Whole milk, cream, cheese, sour cream, condensed milk	Skimmed milk, buttermilk, curds, low-fat paneer
Meat	Organ meat like liver, kidney, heart, red meat, processed meat products such as bacon, ham, sausages, egg yolk	Fish, lean cut of meat with fat trimmed, chicken without skin, egg white
Fats	Saturated fat, butter, vanaspati, ghee	Vegetable oils
Miscellaneous	Sugars, sweets, desserts, chocolates, biscuits, processed foods like jams, fried items such as chips, mixtures, namkeens, samosa	

Dietary treatment of obesity has a critical role, as a part of a comprehensive program of weight control, which includes increased physical activity, lifestyle modification, and behavioral changes. Dietary approaches to obesity management should not be viewed as an independent treatment but, as one of the component of a long-term weight control program to keep weights and risks at healthier levels.

PHYSICAL ACTIVITY INTERVENTION

Introduction

Excess body weight is caused by the imbalance between energy intake and energy expenditure, when energy intake is greater than energy expenditure thus causing a "positive energy balance". Approximately 60% of energy expenditure is contributed by the basal metabolic rate (BMR), 10% by diet induced thermogenesis and about 30% by physical activity, which is the major modifiable component of energy expenditure that has been the target of behavioral interventions to reduce body weight.[61]

Evidence suggests that engaging in regular physical activity prevents development of overweight and obesity. Likewise, once a person becomes overweight or obese, regular physical activity confers several clinical benefits. The contraction of the muscles and the increased heart rate due to physical activity increases the energy expenditure.

Energy expenditure is related to both body size and body composition. The average adult's basal (BMR) or resting metabolic rate (RMR) is approximately 3.5 mL/kg/min oxygen or 1 kcal/kg body weight per hour. The energy cost of activities is expressed as multiples of BMR, otherwise known as metabolic equivalents (METs) and can vary from 2.0 METs for leisurely walking to 8.0 METs for running at 8 km/h or playing football.[62] If a person has to expend about 150 kcals, the duration of time required to expend this amount will depend on the MET of the activity. If the MET value is 3.0, then 150 kcals divided by the MET level of the activity, that is, in this case 3.0, will be 50 minutes. Depending on the intensity, activities with METs less than 3.0 are termed light activities; those with METs ranging between 3.0 to 6.0 are termed moderate, while those over 6.0 are vigorous. Hence to expend the same amount of kilocalories, a person has to engage for a shorter duration of time as the MET value increases. However, it has been reported that low intensity, longer duration exercise is the most suitable form of exercise for the overweight and obese.[63] At the same time, a study[64] has indicated that exercise accumulated to 30 minutes in short bouts rather than in one long bout over a 12 week period significantly increased VO_2 max and decreased BMI and the sum of skinfolds in overweight women.

In recent years, low levels of physical activity and/or high levels of sedentary behavior have become a matter of concern especially with health related problems increasing.[65] Increasing the time spent in sedentary behaviors displaces the time spent on moderate-to-vigorous physical activity.[66] At present, there is a lot of focus on sitting too much, especially with the advent of television, computers, and labor saving devices and transportation trends. Sitting time and nonexercise activity has been linked in epidemiological studies to obesity.[67] Physiologically, sitting induces the loss of local contractile stimulation leading to loss of skeletal muscle lipoprotein lipase (LPL) activity and reduced glucose uptake. LPL is required for triglyceride uptake and for high density lipoprotein (HDL) cholesterol production.[66] Hence, in any weight management program, it is essential to ensure an increase in physical activity and reduce sedentary behavior. Even if the patient does not lose weight, regular physical activity confers certain health related benefits in overweight and obese patients. This must be coupled with adequate decrease in energy intake for the weight management program to be very effective.

In order to promote weight loss, it is essential to create a situation of energy deficit, or in other words, a "negative energy balance".[61] Short-term interventions using exercise alone or exercise in combination with energy restriction have indicated that restriction in energy in combination with exercise have had the greatest impact on weight loss rather than just increases in energy expenditure through exercise, although a decrease in energy intake also results in weight loss.[61] Although physical activity may not contribute significantly to weight loss, it is critical for maintenance of weight loss.[68] Using a combination of diet and physical activity, intervention has shown reductions in body weight and body fat, lipid profile, systolic blood pressure, in general, and cardiometabolic risk factors and improvement in physical fitness in adults[69,70] and in children.[71] Physical activity, (both exercise endurance training and resistance training) has been shown to improve glucose regulation by enhancing insulin action in the skeletal muscle. Lean skeletal muscle mass has an average resting energy expenditure of 17.6 kcal/kg. Through resistance exercise training, an increase or maintenance of fat free mass can be achieved by stimulating skeletal muscle growth[72,73] while aerobic exercise reduces body fat.[73]

Physical activity is essential for weight loss maintenance due to its impact on energy expenditure. With weight loss, the BMR or the total energy expenditure decreases. The more the decline in energy expenditure with weight loss, the lower is the food intake required to maintain the weight loss. Additionally, physical activity enhances fat-free mass which is metabolically more active than fat mass and could increase energy expenditure.[68]

Counseling for Physical Activity

An initial assessment of the physical activity level of the patient is necessary before counseling on physical activity and behavior modification. It also helps to identify those who do not meet the minimal requirement of physical activity per day (over 60 minutes of moderate-to-vigorous physical activity). It is essential to assess and establish weight loss goals. Benefits include, the risk factor reduction for coronary heart disease and related comorbidities. A feasible target is a weight loss of about 10% of body weight over a period of 6 months. Patient concerns on exercising and an understanding of the social barriers, such as feeling uncomfortable while exercising in public, must be taken into account while advising on the exercise schedule so that patient compliance is ensured. In general, the benefits and barriers to physical activity must be discussed.[74] The guidelines for physical activity are provided in table 6.

About 150 minutes per week of moderate intensity physical activity to achieve weight control leads to better health outcomes, although higher levels may be required to achieve long-term weight loss outcomes.[61] About

TABLE 6 : General guidelines for physical activity

Adults	60 minutes of physical activity daily which should include at least 30 minutes of moderate intensity aerobic activity, 15 minutes of work-related activity, and 15 minutes of muscle strengthening exercises
Children and adolescents	Accumulation of a minimum of 60 minutes and up to several hours of at least moderate-to-vigorous physical activity daily which is achieved through sports activities and active transport. Sedentary activities including viewing television and working on computers should be restricted to less than 2 hours per day during leisure time. This should include about 20–30 minutes of muscle strengthening physical activity (e.g., playground equipment, climbing trees, lifting weights, etc.) on at least 3 days a week and 20–30 minutes of bone strengthening exercises (e.g., running, hop-scotch, jumping rope, tennis, etc.)
Pregnancy and lactation	Moderate intensity exercise for at least 30 minutes on most if not all days of the week (~150 min/week) in the absence of any contra-indications is considered safe throughout pregnancy. For lactating women, exercise should be initiated as soon as possible after the birth of the baby
Elderly	Recommended exercise levels are similar to healthy adults with added resistance training for improving strength and physical functioning

TABLE 7: Examples of activities with various physical activity intensities

Light intensity	Watching television, writing, desk work, slow walking (less than 3.2 km/hour), strolling
Moderate intensity	Walking at moderate or brisk pace, roller skating, cycling, driving or maneuvering heavy vehicles, running, home exercise, yoga, dancing, gardening work like digging or raking leaves, scrubbing or mopping the floor, carrying heavy grocery bags, carrying a child or grocery bags, below 12 kgs, up the stairs, manual sweeping and washing of clothes, actively playing with children, pushing the stroller, playing table tennis, tennis, cricket, jumping on trampoline, playing frisbee, playing on school playground equipment, hopscotch
Vigorous intensity	Jogging, running, trekking, uphill bicycling, bicycling more than 10 mph, push-ups and pull-ups, karate, judo, boxing, competitive sports (football, basketball, swimming), skipping, moving or pushing heavy furniture, carrying more than 12 kgs of grocery or a child up the stairs

Reference: www.cdc.gov/nccdphp/dnpa/physical/.../PA_Intensity_table_2_1.pdf

2,500–2,800 kcal/week, that is, 60–90 minutes of daily moderate-intensity physical activity may be required to attain substantial weight losses of approximately 14 kg or more.[68] Table 7 provides examples of activities with different physical activity intensity. Both aerobic and resistance exercise schedules need to be included in the regimen. Additionally, advising intermittent bouts of accumulated exercise would ensure both participation as well as compliance to the exercise schedule.[61] Lifestyle approaches, such as walking instead of using motorized transport and walking up the stairs instead of using the lift and reducing the time spent sitting and watching television or working on the computer, should be used while advising overweight or obese patients. A 2 to 5 minute walking break every hour, instead of continuously sitting for 8 hours, allows a person to expend about 59–132 kcals per day.[75]

For a weight loss program to be successful, it is necessary to have multiple contacts with the patient on behavioral modifications to increase physical activity behaviors, provide advice and motivate on the appropriate exercises to be engaged in, including information on harms and benefits, and decide with the patient a realistic goal to be achieved and the modification in lifestyle required to meet this goal.[76] High impact activities should be avoided as it hinders patient compliance and increases risk of injury.

The present guidelines and recommendations for physical activity for overweight and obese Asian Indians[77] are:
- Gradual initiation and increase in duration of physical activity among sedentary individuals
- At least 150 minutes per week of moderate intensity aerobic physical activity for substantial health benefits and 300 minutes per week of moderate-intensity physical activity for more sustained weight loss
- For prevention of weight regain after weight loss, 60–90 minutes of daily moderate intensity physical activity.

In general, obese individuals should begin with low intensity aerobic exercises for a short duration and increase the duration and intensity to achieve 60 minutes of daily moderate intensity aerobic exercises (e.g., walking, running, jogging, cycling, climbing stairs, swimming, etc.). Once weight loss is achieved the exercise schedule should be maintained.

Overall, lifestyle based changes that increase physical activities over baseline level are most successful in weight loss programs. Patients should be encouraged to increase their physical activity level to gain functional or health benefits even in the absence of substantial reductions in weight. In obese patients in whom cardiovascular fitness is low, the emphasis should be on duration and frequency of physical activity rather than on intensity. Only among those with high cardiovascular fitness should the intensity be increased. It should however be recognized that a single prescription on physical activity may not suit everyone as it is dependent on initial fitness, health status, personal preference and lifestyle. For an individual to sustain the activity, a preferred type of activity is important.

BEHAVIORAL MODIFICATIONS

Introduction

Behavioral modification is a term which describes the use of behavioral techniques to modify or change lifestyle behaviors (diet and physical inactivity) that lead to obesity. Traditional Indian practices like yoga emphasize the necessity to take good care of one's physical body by proper nutrition and exercise in order to achieve what is truly important in life—one's spiritual journey. One could say that the "yoga lifestyle" lists one of the most holistic behavioral guidelines for weight and health management.

The behavioral management of obesity ultimately focuses on helping the patient use various behavioral strategies to modify eating behavior and physical activity levels[78] in order to reduce body weight, improve levels of fitness, and reduce the morbidity and mortality due to obesity and diabetes.[79,80]

The Goal of Behavioral Management

The goal of behavioral management should ideally be to help the obese individual improve their health status and not merely lose weight. As it is not easy for patients to sustain advice which merely states "eat less and exercise more", lifestyle management is all about helping the person make their own road map to weight loss—to identify "obesogenic" eating behaviors and barriers to physical activity in his own life and set about gradually changing them, permanently.

Terminology

Though obesity occurs in all genders, for ease, uniformity, and to avoid gender bias, the obese individual will be referred to as a male in this section. Though the term "client" is sometimes used in weight loss literature, the term "patient" will be used here as it better conveys the nuances of an ethical patient-therapist relationship. The trained therapist might be a clinical psychologist, nutritionist, doctor, or another trained health professional and will be referred to a as a therapist.

This section is written to provide basic information on the topic and should be supplemented with teaching by a suitably trained teacher. The issues in behavioral management have been simplified here and it would be inadvisable for a reader to attempt behavioral modification in a patient unless they are suitably trained by a qualified professional and their work with the patient is supervised. In addition, as many obese individuals may have underlying health problems or may develop new health problems, it is important that their physical and mental health be kept under review by a trained physician.[81] Of course, there may be a few highly self-motivated individuals who can manage this weight loss journey themselves if they have the right information, but even these patients should have ongoing regular medical review.

Principles of Behavioral Management

Since eating behavior influences energy intake and overall levels of physical activity (not merely physical "exercise" for a short period) affects energy expenditure, the fundamental principle of behavioral management is about helping the patient identify his "obesogenic" behaviors (i.e., those eating and activity level behaviors which lead to obesity over a period of time) and set about *gradually* correcting them. One could surmise that the existence of the entire "weight loss" industry proves that though most people start off enthusiastically enough on the weight loss journey, few succeed. The bottom line is not so much about identifying these behaviors (which is an important initial step) and changing these behaviors but *sustaining the behavioral change*.

The assumption in behavioral management is that maladaptive eating and physical inactivity behaviors are "learned" through conditioning (classical and operant) and modelling[82] (Box 1). If alternative adaptive and healthier eating and activity behaviors can be learned and reinforced through the same learning techniques, weight loss will be inevitable.

Box 1 | **Examples of the role of learning in the development of obesogenic eating behaviors and changing them**

Many obesogenic behaviors are "learned" or "unlearned" through:
- Conditioning (learning by association)
  For example:
  - Comfort eating and stress eating associates eating with feeling "good" or "distressed". Unless the individual learns to de-stress without using food, he will automatically turn to eating comfort foods when under stress and this leads to obesity
  - Rewarding desired behavioral changes reinforces the desired behavior. In times the individual associates the desired behavior with the reward and it becomes easier to initiate the desired behavior. Walking for 1 hour daily for 2 weeks can be rewarded with new clothes. The reward should not be obesogenic in itself. It is important to reward behavioral changes and not just weight loss
- Modeling (observational learning)
  - Modeling is especially important in children where parents are also into healthy eating and physical activity, it is easier for children to follow suit

Steps in Behavioral Management

- Assessing readiness to change behavior
- Setting realistic goals
- Self-monitoring
- Stimulus control.

All the above steps lead to enabling the patient make the necessary lifestyle changes and sustaining them.[83]

Assessing Readiness to Change Behavior

While patients might get referred for lifestyle modification to achieve weight loss, it is important to ascertain if the patient is truly ready to make the changes needed. This is part of the ethical management of weight loss. Unless this evaluation is done, one risks not only inevitable failure but demoralizing the patient, which will deter him from making an attempt at weight loss in the future.

The transtheoretical (stages of change model), which has been often used to provide a framework for assessing a patient's readiness to change addictive behavior proposes that at any time a patient can be in one of the following stages—precontemplation, contemplation, preparation, action, maintenance, and relapse.[84] The importance of knowing the stage the patient is in is to ensure that the advice or input given to a patient at a particular time is appropriate to the stage he is in.[85] For example, if a patient is in the precontemplation stage—i.e., a referral for weight loss might have been made at the behest of family members and the patient himself does not feel the need to lose weight at that time. At this time, the right approach would be to focus on establishing rapport with the patient, educating the patient about why weight loss has been recommended, some basic information about treatment strategies and providing information on how the patient can contact the therapist/doctor/nutritionist if he changes his mind about treatment (Box 2).

Box 2	Educating the patient
Educating the patient about energy balance-calorie intake and energy expenditure is crucial. While many obese patients already know a lot about these things, it is important to educate them on the importance of various issues like portion sizes, balanced diet, GI of food items, adequate water intake, adequate sleep, stress management, importance of not dieting, importance of breakfast, strength training (using simple weights) and aerobic exercise.[86-88]	
In diabetic patients, it is important for patients to understand the benefits of improving physical activity levels.	

For many people, the realization that one needs to make the weight loss journey occurs when one is faced with a medical consequence of obesity like diabetes. The inevitable anxiety on dealing with this diagnosis can be turned into something positive—i.e., patients feel better when they realize that something can be done to prevent or delay the consequences of this diagnosis.

Medical and psychiatric fitness have to be ascertained before starting behavioral modification.

If the patient has any existing medical conditions, such as hypertension, then it should be controlled before the patient embarks on behavioral modification. Similarly, in patients with psychiatric illnesses, like depression, psychoses, alcohol/nicotine addiction, binge, or other eating disorders, it is important that the patient is in a stable condition, before starting behavioral modification.

When the patient is under treatment for medical and psychiatric conditions, it is good practice to ensure ongoing medical and psychiatric care and adequate liaison between the various health professionals involved in the care of the patient. As some medications can cause weight gain, it is important to explore if alternative medication is a viable option or not.

Setting Realistic Goals

Setting realistic goals is important as it allows the patient and the therapist to have something to measure progress (or nonprogress) by. Many obese patients have unrealistic goals, which even if possible by drastic means, would be unsafe. Setting realistic goals is important not only for health reasons, but allows for success. This is the key in preventing demoralization in the long journey to sustainable weight loss. Most behavioral therapy regimes attempt a 10% weight loss over a 6 month period. However, most experts suggest that even achieving a 5% weight loss has great medical benefits. Even this small target is not easy to maintain and it is important that the patient does not lose hope, with the inevitable plateaus and occasional weight gains.

It is interesting that many of the medications which had been prescribed for weight loss (most have been subsequently withdrawn from the market for safety reasons), have shown smaller amounts of weight loss in clinical trials.

When patients have unrealistic goals especially if their goal is short-term like weight loss before a wedding ceremony, it is particularly important to educate the patient on appropriate weight loss and assess readiness to change before embarking on behavioral regime. Sometimes, the right thing to do is *not* to take up a patient for behavioral management at that particular time.[89]

Targets of goal setting: In behavioral therapy, it is particularly important to have goals in specific areas like decreasing total calorie intake, abolishing a particular obesogenic eating behavior, increasing duration of physical activity, reduction of duration of inactivity like television watching, and increasing sleep duration (if needed). Setting realistic goals also allows for a sense of accomplishment when a goal is achieved which is a powerful reinforcer of the new alternate behavior. In children, rewarding these achievements allows reinforcing the good behavior. The list of behaviors that can be tackled is discussed in more detail in the section under self-monitoring.[90,91]

Self-monitoring

Self-monitoring is the cornerstone of effective behavior therapy.[83,92] Self-monitoring of obesogenic behaviors by methods, like using a diary, helps the patient identify and keep track of these behaviors. It also helps the obese patient gradually work through their own denial and minimization. Many obese patients do not realize how much they are eating or how often they are not exercising until they write it down.

The importance of self-recording is that it allows the patients to clearly see for themselves the spectrum and frequency of their own obesogenic behaviors. Secondly, if recorded sincerely, it allows for measuring progression or regression clearly. It is important that the therapist allows some time and latitude for the patients to begin to do this effectively and many studies have shown effective self-monitoring is clearly linked to successful weight loss.

Areas of self-monitoring

Other than weight,[93] total calorie intake (by keeping a food diary), water intake, duration of physical activity, overall activity levels, duration of television viewing or other sedentary activity, and sleep duration, it is useful to particularly list all "obesogenic" eating behaviors (behaviors which leads to obesity).[90,91] Some of these are listed in box 3.

Caveats: Each of the eating behaviors listed above does not cause obesity in itself. Its importance is in the fact that in an obese individual if these are *frequently* present, then tackling it can lead to successful weight loss box 4.

Some issues regarding eating may have cultural connotations, as some Indian studies have shown that the study populations studied were not so distressed about being overweight and binging on food commonly not associated with feeling very guilty.[90,95]

Even if some important parameters like BMI, waist measures,[96] and HbA1c levels are monitored by the health professional, it can be motivating for the patient to have a visual record of their measures.

> **Box 3** **Some potentially obesogenic eating behaviors**
> - Craving for certain food items and acting on it
> - Getting out of bed at night to eat (night eating)
> - Buying snacks (high calorie foods) impulsively and eating it
> - Overeating at mealtimes
> - Eating a meal when not hungry
> - Binging (eating large amounts over a short period) with a sense of loss of control
> - Eating till uncomfortably full
> - Eating too fast
> - Eating alone as embarrassed about one's eating behavior
> - Inability to leave food behind in a plate
> - Grazing on food in between meals

> **Box 4** **Tackling the eating behavior of "eating too fast"**
> Many obese individuals eat too fast.[90] Telling them to chew slowly is important. This allows time for the satiety signals from stomach to reach the brain (so less likely to over eat). Other techniques like "mindful eating" allow one to experience the enjoyment of eating small amounts of good food, with the hope that this will prevent them from over eating. Though mindful eating has been much discussed recently, it is interesting to see that even Mahatma Gandhi discussed the importance of eating slowly, as an aid for digestion.[94]

Stimulus Control

Identifying circumstances when obesogenic behaviors are most likely to occur, allows for alternate behavior to be planned. This in turn allows for easier execution of the alternate healthier behavior. In behavioral therapy parlance, handling these triggers is called stimulus control. An honest food and physical activity diary (self-monitoring) will invariably help the patient realize what the potential road blocks to his weight loss journey are. Anticipating these internal or external cues can help the patient either avoid these circumstances or plan an alternate behavior beforehand (Box 5). For example, shopping while hungry or thirsty might lead to unnecessary buys like sugary drinks. Ensuring there is a bottle of water in hand could reduce this risk. Not having a healthy, low calorie meal quickly available when hungry might lead to junk food consumption. If the patient anticipates that on return from work he will be too hungry to wait for the meal, he must plan to have a simple meal ready quickly or keep a bowl of salad in the fridge beforehand.[89] If the patient is prone to overeating at parties, it is wise to ensure having a small healthy snack before going to the party. It would be difficult to avoid over eating if one is hungry.

> **Box 5 Food and physical activity diary**
>
> The most important tool is for the patient to maintain a diary, listing the foods they eat, quantities, circumstances and reasons for the same. It is useful to list physical activity (or inactivity as the case may be). A few lines of narrative is always useful. Even if some days are missed, there is nothing more useful than the diary for the obese patient to overcome their degree of denial and minimization. For example, a narrative account can read like this: "While standing at the queue in the supermarket, I saw the biscuits and samosas. I thought I would buy it for the kids to eat in the evening. Came home and as they had gone out to play, I ate all of it as I did not want to waste it. Felt really guilty afterward".
>
> In view of the above, he can plan that the next time he is in the supermarket, he can ensure the following actions:
> - Do not buy anything that is not in the shopping list—i.e., no impulse buying
> - If samosas are bought and kids are not at home, give them away to someone
> - If craving for samosas, give away all but one. Eat it slowly with enjoyment, (after all it is only a samosa) and walk for some extra time the next day to burn off the extra calories

For patients at the start of weight loss journey, it is easiest to *avoid* situations where they are likely to indulge in obesogenic behaviors, rather than put themselves to the test. For example, cut down on eating out, rather than saying that they will not order dessert.

Spending a few moments at the start of every day and periodically in the course of the day, anticipating potential road blocks in the weight loss journey is a useful exercise. This is important to remind the patient that it is better to plan alternate behaviors than to be caught unawares.

Sometimes, rehearsing scenarios may help. Some patients have difficulty being assertive and saying "No" to food when they don't want it. They can be asked to rehearse how they can refuse food politely if offered. For example, the patient can be taught how to respond when a box of Diwali sweets is passed around at work. Rehearsal tactics has worked in helping patients deal with addictive behaviors like alcohol dependence.

Some individuals just need to be told what to change and they can do it. For some other patients when they regain control over their food choices, they can actually enjoy occasional "treats" without guilt or weight gain. However, for many obese individuals, the most important thing to remember is that often faulty eating behavior and physical activity behaviors have become "habits" for them. If the obesogenic behavior started as a habit (or even as a coping strategy at some point of stress in the past), it is not easy to change it. Changing habits require time, patience, and most importantly perseverance. Many people forget that unless they commit to this change, *continually*, it is impossible to attain the goal. As of now, anyone who claims a quick fix short cut to weight loss is making a wrong claim (even if it is true, it is likely to be unsafe). Replacing obesogenic behaviors with healthier alternatives is the outcome that one is looking for.

As there may be several obesogenic behaviors in a given patient, it is best to start with a behavior which the patient feels is the easiest to change. Once that is successfully changed, one can move onto the next one.

Other Helpful Strategies

For patients who find it particularly difficult to overcome obesogenic eating behaviors or their barriers to physical activity, it is useful to use strategies like problem solving approaches. Social support from family members and key friends is also very helpful. Non-food reward for weight loss is useful (contingency management), but for many adults the weight loss itself is a reward. Other psychological and behavioral interventions which have been tried for weight loss include cognitive behavior therapy (Box 6) and acceptance based behavioral interventions (Box 7).

Box 6 | **Other psychological treatments for obesity**

Cognitive behavioral therapy (CBT) has been used in treatment of obesity and focuses on the following steps:[82]
- Establishing a therapeutic therapist-patient relationship
- Educating the patient
- Self-monitoring by patient
- Identifying maladaptive cognitions (thinking patterns) about eating
- Working on changing these thoughts (cognitive restructuring)
- Handling cues for overeating and binging
- Maintaining change
- Handling relapse

Box 7 | **Newer therapies under evaluation for efficacy in weight loss**

Acceptance based health behavior interventions (ABBT)
One of the important psychological reasons for patients to fail in sustaining lifestyle changes is their difficulty in tolerating distress. It is hypothesized that patients who find it difficult to tolerate uncomfortable sensations, like craving for food, are more likely to relapse into weight gain. Acceptance based therapies focus on helping patients "mindfully accept" these uncomfortable sensations and thereby choose the appropriate healthy alternate behavior.[97]

Special Issues in Managing Children and Adolescents

While the general principles of obesity management are similar in children and adolescents,[98] it is important to tailor the information/management plans to the development stage of the child in order to be effective. Ensuring that children start out with healthy eating and exercise habits are much easier than trying to change them later.

For children and teenagers, education about healthy eating and physical activity is the obvious first step. Tweaking the environment is particularly important with reduction of access to fast foods and sugary drinks. In teenagers, handling obesity is particularly challenging in view of the multiple other issues this age group has to grapple with. Its important is to ensure that underlying depression and stress is not missed.

Generally, studies have shown that when the family is involved in the behavioral regime, there is a more favorable outcome than only involving the child.[99-101] This means that it is important for the therapist to understand the family dynamics that may be involved in a given situation. Parental obesity has been noted to be a risk factor for childhood obesity. Parents should be reminded that children learn a lot by modeling and that their own eating and exercise lifestyle behavior speaks louder to their children than what they say. There is a story of how Gandhiji handled a child brought to him by a mother who requested that he advise him against eating too much sugar. Gandhiji asked the lady to bring the boy back to him the next week. When the lady brought the boy the following week, Gandhiji spoke to him about not eating too much sugar. When the lady asked why he had not given that advice the previous week, Gandhiji replied, "Last week, I too was eating sugar".[102]

Parents need to be consistent with their children and ensure that they focus on health rather than looks. However, it might be useful to point out the beneficial effects of fruits and vegetables on the skin while dealing with adolescents to increase their fruit and vegetable intake. Self-esteem is often reduced in overweight children[103] and health professionals should not inadvertently allow children or the parents to obsess about their weight.

While electronic media like television, video, computer, and the internet have been blamed for contributing to the obesity epidemic in children by reducing physical activity levels, there is mounting evidence that these media also contribute to obesity by increasing their calorie intake.[98,100] Ensuring that children do not watch television and eat a meal is an important behavior to target. Several issues in children, like advertising of junk food, foods available in the school canteen and playground space availability, are very important but can be handled only at a policy level.

Diabetic children need to be able to deal with many issues specific to managing diabetes effectively[104] and may go through particular difficulties in their teens in terms of social skills and peer pressure. Referral to a clinical psychologist would be appropriate.

Special Care Regarding Eating Behaviors in Children

- As some children who subsequently develop eating disorders like anorexia nervosa and bulimia are initially overweight, it is important that the advice to children focuses more on health than body shape. If the child shows signs of an eating disorder, there should be a referral to a child psychologist
- When rewarding children, it is advisable that the reward does not reinforce another obesogenic behavior. For example, cycling for half an hour being rewarded with half an hour of TV viewing. However, if the child is usually allowed half an hour of TV per day, it can be made conditional on the half hour of cycling. Often sincere praise for the child's efforts acts as a good reward
- While the growth spurts in obese children allow for normalization of BMI even without weight loss,[98] it is important to ensure that the children do not develop food fads and nutritional deficiencies.

Special Precautions

Watch for Unmasking of Other Problems

Sometimes, issues which may not have been picked up at screening may become evident once rapport with the patient improves and patient discloses more information.[89] One should watch for undue preoccupation with calorie counting, exercise, and weight loss which can signal an eating disorder like bulimia. Sometimes, clinical depression may become evident and would warrant referral to a psychiatrist. As mentioned earlier, the physical health of the obese patient warrants regular monitoring.

Modalities of Delivery of Behavioral Treatment

Group therapy has been shown to be more effective than individual sessions in ensuring weight loss, not to mention being cost-effective.[83] Behavioral treatment is usually provided in weekly and later bimonthly sessions, over some 10–12 sessions or so. Sometimes, weekly sessions are offered over 4–6 months. The internet has also been used as a medium to deliver behavioral counseling.

Effectiveness of Behavioral Regimes

Several studies have shown that while approximately one-third of patients lose 10 % body weight over 6 months, another one-third about 5%, and the last one-third—less than that.[83] Within 5 years, nearly half of the patients regain the lost weight, which means maintenance of the weight loss is a challenge. It has been noted that if there is continued contact with the therapist,[105] there is better chance of keeping the weight off. A review article by Butyryn et al.[83] on the behavioral treatment of obesity discusses these issues in more detail.

Conclusion

It has been said that successful weight loss is all about "skill power and not will power".[106] The role of the nutritionist is to ensure the patient has the knowledge and the skills to ensure successful weight loss. If there are behavioral difficulties which get in the way of ensuring weight loss, they need to be identified and handled by a referral to a trained counselor if needed.

DRUG OR PHARMACOTHERAPY AND SURGERY

Introduction

Weight loss drugs approved by the FDA can be used as part of a comprehensive weight loss program for patients with a BMI equal to or above 30 kg per m^2 with no accompanying obesity-related risk factors or diseases, or for patients with a BMI equal to or above 27 kg per m^2 with accompanying obesity related comorbidity. Weight loss medication in combination with a weight loss regimen leads to about 4–5 kg weight loss more than dietary measures alone.[107] However, drugs are not likely to be effective without a calorie restricted diet, and thus are only adjuncts to, rather than substitutes for, reducing diets. It is crucial to assess the efficacy and safety of the drug and it should be immediately discontinued if there are adverse effects. The use of medications, such as orlistat, inhibits gastric and pancreatic lipase production and decreases fat absorption. There are many drugs that have been approved by FDA for short-term, but this chapter will not deal with the various mechanism, advantages and side-effects. It should be remembered that weight loss drugs are expensive, have side-effects, and about 25% of individuals who are prescribed medications may not have the expected response.[8] If patients do not lose about 1.8 kg in the first 4 weeks after the use of the drug, then it may be appropriate to discontinue its use. A weight loss of 1.8 kg, within the first 4 weeks predicts at least 5% weight loss by 6 months of therapy, with continued use of diet and drug.[8] The data for the use of pharmacotherapy in adolescents is limited and thus the use should be reserved for morbidly obese adolescents, and used only after conservative therapy has failed. The physician and the patient must have realistic expectations regarding response to the therapy.

Weight loss surgery is an option in carefully selected patients with severe obesity (BMI equal to or above 40 kg/m^2 or with a BMI equal to or above 35 kg/m^2 with comorbid conditions), when conservative therapy has failed and the patient is at high risk for obesity-related morbidity and mortality. Bariatric surgery (gastric restrictive surgery) is a well-established technique to help attain weight loss. Food intake of the patient is considerably altered as the gastric capacity of the patients is after surgery.[108] Post-surgery, it is important to continue long-term dietary restrictions and supplementation of vitamins and mineral to avoid deficiencies. Malnutrition is a risk that is associated with bariatric surgery. Patients should be provided with preoperative and postoperative nutritional education to reduce food intolerances, regurgitation, help in selecting more nutrient-dense foods and use appropriate supplements to avoid most deficiencies.

In case of adolescents, the recommendations are that bariatric surgery should be restricted to individuals with BMI equal to or above 40 kg/m^2 with major complications, such as overweight, type 2 diabetes,[109] and those individuals for whom there has been failure for at least 6 months of conservative therapy. The mean weight loss was about 30 kg, when surgery was used in the pediatric age group.[109,110]

Treatment for Childhood Obesity

The involvement of family is crucial in the treatment of childhood and adolescent obesity since purchasing, preparing, and serving of food is not within the capacity of the child. Reduced calorie intake remains the cornerstone of weight reducing strategy in children and dietary history is important to identify foods that can be altered or eliminated. The primary goal of treatment for a child with obesity should focus on achieving healthy eating and physical activity habits rather than attainment of an ideal body weight.[111] Dietary management should aim at weight maintenance or weight loss without compromising appropriate calorie intake and normal nutrition. After completing an initial weight management program, the child and family must continue to work to maintain a desired weight as the child develops. Successful treatment requires long-term follow-up, with frequent physician visits, continual monitoring and reinforcement. Throughout these encounters, physicians must remain sensitive, compassionate, and supportive of the patient and family to foster necessary improvements, and lifestyle changes. In children and adolescents, tailored messages should emphasize the importance of regular physical activity accompanied by a properly balanced diet so that growth is not impaired.

Conclusion

Effective measures for achieving a desired weight include promoting healthy diets of lower energy density, regular physical activity and behavioral change, with emphasis on long-term weight management rather than short-term, extreme weight reduction. To maintain a healthy weight, good dietary habits must be coupled with increasing physical activity, and these must become permanent lifestyle changes. A moderate calorie restriction (500 kcal/day), along with increased physical activity and behavioral modifications appears to help maintain weight loss in the long-term. Nutritional approach to weight loss should emphasize first on good overall nutritional practice.

Courtesy

The authors acknowledge

Dr Sumathi Swaminathan, Assistant Professor, St John's Research Institute, Bengaluru for contributing the section on "Physical Activity Intervention"

Dr Sunita Simon Kurpad, Professor and Head, Department of Psychiatry, Professor, Department of Medical Ethics, St John's Medical College Hospital, Bengaluru for contributing the section on "Behavioral Modifications" in this chapter.

References

1. Cummings S, Parham ES, Strain GW. Position of the American Dietetic Association: weight management. J Am Diet Assoc. 2002;102(8):1145-55.
2. National Institutes of Health Obesity Education Initiative. The Practical Guide Identification, Evaluation, and Treatment of Overweight and Obesity in Adults. National Institutes of Health, U.S Department of Health and Human Services, Public Health Services, National Institutes of Health, National Heart, Lung, and Blood Institute. NIH Publication No. 00-4084. October 2004.
3. Pontiroli AE, Folli F, Paganelli M, Micheletto G, Pizzocri P, Vedani P, et al. Laparoscopic gastric banding prevents type 2 diabetes and arterial hypertension and induces their remission in morbid obesity: a 4-year case-controlled study. Diabetes Care. 2005;28(11):2703-9.
4. Foster GD, Wadden TA, Phelan S, Sarwer DB, Sanderson RS. Obese patients' perceptions of treatment outcomes and the factors that influence them. Arch Intern Med. 2001;161(17):2133-9.
5. Galuska DA, Will JC, Serdula MK, Ford ES. Are health care professionals advising obese patients to lose weight? JAMA. 1999;282(16):1576-8.
6. National Institute of Health. Talking with Patients about weight loss. Tips for primary care professionals. (NIH Publication -07-5634) 2007. Bethesda, MD:Author.
7. Van Dorsten B, Lindley EM. Cognitive and behavioral approaches in the treatment of obesity. Endocrinol Metab Clin North Am. 2008;37(4):905-22.
8. American Dietetic Association (ADA). Adult Weight Management Guideline: Major Recommendations. ADA Evidence Analysis Library. 2009.
9. Marinilli Pinto A, Gorin AA, Raynor HA, Tate DF, Fava JL, Wing RR. Successful weight-loss maintenance in relation to method of weight loss. Obesity (Silver Spring). 2008;16(11):2456-61
10. Estruch R, Martinez-Gonzalez MA, Corella D, Salas-Salvadó J, Ruiz-Gutierrez V, Covas MI, et al. Effects of a Mediterranean-style diet on cardiovascular risk factors: a randomized trial. Ann Intern Med. 2006;145(1):1-11.

11. Fairburn CG, Brownwell KD. Eating Disorders and Obesity: A Comprehensive Handbook. New York: Guilford Press; 2005.
12. Lean ME, James WP. Prescription of diabetic diets in the 1980s. Lancet. 1986;1(8483):723-5.
13. U.S.Department of Health and Human Services, National Institutes of Health, National Heart, Lung, and Blood Institute. Aim for a Healthy Weight. NIH Publication No. 05-5213. 2005.
14. Chaston TB, Dixon JB, O'Brien PE. Changes in fat-free mass during significant weight loss: a systematic review. Int J Obes (Lond). 2007;31(5):743-50.
15. Misra A, Chowbey P, Makkar BM, Vikram NK, Wasir JS, Chadha D, et al. Consensus statement for diagnosis of obesity, abdominal obesity and the metabolic syndrome for Asian Indians and recommendations for physical activity, medical and surgical management. J Assoc Physicians India. 2009;57:163-70.
16. Jeffrey RW, Wing RR, Thornson C, Burton LR, Raether C, Harvey J, et al. Strengthening behavioral interventions for weight loss: a randomized trial of food provision and monetary incentives. J Consult Clin Psychol. 1993;61(6): 1038-45.
17. Heymsfield SB, van Mierlo CA, van der Knaap HC, Heo M, Frier HI. Weight Management using a meal replacement strategy: meta and pooling analysis from six studies. Int J Obes Relat Metab Disord. 2003;27(5):537-49.
18. Fletchner-Mors M, Ditschuneit HH, Johnson TD, Suchard MD, Adler G. Metabolic and weight loss effects of long-term dietary intervention in obese patients: four-year results. Obes Res. 2000;8(5): 399-402.
19. American Dietetic Association. Managing Obesity: A Clinical Guide. Second ed. Diana Faulhaber, American Dietetic Association, 2009.
20. Kushner RF, Kushner N, Jackson Blatner D. Counseling Overweight Adults: The Lifestyle Patterns Approach and Toolkit. Chicago: American Dietetic Association, 2009.
21. Ryttig KR, Flaten H, Rössner S. Long-term effects of a very low calorie diet (Nutrilett) in obesity treatment. A prospective, randomized, comparison between VLCD and a hypocaloric diet+behavior modification and their combination. Int J Obes Relat Metab Disord. 1997;21(7):574-9.
22. Torgerson JS, Lissner L, Lindroos AK, Kruijer H, Sjostrom L. VLCD plus dietary and behavioural support versus support alone in the treatment of severe obesity. A randomised two-year clinical trial. Int J Obes Relat Metab Disord. 1997;21(11):987-94.
23. National Task Froce on the Prevention and Treatment of Obesity. Very low-calorie diets. JAMA. 1993;270(8):967-74.
24. Tsai AG, Wadden TA. Systematic review: an evaluation of major commercial weight loss programs in the United States. Ann Intern Med. 2005;142(1):56-66.
25. Varady K, Bhutani S, Church EC, Klempel MC. Short-term modified alternate-day fasting: a novle dietary strategy for weight loss and cardioprotection in obese adults. Am J Clin Nutr. 2009;90(5):1138-43.
26. Pirozzo S, Summerbell C, Cameron C, Glasziou P. Advice on low-fat diets for obesity. Cochrane Database Syst Rev. 2002;(2):CD003640.
27. Astrup A, Grunwald GK, Melanson EL, Saris WH, Hill JO. The role of low-fat diets in body weight control: a meta-analysis of ad libitum dietary intervention studies. Int J Obes Relat Metab Disord. 2000;24(12):1545-52.
28. Meckling KA, Sherfey R. A randomized trial of a hypocaloric high-protein diet, with and without exercise, on weight loss, fitness, and markers of the metabolic syndrome in overweight and obese women. Appl Physiol Nutr Metab. 2007;32(4):743-52.
29. Nordmann AJ, Nordmann A, Briel M, Keller U, Yancy WS Jr, Brehm BJ, et al. Effects of low-carbohydrate vs low-fat diets on weight loss and cardiovascular risk factors: a meta-analysis of randomized controlled trials. Arch Intern Med. 2006;166(3):285-93.
30. Bray GA, Popkin BM. Dietary fat intake does affect obesity! Am J Clin Nutr. 1998;68(6):1157-73.
31. Dunn CL, Hannan PJ, Jeffery RW, Sherwood NE, Pronk NP, Boyle R. The comparative and cumulative effects of a dietary restriction and exercise on weight loss. Int J Obes (Lond). 2006;30(1):112-21.
32. Peters JC. Dietary fat and body weight control. Lipids. 2003;38(2):123-7.

33. Simopoulos AP: The importance of the omega-6/omega-3 fatty acid ratio in cardiovascular disease and other chronic diseases. Exp Biol Med (Maywood). 2008;233(6):674-88.
34. Diekman C, Elmadfa I, Koletzko B, Puska P, Uauy R, Zevenbergen H: Summary statement of the International Expert Meeting: health significance of fat quality of the diet. Barcelona, Spain, February 1–2, 2009. Ann Nutr Metab. 2009;54 Suppl 1:39-40.
35. Willet WC: The role of dietary n-6 fatty acids in the prevention of cardiovascular disease. J Cardiovasc Med (Hagerstown). 2007;8 Suppl 1:S42-5.
36. Misra A, Sharma R, Gulati S, Joshi SR, Sharma V, Ghafoorunissa, et al. Consensus dietary guidelines for healthy living and prevention of obesity, the metabolic syndrome, diabetes, and related disorders in Asian Indians. Diabetes Technol Ther. 2011;13(6):683-94.
37. Atkins RC. Dr. Atkins' New Diet Revolution. (expanded edition). New York: M.Evans and Company, Inc.; 2003.
38. Gardner CD, Kiazand A, Alhassan S, Kim S, Stafford RS, Balise RR, et al. Comparison of the Atkins, Zone, Ornish, and LEARN diets for change in weight and related risk factors among overweight premenopausal women: the A TO Z Weight Loss Study: a randomized trial. JAMA. 2007;297(9):969-77.
39. Stern L, Iqbal N, Seshadri P, Chicano KL, Daily DA, McGrory, J et al. The effects of low-carbohydrate versus conventional weight loss diets in severely obese adults: one-year follow-up of a randomized trial. Ann Intern Med. 2004;140(10):778-85.
40. Seagle HM, Strain GW, Makris A, Reeves RS, American Dietetic Association. Position of the American Dietetic Association: weight management. J Am Diet Assoc. 2009;109(2):330-46.
41. Thomas DE, Elliott EJ, Baur L. Low glycaemic index or low glycaemic load diets for overweight and obesity. Cochrane Database Syst Rev. 2007;(3):CD005105.
42. Franz MJ. The argument against glycemic index: what are the other options? Nestle Nutr Workshop Ser Clin Perform Programme. 2006;11:57-68 discussion: 69-72.
43. Reid M, Hammersley R, Hill AJ, Skidmore P. Long-term dietary compensation for added sugar: effects of supplementary sucrose drinks over a 4-week period. Br J Nutr. 2007;97(1):193-203.
44. Alfenas RC, Mattes RD. Influence of glycemic index/load on glycemic response, appetite, and food intake in healthy humans. Diabetes Care. 2005;28(9):2123-9.
45. American Diabetes Association, Bantle JP, Wylie-Rosett J, Albright AL, Apovian CM, Clark NG, et al. Nutrition recommendations and interventions for diabetes: a position statement of the American Diabetes Association. Diabetes Care. 2008;31 Suppl 1:S61-78
46. Whybrow S, Harrison CL, Mayer C, James Stubbs R. Effects of added fruits and vegetables on dietary intakes and body weight in Scottish adults. Br J Nutr. 2006;95(3):496-503.
47. Ello-Martin JA, Ledikwe JH, Rolls BJ. The influence of food portion size and energy density on energy intake: implications for weight management. Am J Clin Nutr. 2005;82(1 Suppl):236S-241S.
48. Ello-Martin JA, Roe LS, Ledikwe JH, Beach AM, Rolls BJ. Dietary energy density in the treatment of obesity: a year-long trial comparing 2 weight-loss diets. Am J Clin Nutr. 2007;85(6):1465-77.
49. Rolls BJ, Roe LS, Beach AM, Kris-Etherton PM. Provision of foods differing in energy density affects long-term weight loss. Obes Res. 2005;13(6):1052-60.
50. Loos RJ, Rankinen T, Leon AS, Skinner JS, Wilmore JH, Rao DC, et al. Calcium intake is associated with adiposity in Black and White men and White women of the HERITAGE Family Study. J Nutr. 2004;134(7):1772-8.
51. Soares MJ, Binns C, Lester L. Higher intakes of calcium are associated with lower body mass index and waist circumference in Australian adults. A examination of the 1995 National Nutrition Survey. Asia Pacific Journal of Clinical Nutrition 2004;13(Suppl) S85.
52. Teegarden D, Zemel MB. Dairy product components and weight regulation: symposium overview. J Nutr. 2003;133(1):243S-244S.
53. Ping-Delfos WC, Soares MJ. Cummings NK. Acute suppression of spontaneous food intake following dairy calcium and vitamin D. Asia Pacific Journal of Clinical Nutrition 2004;13(Suppl) S82.
54. Soares MJ, Chan She Ping-Delfos W, Ghanbari MH. Calcium and vitamin D for obesity: a review of randomized controlled trials. Eur J Clin Nutr. 2011;65(9):994-1004.

55. Kleiner SM. Water: an essential but overlooked nutrient. J Am Diet Assoc. 1999;99(2):200-6.
56. Rolls B, Barnett RA. The Volumetrics Weight-Control Plan: feel full on fewer calories. New York: HarperTorch; 2003.
57. Rolls B. The Volumetrics Eating Plan. New York: Harper Collins Publishers; 2005.
58. Greenwood JL, Stanford JB. Preventing or improving obesity by addressing specific eating patterns. J Am Board Fam Med. 2008;21(2):135-40.
59. Groff JL, Gropper SS, Hunt SM. Advanced Nutrition and Human Metabolism. St Paul, Minnesota: West Publishing Co; 1990.
60. Ma Y, Bertone ER, Stanek EJ, Reed GW, Hebert JR, Cohen NL, et al. Association between eating patterns and obesity in a free-living US adult population. Am J Epidemiol. 2003;158(1):85-92.
61. Jakicic JM, Otto AD. Physical activity considerations for the treatment and prevention of obesity. Am J Clin Nutr. 2005;82(1 Suppl):226S-229S.
62. Saris WH. Fit, fat and fat free: the metabolic aspects of weight control. Int J Obes Relat Metab Disord. 1998;22 Suppl 2:S15-21.
63. Tremblay A, Simoneau JA, Bouchard C. Impact of exercise intensity on body fatness and skeletal muscle metabolism. Metabolism. 1994;43(7):814-8.
64. Schmidt WD, Biwer CJ, Kalscheuer LK. Effects of long versus short bout exercise on fitness and weight loss in overweight females. J Am Coll Nutr. 2001;20(5):494-501.
65. Katzmarzyk PT. Physical activity, sedentary behavior, and health: paradigm paralysis or paradigm shift? Diabetes. 2010;59(11):2717-25.
66. Owen N, Healy GN, Matthews CE, Dunstan DW. Too much sitting: the population health science of sedentary behavior. Exerc Sport Sci Rev. 2010;38(3):105-13.
67. Hamilton MT, Hamilton DG, Zderic TW. Role of low energy expenditure and sitting in obesity, metabolic syndrome, type 2 diabetes, and cardiovascular disease. Diabetes. 2007;56(11):2655-67.
68. Hill JO, Wyatt HR. Role of physical activity in preventing and treating obesity. J Appl Physiol (1985). 2005;99(2):765-70.
69. Fett C, Fett W, Fabbro A, Marchini J. Dietary Re-education, Exercise Program, Performance and Body Indexes Associated with Risk Factors in Overweight/Obese Women. J Int Soc Sports Nutr. 2005;2:45-53. doi: 10.1186/1550-2783-2-2-45.
70. Saremi A, Shavandi N, Parastesh M, Daneshmand H. Twelve-week aerobic training decreases chemerin level and improves cardiometabolic risk factors in overweight and obese men. Asian J Sports Med. 2010;1(3):151-8.
71. Sabia RV, dos Santos AE, Ribeiro RPP. Effect of physical activity associated with nutritional orientation for obese adolescents: comparison between aerobic and anaerobic exercise. Rev Bras Med Sporte. 2004;10:356-61.
72. Tresierras MA, Balady GJ. Resistance training in the treatment of diabetes and obesity: mechanisms and outcomes. J Cardiopulm Rehabil Prev. 2009;29(2):67-75.
73. Poehlman ET, Turturro A, Bodkin N, Cefalu W, Heymsfield S, Holloszy J, et al. Caloric restriction mimetics: physical activity and body composition changes. J Gerontol A Biol Sci Med Sci. 2001;56 Spec No 1:45-54.
74. McInnis KJ, Franklin BA, Rippe JM. Counseling for physical activity in overweight and obese patients. Am Fam Physician. 2003;67(6):1249-56.
75. Swartz AM, Squires L, Strath SJ. Energy expenditure of interruptions to sedentary behavior. Int J Behav Nutr Phys Act. 2011;8:69.
76. Ainsworth BE, Youmans CP. Tools for physical activity counseling in medical practice. Obes Res. 2002;10 Suppl 1:69S-75S.
77. Misra A, Nigam P, Hills AP, Chadha DS, Sharma V, Deepak KK, et al. Consensus physical activity guidelines for Asian Indians. Diabetes Technol Ther. 2012;14(1):83-98
78. Foster GD. Clinical implications for the treatment of obesity. Obesity (Silver Spring). 2006;14 Suppl 4:182S-185S.

79. Leblanc ES, O'Connor E, Whitlock EP, Patnode CD, Kapka T. Effectiveness of Primary Care–Relevant Treatments for Obesity in Adults: A Systematic Evidence Review for the U.S. Preventive Services Task Force. Ann Intern Med. 2011;155(7):434-47.
80. Wadden TA, Butryn ML, Wilson C. Lifestyle modification in the management of obesity. Gastroenterology. 2007;132(6):2226-38.
81. Kushner RF. Roadmaps for Clinical Practice Case Studies in Disease Prevention and Health Promotion. In: Assessment and Management of Adult Obesity. A Primer for Physicians. Chicago: American Medical Association; 2003.
82. Sadock BJ, Sadock VA, Ruiz P. Kaplan and Sadock's Comprehensive Textbook of Psychiatry. Volume 2, 9th edition. Philadelphia: Wolters Kluwer Health/ Lippincott Williams & Wilkins; 2009.
83. Butryn ML, Webb V, Wadden TA. Behavioral management of obesity. Psychiatr Clin North Am. 2011;34(4):841-59.
84. Prochaska JO, Diclemente CC. Towards a comprehensive model of change. In: Miller WR, editor. Treating addictive behaviors. New York: Plenum; 1986. pp. 2-27.
85. Kushner RF, Sarwer DB. Medical and behavioral evaluation of patient with obesity. Psychiatr Clin North Am. 2011;34(4):797-812.
86. Bijlani R. Eating Wisely and Well. New Delhi: Rupa publications; 2012.
87. Norris SL, Engelgau MM, Narayan KM. Effectiveness of self-management training in type 2 diabetes. a systematic review of randomized controlled trials. Diabetes Care. 2001;24(3):561-87.
88. Funnel MM, Anderson RM. Empowerment and self-management of diabetes. Clinical diabetes. 2004;22(3):123-7.
89. Simon Kurpad S, Kuriyan R. Weight Loss and its Challenges. (Manuscript under preparation).
90. Kurpad SS, George SA, Srinivasan K. Binge eating and other eating behaviors among patients on treatment for psychoses in India. Eat Weight Disord. 2010;15(3):e136-43.
91. DSM V. American Psychiatric Association. (2013). Diagnostic and Statistical Manual of mental disorders. 5th edition. Washington, DC.
92. Wadden TA, Berkowitz RI, Womble LG, Sarwer DB, Phelan S, Cato RK, et al. Randomized trial of lifestyle modification and pharmacotherapy for obesity. N Engl J Med. 2005;353(20):2111-20.
93. Butryn ML, Phelan S, Hill JO, Wing JR. Consistent self-monitoring of weight: a key component of successful weight loss maintenance. Obesity (Silver Spring). 2007;15(12):3091-6.
95. Simon Kurpad S, Tandon H, Srinivasan K. Prevalence of obesity amongst psychiatrically ill patients. Indian J Psychiatry 2001;43:138–46.
94. Gandhi MK. Diet and Diet Reform. Ahmedabad: Navajivan Publishing House; 1949.
96. Kurpad SS, Tandon H, Srinivasan K. Waist circumference correlates better with body mass index than waist-to-hip ratio in Asian Indians. Natl Med J India. 2003;16(4):189-92.
97. Goodwin CL, Forman EM, Herbert JD, Butryn ML, Ledley GS. A pilot study examining the initial effectiveness of a brief acceptance-based therapy for modifying diet and physical activity among cardiac patients. Behav Modif. 2012;36(2):199-217.
98. Vos M, Barlow SE. Update in childhood and adolescent obesity. Pediatr Clin North Am. 2011 Dec;58(6):xv-xvii. doi: 10.1016/j.pcl.2011.09.016.
99. Wilfley DE, Kass AE, Kolko RP. Counselling and behavior change in Paediatric Obesity. Pediatr Clin North Am. 2011;58(6):1403-24.
100. Vandewater EA, Denis LM. Media, social networking and pediatric obesity. Pediatr Clin North Am. 2011;58(6):1509-19.
101. Epstein LH, Valoski A, Wing RR, McCurley J. Ten year outcomes of behavioral family based treatment for childhood obesity. Health Psychol. 1994;13(5):373-83.
102. Eknath Easwaran. Gandhi the Man (Centenary edition). New Delhi: Jaico Publishing House;1997. pp. 170-1.
103. Whitlock E, O'Connor EA, Williams S, Beil T, Lutz K. Effectiveness of Weight Management Programs in Children and Adolescents. Evid Rep Technol Assess (Full Rep). 2008;(170):1-308.

104. Wysocki T. Behavioral assessment and intervention in pediatric diabetes. Behav Modif. 2006;30(1):72-92.
105. Tate DF, Jackvony EH, Wing RR. Effects of Internet behavioral counseling on weight loss in adults at risk of type 2 diabetes: a randomized trial. JAMA. 2003;289(14):1833-6.
106. Foster GD, Makris AP, Bailer BA. Behavioral treatment of obesity. Am J Clin Nutr. 2005;82(1 Suppl):230S-235S.
107. Weight-control Information Network, National Institute of Diabetes and Digestive and Kidney Diseases, U.S.Department of Health and Human Services, National Institutes of Health. Prescription Medications for the Treatment of Obesity. 2007.
108. Kolasa KM, Kay C, Henes S, Sullivan C. The clinical nutritional implications of obesity and overweight. N C Med J. 2006;67(4):283-7.
109. Inge TH, Zeller M, Garcia VF, Daniels SR. Surgical approach to adolescent obesity. Adolesc Med Clin. 2004;15(3):429-53.
110. Strauss RS, Bradley LJ, Brolin RE. Gastric bypass surgery in adolescents with morbid obesity. J Pediatr. 2001;138(4):499-504.
111. Barlow SE, Dietz WH. Obesity evaluation and treatment: expert committee recommendations. Pediatrics 1998; 102:E29. [Retrieved September 2000] Available from: http://www.pediatrics.org/cgi/content/full/102/3/e29.

CHAPTER **6**

Nutrition in Type 1 Diabetic Children

> **Abstract**
>
> The nutritional management of type 1 diabetes (T1DM) includes education of the individual and family, focus on dietary, and lifestyle changes which promote diabetes self-care. This chapter discusses the existing evidence on the amount and type of carbohydrate intake, fiber intake, and glycemic index in type 1 diabetic patients. Sample diet plan along with nutritional recommendations are summarized. The chapter also stresses on the importance and evidence of physical activity, behavioral management, and education of family in T1DM.

Introduction

Children and adolescents with type 1 diabetes mellitus (T1DM) have special needs that dictate different standards of care. While caring for children with diabetes, it is important to involve adults (parents/guardians) in the child's diabetes management and the education on the care of a child or adolescent with diabetes must be provided to the entire family. Appropriate self-care can be integrated into the child's diabetes management with increasing age of the child. The goal should be a gradual transition toward independence as the child continues to grow and adult supervision is crucial throughout the transition.

Education of the Individual and Family

Immediately after diagnosis, regardless of the severity, the child or young adult requires medical treatment along with appropriate education to provide the child and family the necessary knowledge and skills for self-management. The education should be a planned life-long process, starting at diagnosis and continuing as an essential component of diabetes care. The education program should be personalized to the needs of the child or young adult, family, and be culture specific. The education should ideally be provided by a team of certified professionals such as physician, nurse, dietician, and psychologist. The educator should possess skills such as good communication, compassion, and sensitivity. While dealing with a growing child it is very important that behavior change approaches, motivational interviewing, and counseling should be regularly reviewed to meet the constantly changing needs and requirements in this condition. Therefore, the education should not be a one-time event but an ongoing process as the child grows. Indeed, educational interventions that provide frequent telephonic contact and in person care has shown to improve glycosylated hemoglobin (HbA1c) levels and to decrease hospitalization rates for acute diabetes complications.[1,2] The dietician needs to develop a consistent, trusting, and supportive relationship with the individual and the family.

Nutritional Management of Children and Adolescents

Medical nutrition therapy (MNT) plays a major role in the management of T1DM and the dietary plan should be individualized to accommodate food preferences, cultural influences, physical activity patterns, family eating patterns, and habits. MNT with its focus on dietary and lifestyle changes provides an important foundation for diabetes self-care. The nutrition guidelines for children or young adults with T1DM does not advocate a specific diet or restriction of particular foods but instead focuses on healthy eating habits suitable for children and adults and, therefore, for the whole family. Healthy eating habits should be adopted by the children or young adults to ensure adequate intake of essential vitamins and minerals. In order to provide optimum diabetes care, it is important to provide individuals with evidence-based nutrition care. Since the energy requirements change with age, physical activity, and growth rate, it is important to conduct a nutritional assessment of the individual at least every year [measurement of height, weight, body mass index (BMI)]. Good metabolic control is essential for normal growth and development and BMI should be monitored regularly and calories restricted if the child becomes overweight. The nutritional advice should be provided keeping in mind the cultural, ethnic, family traditions, and the psychosocial needs of the individual child. Advice on planning, content and the timing of snacks/meals, and lifestyle changes should be provided by the dietician. It is important to involve the whole family in making appropriate changes based on healthy eating principles. The aims of nutritional management in T1DM are summarized in box 1.

Nutrition in Type 1 Diabetic Children

> **Box 1   Aims of nutritional management**
> - Encourage sustainable healthy eating and behavior habits
> - Maintain a healthy weight appropriate for age
> - Provide adequate energy and nutrients to promote normal growth and development
> - Encourage regular physical activity but provide education on handling complications
> - Build a trusting, supportive relationship with the child or young adult to facilitate behavior change and long-term lifestyle modifications
> - Maintain and preserve quality of life
> - Prevent and treat complications such as hypoglycemia, hyperglycemia
> - Reduce the risk of long-term complications

Energy Balance and Weight Maintenance

It is important to consider the appetite of the child or young adult while determining energy requirements and it is possible that in order to restore catabolic weight loss, they may have excess appetite and energy intake at the time of diagnosis. This should, however, be reduced when appropriate weight has been gained. Further, regular monitoring is needed to assess appropriate weight gain. Energy intake should be sufficient to achieve optimal growth and maintain an ideal body weight. Forcing a child or young adult to eat without an appetite or withholding food in order to control blood glucose is not advisable as this may adversely affect growth and development. Constant guidance on self-discipline, energy content of foods, appropriate portion sizes, regular meals, fat and sugar intake, and physical activity should be provided. Since energy intake and nutritional demands increase substantially in puberty, regular monitoring is necessary. Although there are no clear Indian guidelines on the distribution of macronutrients for individuals with T1DM, the following could be used, since they are sensible and pose no risk (Table 1).

TABLE 1: Guidelines on the distribution of macronutrients for individuals with type 1 diabetes mellitus

Carbohydrate	60–65%
	Complex carbohydrates such as whole grain cereals, fresh fruits, vegetables
Protein	12–15% or 0.8 g/kg body weight
	Skimmed milk and milk products, legumes, lean meat, and fish
Fat	20–25%

Carbohydrate Intake

Carbohydrate intake monitoring and balancing carbohydrate intake with insulin is central to the dietary management of T1DM and a mismatch between carbohydrate intake and insulin can result in immediate and long-term complications. In these individuals, carbohydrate counting and exchange lists are useful in maintaining the blood glucose levels. Carbohydrate counting involves counting food portions of 15 g carbohydrates, regardless of the source, and examples are provided in Appendix 2.

It is important to maintain meal and snack carbohydrate intake consistently distributed throughout the day on a regular basis and studies have demonstrated that day-to-day consistency in distribution of carbohydrate intake improved glycemic control.[3] Another study showed that while consistency in the amount and source of carbohydrate was associated with better glycemic control, this may not apply to individuals on intensified insulin therapy. In this situation, it may be necessary to adjust insulin doses based on the carbohydrate intake at each meal.[4] Type 1 diabetic individuals who adjusted mealtime insulin to match planned carbohydrate intake have reported improved glycemic control.[5] Individuals or care givers can be trained to adjust the insulin to carbohydrate intake by appropriate education and counseling on interpretation of blood glucose patterns and nutrition-related medication management.

The studies currently available on the differing percentage of carbohydrate intake have limitations, such as short duration, small sample sizes, being predominately nonrandomized trials, with no assessment of actual dietary intake. The evidence is not conclusive with some studies which substituted monounsaturated fats (MUFA) for carbohydrate, reported mixed results on glycemia and lipids,[6] while other studies reported benefits, when comparing low-carbohydrate (20%) diet to a higher-carbohydrate diet.[3] When T1DM individuals were provided with diets lower in carbohydrate and higher in total and saturated fats, it was observed that there was worsening in the glycemic control, independent of exercise, and BMI.[7] Diets too low in carbohydrate should be avoided as this would eliminate many foods that are important sources of vitamins, minerals, fiber, and energy. Comprehensive nutrition education and counseling can help individuals with T1DM to adjust insulin doses to match carbohydrate intake. Adjusting insulin doses based on planned carbohydrate intake has been shown to improve glycemic control and quality of life without any adverse effects. However, protein and fat content (total energy intake) cannot be ignored as excessive energy intake may lead to weight gain.

Studies examining the effects of sucrose in the diet of diabetic individuals have consistently reported that the total amount of carbohydrate consumed at meals is the main determinant of postprandial glucose levels, regardless of whether it is sucrose or starch. Studies with duration from 2 days to 4 months and sucrose intake ranging from 19 g/day to 42 g/day (5–35% of daily energy), reported no effect of sucrose intake on glycemic control, when compared to a lower sucrose intake, while total carbohydrate intake was similar.[8,9] However, another study observed that the addition of sucrose resulted in increased hyperglycemia and serum lipid levels.[10] The literature on the effect of sucrose is still limited as it is not known whether diabetics who substitute excessive amounts of sucrose, which is empty of other nutrients for starches will have inadequate intake of essential nutrients, and if regular consumption of foods rich in sucrose will lead to excessive energy intake and weight gain. Substitution of sucrose containing foods with other carbohydrate foods should be recommended for diabetic individuals who choose to sometimes consume foods with sucrose in moderation. Sucrose containing beverages may cause high glucose levels and excessive weight gain and thus should be avoided unless being used as treatment for hypoglycemia. However, sucrose should not be totally avoided as it may have psychological implications, and a careful assessment of the possibility must be made.

Fiber Intake

Evidence is inconclusive with regards to the influence of increasing dietary fiber on glycemic outcomes in individuals with diabetes. Individuals with T1DM consuming a 50 g fiber diet showed a modest 2% reduction in HbA1c levels.[11] A high fiber diet as compared to a low fiber diet showed beneficial effects on 24 hour glycemic profile of type 1 diabetic individuals.[12] On the other hand, studies have found no differences in HbA1c and fasting blood glucose between high and low fiber diets.[13,14] Conclusive evidence is available for the cholesterol lowering effect of high fiber when compared to low fiber diets in insulin dependent diabetic individual.[14] The recommendations for diabetic individuals will be to include about 25–30 g of fiber per day with inclusion of foods rich in soluble fiber such as fruits, vegetables, and legumes. Evidence is limited on the effect of long-term high fiber diet on diabetics and also whether diets with 45–50 g of fiber are achievable and sustainable in a free living condition.

Glycemic Index and Glycemic Load

There is conflicting and limited evidence for the effectiveness of using glycemic index (GI) in planning the meal of diabetics. Studies in type 1 diabetic individuals show that a low GI diet versus a high GI was found to lower HbA1c in type 1 diabetic individuals,[15] while there was no difference in HbA1c levels in another study.[16] The studies available have different definitions of high-GI or low-GI diets and confounding dietary factors and more studies are needed before firm conclusions can be made. Glycemic load is obtained by multiplying the GI of a food by the amount of carbohydrate in the portion size actually consumed. Using a low-GI diet as the only approach to nutrition management of T1DM is not recommended. A food with low-GI and glycemic load, but high in fat and low in micronutrients is not a healthy option. Individuals with T1DM can be provided additional guidance on how to lower the GI of the diet after he/she has got used to the concept of distributing carbohydrate throughout the day and matching carbohydrate intake to insulin intake. Table 2 provides a list of foods with the GI.

Non-nutritive Sweeteners (Artificial Sweeteners)

The sweeteners that are approved by the US Food and Drug Administration (FDA) are aspartame, saccharin, acesulfame K, neotame, and sucralose. The sweetener acceptable daily intake (ADI) is the level a person can safely consume on average everyday over a lifetime without risk.[18] The approved ADI levels are 50 mg/kg body weight for aspartame, 15 mg/kg body weight for acesulfame K, 18 mg/kg body weight for neotame, 5 mg/kg body weight for sucralose,[19] and 0-5 mg/kg body weight for saccharin.[20] A recent addition to be considered safe by the FDA as a food additive is rebaudioside A (derived from *Stevia*). The recommendation for diabetic individual using FDA approved artificial sweeteners should be to use it within the ADI level and to be aware that some of the products containing these sweeteners will contain energy and carbohydrate from other sources. More studies are warranted to determine the amount consumed and to assess the long-term metabolic outcomes and effects on appetite on individuals with diabetes.

Protein Intake

The protein requirement for children or young adults with diabetes is the same as the normal children or young adults. Type 1 diabetic individuals with normal renal function can consume about 0.8-1 g/kg body weight of protein. Protein can be obtained by both vegetable and animal source. Good sources of protein include milk and milk products, legumes, whole grains, meat, fish, and soya. Whole milk, high fat dairy products, and red meat should be used in moderation in order to reduce the intake of saturated fat. In individuals with diabetic nephropathy, a protein intake below 1 g/day is recommended as it has shown to improve albuminuria. Albumin levels and energy intake should be regularly monitored in individuals with advanced diabetic nephropathy and changes in energy and protein intake should be made to prevent undernutrition.

TABLE 2: The glycemic index (GI) chart[17]

Food items	Low GI (<55)	Medium GI (56–69)	High GI (>70)
Cereals and its products	Whole wheat, barley, millet, rye, all bran cereal, wheat tortilla	Oats bran, macaroni, wheat tortilla	Whole wheat bread, white flour bread, rice noodles, parboiled rice, oat meal, oat bran cereal, millets (boiled), multigrain bread, corn yellow, idli, dosa, upma, semolina, pongal, poori, pancakes, bagel (white frozen), cornflakes, spaghetti, rice and curry, corn tortilla
Pulses and legumes	Beans, peas, channa, rajma, green gram, soya bean, lentils (red, green cooked), kidney beans, split peas (yellow cooked), soy milk, dhokla	Baked beans (canned	
Vegetables	Spinach, lettuce, lady's finger, cabbage, celery, cucumber, radish, brinjal, broccoli, onions, cauliflower, tomatoes, capsicum, peas, squash		
Fruits	Grapes, apples, pears, plums, apricots, cherries	Oranges, pine apple, bananas, strawberries	Watermelon, muskmelon, raisins, papaya, lychee, dates dried, figs dried, mango
Juices		Apple juice, carrot juice, grapefruit juice, orange juice, pineapple juice	Cranberry juice
Starchy vegetables	Yam	Carrots	Potatoes (boiled, baked, mashed)
Dairy and its products	Curds (low fat, plain, with fruit), whole fat milk, skim milk		Ice cream
Sweeteners			Honey, sugar
Beverages			Carbonated/sweetened beverages
Miscellaneous		Sponge cake	Angel food cake, croissant, doughnut, pastry, scones, waffles, pizza

Source: Kaye Foster-Powell, Susanna HA Holt, Janette C Brand-Miller. International table of glycemic index and glycemic load values. Am J Clin Nutr. 2002;76(2)5-56.

Fat Intake

Atherosclerosis is one of the leading causes of morbidity and mortality in adults with T1DM and there is adequate evidence that atherosclerosis is often present in some individuals by adolescence.[21] Studies assessing carotid artery intima-media thickness (IMT) in children and youth with diabetes indicated a significant increase in IMT, which correlated with low-density lipoprotein (LDL) cholesterol levels in youth with diabetes compared with age and sex matched children.[22,23] Total fat and saturated fat intake of children with T1DM were higher than healthy children.[24,25] One of the reasons could be that the focus on carbohydrate counting could cause a shift toward lower carbohydrate but higher fat. Youth with diabetes considered healthy foods to be those which control blood sugar levels best and reported controlling carbohydrate consumption by substituting foods high in saturated fat for carbohydrate containing foods.[26] Thus the education provided should emphasize that consumption of carbohydrate from healthy foods such as fruits, vegetables and nuts should not be restricted too much and that a high saturated and cholesterol diet could lead to cardiovascular disease.

The dietary management of elevated lipid levels includes reduction in total fat, saturated fat, and cholesterol for children greater than 2 years of age with lifestyle modifications for weight control and increased physical activity to optimize lipid levels. Young people with T1DM should consume less than 7% of calories from saturated fat.[27] MUFA found in peanut, olive, sesame, and rapeseed oils and nuts should be 10–20% of the total energy as they may be beneficial in controlling lipid levels and protecting against cardiovascular disease. Polyunsaturated fatty acids (PUFA) sources such as corn, sunflower, safflower, and soybean or from oily marine fish may assist in the reduction of lipid levels when substituted for saturated fat. Oily fish such as tuna, sardines, and mackerel should be recommended to be consumed once or twice weekly.[28,29]

Vitamin and Micronutrients

The vitamin and mineral requirement of children or young adults with T1DM is the same as healthy children or young adults. Fresh fruits and vegetables should be recommended as they are rich sources of vitamins and minerals. Vitamins and minerals need not be supplemented unless there is deficiency, or a suspicion of deficient intakes.

Salt

The intake of processed foods which are rich in salt should be discouraged.

A summary of the recommendations for T1DM individuals are given in table 3.

TABLE 3: Recommendations for type 1 diabetes mellitus individuals

Parameters	Recommendations
Education	• Provide necessary knowledge and skill to individual with T1DM and family • Continuous ongoing process with modification based on changing needs and requirement of the growing child • Educator should build a trusting and supporting relationship
Energy	• Sufficient energy intake to optimize growth and maintain ideal body weight • Regular monitoring of energy intake to assess appropriate weight gain
Carbo-hydrate	• Balancing carbohydrate intake with insulin is important in the dietary management of T1DM • Carbohydrate counting is central to maintain optimal blood glucose levels • Maintenance of consistent meal and snack carbohydrate intake on a regular basis • Very low carbohydrate intake is not advised • Sucrose need not be totally avoided, but can be consumed on occasions, by substituting sucrose containing foods with other carbohydrate foods • Fiber intake should be 25–30 g with inclusion of adequate soluble fiber • Guidance to lower GI of the diet can be provided, once the diabetic individual is comfortable with the concept of matching, distributing carbohydrate throughout the day
Protein	• Requirement is similar to normal children/young adults • In diabetic nephropathy, requirement may be lower based on the severity of the condition
Fat	• Foods high in saturated fat and cholesterol should be limited • Educate that high fat foods should not replace healthy carbohydrate such as fruits, vegetables, and whole grains
Salt	• Excessive intake of processed foods which are rich in sodium should be discouraged
Vitamins and minerals	• Adequate intake is recommended with sufficient intake of fresh fruits and vegetables • Supplements are not necessary unless there is deficiency or signs of deficient intake
Physical activity and exercise	• Individuals with T1DM can enjoy the benefits of exercise with sufficient planning of nutrition, hydration, and insulin management • Overweight diabetic children/young adults need exercise to control/reduce body weight • Adequate care should be taken to prevent hypoglycemia
Behavioral modification	• Education for behavioral modification should be provided to both children/young adults with T1DM and their parents

GI, glycemic index; T1DM, type 1 diabetes mellitus.

Formulating a Meal Plan (Table 4)

Children usually have three meals and 2–3 snacks depending on the age of the child, level of physical activity, and length of time between meals. Since the energy needs of children keep changing, the food intake should be re-evaluated often and if there is a change in carbohydrate intake then the insulin dose should be reviewed. It is not advisable to provide additional servings of protein and fat rich foods to satisfy hunger.

TABLE 4: Sample diet for a day—Menu plan with 15 servings of carbohydrate

Meal	Carbohydrate servings
Early morning	
Coffee/milk: One glass (without sugar)	
Breakfast	
Vegetable upma: 1¼ cup	3½ serving
Vegetable chutney: 3 tbsp	
Egg white: One	
Midmorning snack	
Apple: One	
Buttermilk: One glass	1 serving
Lunch	
Rice: 1½ cup	3½ serving
Sambhar: ¾ cup	½ serving
Cauliflower potato curry: 6 tbsp	1 serving
Fresh vegetable salad: ½ cup	½ serving
Skimmed curd: ½ cup	
Skinless grilled chicken: Three small pieces (25 g each)	
Evening snack	
Green tea: One glass (without sugar)	
Sprouts with vegetable: ½ cup	1 serving
Dinner	
Chapattis: 3 piece	2 serving
Corn spinach: ¾ cup	1½ serving
Vegetable salad: ½ cup	½ serving
Bedtime	
Milk: One glass (without sugar)	

Note: This sample diet provides 1,800 kcal of energy and has been calculated using carbohydrate counting provided in Appendix 2. The diet must be modified according to individual needs and requirements.

Adherence to Diet and Predictors of Adherence

A high level of cooperation between the parent and child or young adult is needed to achieve optimal dietary adherence and overcome barriers in T1DM. Individuals with T1DM who adhere to recommendations of dietary management have shown to have better glycemic control[30] and following the recommendations of healthy eating may be the best method for preventing or treating comorbidity.[27] Awareness of the predictors of dietary adherence is important because it is the key to identifying risk factors for poor adherence and planning interventions. The mealtime interaction between parent-child has shown to be a predictor of dietary adherence in young children below 8 years with T1DM.[30] T1DM youth with better carbohydrate counting skills had better glycemic control.[31,32] Two studies used focus groups to gather data on youth and parents' perceptions of healthy eating for diabetes which have explored whether knowledge deficits predict adherence to healthy eating behaviors in youth with T1DM[26,31] and identified misperceptions of healthy eating practices in T1DM among youth and parents. Youth commonly reported "free" foods (foods high in fat, but low in carbohydrates) as good for diabetes management. Mehta et al. found that youth and parents identified food as "healthy" and "unhealthy" foods based on their effect on glycemic control and categorized fruits as "unhealthy" because they can lead to higher postprandial glucose levels, suggesting that a lack of knowledge or misunderstanding of diabetes dietary management may be a risk factor for poorer adherence for some youth.[26]

Thus, in order to facilitate optimal dietary adherence, the dietician must take care to not just provide guidance on carbohydrate counting and distribution but also to discuss the intake of all other foods and clear any misperceptions/myths that the child or young adults with T1DM or their parents could have.

Exercise and Lifestyle Modification

A sense of well-being, weight control, improved physical fitness, cardio-vascular fitness, lower blood pressure, and improved lipid profile are some of the benefits of exercise in T1DM children and adults. With adequate planning, children with diabetes can enjoy the benefits of physical activity. In diabetic children who are overweight, exercise is an important component of weight management.

Type 1 diabetic individuals have the risk of hypoglycemia occurring due to exercise and the incidence of hypoglycemia has found to depend on pre-exercise blood glucose levels.[33] Additionally, in comparison to sedentary night, participants developed hypoglycemia overnight more on exercise nights. The risk of hypoglycemia during exercise and for up to 31 hours after exercise was higher for participation in continuous moderate intensity exercise (between 40% and 59% aerobic activity) as compared to sustained high intensity exercise with more than 80% of maximum oxygen uptake.[34,35] The recommendations for individuals with T1DM are to encourage them to engage in regular physical activity. Even though no improvement in glycemic control has been observed in individuals with T1DM, it is possible that they could benefit with decreased risk of cardiovascular disease and a better sense of well-being. Monitoring of blood glucose levels before exercise is recommended with suggested intake of 15 g of carbohydrate to maintain the blood glucose levels below target range.

The blood glucose at the beginning of the exercise, the intensity of exercise, existing insulin level, and the insulin regime together determines the amount of carbohydrate needed. Readily absorbed carbohydrate (glucose, sucrose sweets) needs to be available for children with unplanned exercise and for sudden short duration exercise. Care should be taken that these snacks are low in fat and do not provide excessive energy intake (dried fruits, fruit, and cereal bars). Additional carbohydrate (1.0–1.5 g/kg) may be needed during moderate exercise to prevent hypoglycemia, however, this could vary depending on the type of physical activity.[36] Blood glucose testing after the unplanned physical activity will help in managing the variations in blood glucose levels.

Careful individualized planning in nutrition and insulin management is necessary for regular participation in competitive sports. Optimal amounts of carbohydrate are needed for good sports performance. In order to guarantee adequate glycogen stores and make carbohydrate available, low GI, low fat meal should be consumed 1–3 hours prior to the sports.[37] About 1.0–1.5 g/kg of quick acting carbohydrates are needed before and during strenuous exercise to maintain performance.[38] Amounts greater than 60 g of carbohydrate are not recommended as they do not have any added benefits and could cause gastrointestinal disturbances.[39] Fluid intake should be optimal to maintain adequate hydration. Following the exercise, adequate carbohydrate should be provided to replace muscle and hepatic glycogen stores and prevent hypoglycemia caused by increased insulin sensitivity during muscle recovery.[40] Readily digestible form of carbohydrate should be available for consumption immediately post and within 1 hour of completing the exercise.

Behavioral Modification

Dietary change has shown to be more successful in nutrition programs with focus on behavioral modification, rather than knowledge based programs.[41] Successful dietary change in children with obesity has been promoted through behavioral modification techniques for children and their parents. Behavior disorders, depression, eating disorders, and nonadherence to diabetic schedule are higher in children or young adults with diabetes and this is associated with poor control of glycemic levels.[42] Parents play a key role on children's eating behavior by providing the food and also by helping to shape food attitudes and preference through their own eating behavior. Regular family meals with better eating practices and monitoring of food intake have been associated with better glycemic outcomes.[25] Family-focused approach to nutrition intervention, rather than targeting only the child with diabetes may improve the chance for successful dietary change.[43] Practical advice on how to effectively plan and prepare meals should be provided to the individual's family in order to address issues of limited time and busy family schedules. Nutrition interventions should incorporate the perceived benefits of family meals that extend beyond diet quality and include strengthening family bonds.

Adequate training in behavioral and psychological skills could help in the early detection of children struggling with weight control and diabetes.

Conclusion

The use of flexible insulin injection plans has made the dietary prescription for individuals with T1DM less restrictive. The dietary management of T1DM is set within the context of the family, social system, care givers, peer pressure, and emerging independence. Education should be targeted to promote healthy dietary choices that maintain normal body weight and decrease the risk for cardiovascular disease. Parents should be encouraged to be involved in the children's food choices. Nutrition therapy should be individualized, keeping in mind the habitual eating pattern and other lifestyle factors. A trusting relationship between the child, health professional and parents, promoting behavior change during the challenging and disturbing years of childhood and adolescence is fundamental to a successful dietary outcome.

References

1. Svoren BM, Butler D, Levine BS, Anderson BJ, Laffel LM. Reducing acute adverse outcomes in youths with type 1 diabetes: a randomized, controlled trial. Pediatrics. 2003;112:914-22.
2. Beck JK, Logan KJ, Hamm RM, Sproat SM, Musser KM, Everhart PD, et al. Reimbursement for pediatric diabetes intensive case management: a model for chronic diseases? Pediatrics. 2004;113:e47-50.
3. Boden G, Sargrad K, Homko C, Mozzoli M, Stein TP. Effect of a low-carbohydrate diet on appetite, blood glucose levels, and insulin resistance in obese patients with type 2 diabetes. Ann Intern Med. 2005;142(6):403-11.
4. Wolever TM, Hamad S, Chiasson JL, Josse RG, Leiter LA, Rodger NW, et al. Day-to-day consistency in amount and source of carbohydrate intake associated with improved glucose control in type 1 diabetes. J Am Coll Nutr. 1999;18:242-7.

5. DAFNE Study Group. Training in flexible, intensive insulin management to enable dietary freedom in people with type 1 diabetes: dose adjustment for normal eating (DAFNE) randomised controlled trial. Br Med J. 2002;325:746-51.
6. Gerhard GT, Ahmann A, Meeuws K, McMurry MP, Duell PB, Connor WE. Effects of a low fat diet on body weight, plasma lipids and lipoproteins and glycemic control in type 2 diabetes. Am J Clin Nutr. 2004;80:668-73.
7. Delahanty LM, Nathan DM, Lachin JM, Hu FB, Cleary PA, Ziegler GK, et al. Association of diet with glycated hemoglobin during intensive treatment of type 1 diabetes in the Diabetes Control and Complications Trial. Am J Clin Nutr. 2009;89:518-24.
8. Malerbi DA, Paiva ES, Duarte AL, Wajchenberg BL. Metabolic effects of dietary sucrose and fructose in type II diabetic subjects. Diabetes Care. 1996;19(11):1249-56.
9. Nadeau J, Koski KG, Strychar I, Yale JF. Teaching subjects with type 2 diabetes how to incorporate sugar choices into their daily meal plan promotes dietary compliance and does not deteriorate metabolic profile. Diabetes Care. 2001;24(2):222-7.
10. Coulston AM, Hollenbeck CB, Donner CC, Williams R, Chiou YA, Reaven GM. Metabolic effects of added dietary sucrose in individuals with noninsulin-dependent diabetes mellitus (NIDDM). Metabolism. 1985;34(10):962-6.
11. Giacco R, Parillo M, Rivellese AA, Lasorella G, Giacco A, D'Episcopo L, et al. Long term dietary treatment with increased amounts of fiber-rich low-glycemic index natural foods improves blood glucose control and reduces the number of hypoglycemic events in type 1 diabetic patients. Diabetes Care. 2000;23:1461-6.
12. Kinmonth AL, Angus RM, Jenkins PA, Smith MA, Baum JD. Whole foods and increased dietary fibre improve blood glucose control in diabetic children. Arch Dis Childhood. 1982;57:187-94.
13. Lindsay AN, Hardy S, Jarrett L, Rallison ML. High-carbohydrate, high-fiber diet in children with type 1 diabetes mellitus. Diabetes Care. 1984;7:63-7.
14. Anderson JW, Zeigler JA, Deakins DA, Floore TL, Dillon DW, Wood CL, et al. Metabolic effects of high-carbohydrate, high-fiber diets for insulin-dependent diabetic individuals. Am J Clin Nutr. 1991;54:936-43.
15. Buyken AE, Toeller M, Heitkamp G, Karamanos B, Rorriers R, Muggeo M, et al. Glycemic index in the diet of European outpatients with type 1 diabetes: relations to glycated hemoglobin and serum lipids. Am J Clin Nutr. 2001;73:574-81.
16. Fontvieille AM, Rizkalla SW, Penfornis A, Acosta M, Bornet FRJ, Slama G. The use of low glycemic index foods improves metabolic control of diabetic patients over five weeks. Diabet Med. 1992;9:444-50.
17. Kaye Foster-Powell, Susanna HA Holt, and Janette C Brand-Miller. International table of glycemic index and glycemic load values: 2002. Am J Clin Nutr. 2002;76:5-56.
18. American Dietetic Association. Position of the American Dietetic Association: Use of nutritive and nonnutritive sweeteners. J Am Diet Assoc. 2004;104:255-75.
19. Fitch C, Keim KS. Position of the Academy of Nutrition and Dietetics: use of nutritive and nonnutritive sweeteners. J Acad Nutr Diet. 2012;112(5):739-58.
20. Joint FAO/WHO expert committee on food additives (41st report). Evaluation of certain food additives and contaminants. WHO Technical Report Series No 837; Geneva: World Health Organization; 1993.
21. Jarvisalo MJ, Putto-Laurila A, Jartti L, Lehtimaki T, Solakivi T, Ronnemaa T, et al. Carotid artery intima-media thickness in children with type 1 diabetes. Diabetes. 2002;51:493-8.
22. Parikh A, Sochett EB, McCrindle BW, Dipchand A, Daneman A, Daneman D. Carotid artery distensibility and cardiac function in adolescents with type 1 diabetes. J Pediatr. 2000;137:465-9.
23. Raitakari OT, Juonala M, Kahonen M, Taittonen L, Laitinen T, Maki-Torkko N, et al. Cardiovascular risk factors in childhood and carotid artery intima-media thickness in adulthood: the Cardiovascular Risk in Young Finns Study. JAMA. 2003;290:2277-83.
24. Helgeson VS, Viccaro L, Becker D, Escobar O, Siminerio. Diet of adolescents with and without diabetes: trading candy for potato chips? Diabetes Care. 2006;29(5):982-7.

25. Overby NC, Flaaten V, Veierod MB, Bergstad I, Margeirsdottir HD, Dahl-Jorgensen K. Children and adolescents with type 1 diabetes eat a more atherosclerosis-prone diet than healthy control subjects. Diabetologia. 2007;50(2): 307-16.
26. Gellar LA, Schrader K, Nansel TR. Healthy eating practices: perceptions, facilitators, and barriers among youth with diabetes. Diabetes Educ. 2007;33:671-9.
27. Bantlc JP, Wylie-Rosett J, Albright AL, Apovian CM, Clark NG, Franz MJ, et al. Nutrition recommendations interventions for diabetes: a position statement of the American Diabetes Association. Diabetes Care. 2008;31:S61-78.
28. Friedberg CE, Janssen MJ, Heine RJ, Grobbee DE. Fish oil and glycemic control in diabetes: a meta-analysis. Diabetes Care. 1998;21:494-500.
29. De Deckere CA, Korver O, Versahuren PM, Katan MB. Health aspects of Fish and n-3 polyunsaturated acids from plant and marine origin. Eur J Clin Nutr. 1998;52:749-54.
30. Patton SR, Dolan LM, Powers SW. Mealtime interactions relate to dietary adherence and glycemic control in young children with type 1 diabetes. Diabetes Care. 2006;29:1002-6.
31. Mehta SN, Quinn N, Volkening LK, Laffel LM. Impact of carbohydrate counting on glycemic control in children with type 1 diabetes. Diabetes Care. 2009;32:1014-6.
32. Koontz MB, Cuttler L, Palmert MR, O'Riordan M, Borawski EA, McConnell J, et al. Development and validation of a questionnaire to assess carbohydrate and insulin-dosing knowledge in youth with type 1 diabetes. Diabetes Care. 2010;33:457-62.
33. Tsalikian E, Mauras N, Beck RW, Tamborlane WV, Janz KF, Chase HP, et al. Diabetes Research in Children Network Direcnet Study Group. Impact of exercise on overnight glycemic control in children with type 1 diabetes mellitus. J Pediatr. 2005;147:528-34.
34. Guelfi KJ, Jones TW, Fournier PA. New insights into managing the risk of hypoglycaemia associated with intermittent high-intensity exercise in individuals with type 1 diabetes mellitus: Implications for existing guidelines. Sports Med. 2007;37:937-46.
35. Rachmiel M, Buccino J, Daneman D. Exercise and type 1 diabetes mellitus in youth: review and recommendations. Pediatr Endocrinol Rev. 2007;5:656-65.
36. Riddell MC, Iscoe KE. Physical Activity, sport and pediatric diabetes. Pediatr Diabetes. 2006:7:60-70.
37. Perone C, Laitano O, Meyer, F. Effect of carbohydrate ingestion on the glycemic response of type diabetic adolescents during exercise. Diabetes Care. 2005:28:2537-8.
38. Riddell MC, Bar-Or O, Ayub BV, Calvert RE, Heigenhauser GJ, et al. Glucose ingestion matched with total carbohydrate utilization attenuates hypoglycaemia during exercise in adolescents with IDDM. Int J Sport Nutr. 1999:9:24-34.
39. Coyle EF. Fluid and fuel intake during exercise. J Sports Sci. 2004:22:39-55.
40. Peirce NS. Diabetes and Exercise. Br J Sports Med. 1999:33:161-73.
41. Hoelscher DM, Evans A, Parcel GS, Kelder SH. Designing effective nutrition interventions for adolescents. J Am Diet Assoc. 2002;102(3):S52-63.
42. Sherman AM, Bowen DJ, Vitolins M, Perri MG, Rosal MC, Sevick MA, et al. Dietary adherence: characteristics and interventions. Control Clin Trials. 2000;21(5):206S-11S.
43. Rovner AJ, Mehta SN, Haynie DL, Robinson EM, Pound HJ, Butler DA, et al. Perceived benefits, barriers, and strategies of family meals among children with type 1 diabetes mellitus and their parents: focus-group findings. J Am Diet Assoc. 2010;110(9):1302-6.

CHAPTER 7

Type 2 Diabetes Mellitus

Abstract

The goal of this chapter is to provide the reader evidence based information on nutritional management of type 2 diabetic patients, while keeping in mind their cultural preferences, beliefs, and lifestyle. The key goals of nutritional therapy in diabetes are to achieve good glycemic control, maintain optimal body weight, serum lipids levels, and reduce risk of metabolic and microvascular complications. This chapter describes the various strategies to achieve the goals though dietary, physical activity, and education interventions.

Introduction

Type 2 diabetes is a major public health problem in India with the numbers expected to rise to 69 million diabetic individuals by 2025. Additionally, India has the second largest population with impaired glucose tolerance.[1] Managing patients with diabetes effectively requires time, effort, and education that increases awareness of the importance of diabetes management in reducing and preventing complications of diabetes. Diabetes self-management approach, where the individual with diabetes takes responsibility for the day-to-day management of their disease is an important strategy in improving metabolic control and preventing complications. Medical nutrition therapy (MNT) is fundamental for the effective management of type 2 diabetes. The nutritional advice provided should be based on scientific evidence and eventually adjusted for the individual, keeping in mind their cultural preferences, beliefs, and lifestyle. Guidance in making appropriate food choices to reduce risk, improve metabolic control, and quality of life should be provided (Box 1). The advice

> **Box 1** **Nutritional goals for type 2 diabetes**
> - Achieve and sustain optimal metabolic outcomes
> - Make dietary and lifestyle modifications to prevent and treat
>   - Obesity
>   - Dyslipidemia
>   - Cardiovascular disease
>   - Hypertension
>   - Nephropathy
> - Promote quality of life and healthy lifestyles by making healthy food choices and increased physical activity

needs to be on-going, regularly reviewed, and modified according to the individual's changing situations and circumstances. A multidisciplinary team needs to work together with the dietician taking the lead role in achieving nutrition related goals.

Nutritional Recommendations for Patients with Type 2 Diabetes

Weight Management

In overweight or obese individuals with type 2 diabetes, weight loss is an important primary management strategy. Weight loss is associated with 25% reduction in mortality and weight management is the most effective treatment for overweight and obese people with type 2 diabetes.[2] Insulin resistance increases with increasing weight, while weight loss improves insulin sensitivity, metabolic syndrome, and decreases serum triglycerides levels.[3-5] Moderate weight loss (5% of body weight) was associated with decreased insulin resistance, glucose and lipid levels, and reduced blood pressure. Different types of strategies, such as low-fat diets, low carbohydrate diets, very low-calorie liquid diets (VLCLD), meal replacements, commercial diets, and increased physical activity have been used in studies investigating the effect of weight loss on glycemic control in type 2 diabetes. The strategies and the evidence used for weight loss are summarized in table 1.

TABLE 1: Summary of strategies used for weight loss in patients with type 2 diabetes

Strategy	Evidence
Low fat diet	- Significantly reduced body weight, glycosylated hemoglobin (HbA1c) and cardiovascular risk factors and these positive effect were sustained over 4 years[6]

Continued

Continued

Strategy	Evidence
Low carbohydrate diet	• Significant improvement in body weight and glycemic control[7,8] • Main mode of action is through a reduction in energy intake due to carbohydrate restriction[9] • Evidence is limited in people without diabetes showing benefit over the longer term[10] • No evidence of harm when used short-term[11]
Very low-calorie liquid diet	• Should be used for a maximum of 12 weeks continuously or intermittently with a low-calorie diet or if longer should be with adequate support and supervision • May be more effective than other strategies for weight loss in people with type 2 diabetes[12]
Meal replacement	• Partial meal replacements produced greater weight loss than a reduced energy diet over 6 month period[13]
Physical activity	• In isolation, physical activity is not an effective strategy for weight loss in people with type 2 diabetes[14] unless it is for a duration of 60 minutes/day[15] • A combination of diet and physical activity results in greater weight reduction than diet or physical activity alone[16] • Regular physical activity leads to significant reductions in diastolic blood pressure, triglycerides, fasting glucose,[16] and HbA1c[17]

Tips for Diabetic Individuals to Achieve and Sustain Weight Loss

- Have regular meal times and avoid skipping meals
- Start by making small changes in the diet to reduce calories
- Control food intake by preportioning servings
- Eat sensibly and control calories when eating out
- Choose items with less cheese, oily salad dressings, cream, ghee, sugar, and coconut while eating out
- Avoid eating while watching television, reading, or driving
- Eat only when hungry and not when bored.

Diet

The ideal macronutrient composition of the diet in the management of hyperglycemia in type 2 diabetes is still not clear with studies showing contradictory results, but the importance of total energy intake and weight loss is significant. Total calorie intake should be appropriate for weight management with the macronutrient composition varying based on individual's lipid profile, renal functions, and food preferences. The general

TABLE 2: Guidelines for planning a diet in diabetes

Nutrient	Recommendation
Energy	• 25–30 kcal/kg ideal body weight • Needs to be reduced in obesity and increased in underweight
Protein	• 0.8 g/kg body weight • Additional needs to be met during pregnancy, lactation, and period of growth
Fat	• 20–25% of total calories • Saturated fatty acids—6–7% of total calories • Polyunsaturated fatty acid—6–7% of total calories • Mono unsaturated fatty acids—6–7% of total calories • Ratio of omega 6:omega 3—4:1 • Cooking oil—0.5 kg/person/month • Cholesterol intake—300 mg/day • The choice of cooking oil should be either 　○ One with moderate quantity of linoleic acid (groundnut/rice bran/sesame oil) 　○ One with high amounts of linoleic acid (safflower/sunflower/cotton seed/corn oil) along with an oil low in linoleic acid (palm oil) 　○ Use any of the above oils with oils containing alpha linoleic acid (mustard/soya bean oil)
Carbohydrates	• 55–60% of total calories • Encourage complex carbohydrates such as cereals, pulses, and whole grains • Restrict refined carbohydrates such as sugar, honey, and jaggery
Dietary fiber	30–40 g/day
Salt	• Below 6 g/day • Needs to be reduced to 4 g/day in case of hypertension, renal failure, and heart problems
Alcohol	Restrict

Adapted from API-I7CP Guidelines on Diabetes 2007. J Assoc Physicians India. 2007;55:1-50.

guidelines for planning a diet for an individual with diabetes mellitus is provided in table 2.

Carbohydrates

While the evidence to support specific recommendations of carbohydrates in type 2 diabetes is limited, it is clear that the total amount of carbohydrate consumed is the primary determinant of postprandial blood glucose. Effective management of carbohydrate intake should be the primary strategy for optimal glycemic control. Carbohydrates should be about 55–65% of total energy intake. A modest reduction in carbohydrate intake is associated with improvements in glycemic control and low-carbohydrate diets can be particularly effective if associated with weight loss. Day to day consistency in carbohydrate intake results in improved glycemic control and diets very low in carbohydrate should be discouraged since this could eliminate foods rich in vitamins, minerals, fiber, and energy.

Glycemic Index and Glycemic Load

The glycemic index (GI) is defined as the incremental positive area under blood glucose curve of 50 g of carbohydrate from a test food divided by the incremental area of 50 g of reference food. A high GI is above 70, medium GI is 56–69, and low GI below 55. The role of GI in type 2 diabetes is controversial with evidence of low GI diets reducing glycosylated hemoglobin (HbA1c) by 0.5 %,[19] while recent randomized controlled trials suggests no evidence of benefit of low GI diet.[20,21] The studies on effects of GI on blood glucose levels are limited by confounding dietary factors and differing definitions for high and low GI diets. The glycemic load (GL) of a food is obtained by multiplying the GI of a food by the number of grams of available carbohydrate in the food. A high GL is above 20, medium 11–19, and low below 10. The long-term sustainability of low GL diet is still not known.

Dietary Fiber

High-fiber diets (greater than 20 g/1,000 kcal) have reduced postprandial glucose levels but did not have any effect on fasting glucose,[22] while short-term studies have reported minimal or no beneficial effect on blood glucose, insulin and HbA1c.[23,24] Individuals with diabetes can be advised to include 25–30 g of fiber per day, with adequate inclusion of soluble fiber.

Sucrose

Sucrose intake in the diet ranging from 10% to 35% of the total energy was not associated with negative effect on glycemic response when substituted for isocaloric amounts of starch.[25,26] Food and Drug Association (FDA) approved non-nutritive sweeteners can used as long as it is within the accepted daily limits.

Protein

Protein intake has minimal effect on blood glucose and lipid levels and does not alter long-term insulin requirements.[27,28] Thus the recommendations for protein intake in a diabetic individual is similar to a normal person, except when the protein choice is high in saturated fatty acids or in patients with diabetic nephropathy, where a protein intake of less than 0.8 g/kg/day is recommended. It is important to monitor hypoalbuminemia and energy intake in advanced stage of diabetic nephropathy in order to prevent potential risk of malnutrition.

Dietary Fat

Interventional studies have not showed any association between post-prandial glucose response and the type and amount of fat in meals,[29,30,7,31] while epidemiological studies have shown a relationship between high fat intake, high saturated fat intake, and elevated HbA1c levels.[32] Additionally, since diabetic patients are at increased risk for cardiovascular diseases (CVD), it is important to consider this in the dietary plan and nutrition interventions for the prevention and treatment of CVD such as reduction in saturated and transfatty acid and dietary cholesterol should be initiated. The maintenance of serum lipid levels is one of the important goals in diabetes management. Short-term studies of 2-week duration have indicated that monounsaturated fats can be substituted for carbohydrate in the diet without adverse effects on glycemic control or serum lipids,[33] but the long-term effect is not known. The intake of monounsaturated fats, such as nuts and olive oil, should be encouraged with vegetable oils being used in moderation, while saturated fats, trans fat, and dietary cholesterol should be minimized. Weekly consumption (twice a week) of fish decreased risk for coronary heart disease in nondiabetic individual[34] and may also help in diabetic patients.

Micronutrients and Vitamins

Multiple micronutrient deficiencies are likely to exist in individuals with poorly controlled diabetes.[35] Deficiencies of certain minerals, such as potassium, magnesium, zinc, and chromium may predispose to carbohydrate intolerance.[36] Studies on chromium supplementation in diabetes management has mixed results and thus should not be recommended in diabetes management. Similarly, the clinical trials with zinc supplementation in diabetic patients are few and have yielded inconsistent results. The evidence for calcium and vitamin D intake does not suggest higher intake for people with diabetes. Available evidence also suggests that diabetic patients do not have additional requirements for vitamins such as vitamin A, B, C, and E. Thus diabetic patients should be educated on the importance of acquiring daily vitamin and mineral requirements from food sources, unless there is an underlying deficiency. In the case of high-risk groups, such as elderly, pregnant, and lactating women, it may be necessary to supplement with vitamins and minerals based on individual needs.

Alcohol Intake

Physicians need to advise patients with diabetes on alcohol intake on an individual basis. The limit for alcohol intake in diabetic patient is similar to nondiabetic patients, but should not be given to pregnant women, patients with pancreatitis, or severe hypertriglyceridemia. However, it should be remembered that alcohol intake may cause hyper- or hypoglycemia depending on the amount consumed and whether consumed with or without food and medications. Additional care should be taken of the potential adverse interactions of alcohol with medications.

Physical Activity

Regular physical activity is an important component in the management of an individual with type 2 diabetes. It is, however, important to have prior assessment of the anticipated benefits and associated risk of the physical activity schedule while incorporating the program in the treatment plan. Physical activity has proven benefits on cardiovascular risk reduction and glycemic control in individuals with type 2 diabetes, and studies have reported a mean weighted reduction of 0.45–0.65% in HbA1c.[37,38] Additional benefits include improved insulin sensitivity and decreased risk for all-cause mortality.[39,14] About 90–150 minutes/week of accumulated moderate intensity aerobic physical activity along with resistance/strength training is recommended for type 2 diabetic patients. Improved glycemic control has been observed with both aerobic and resistance exercise. Aerobic exercise improves blood glucose levels and reduces low-density lipoprotein (LDL) cholesterol by 5%, with little effect on other lipid levels,[40] while resistance training has effects on both blood glucose levels and cardiovascular risk factors effects.[41] Individuals with type 2 diabetes, managed either by only diet or in combination with oral hypoglycemic agents, can exercise in both the fasting and post-meal state,[42] and blood glucose level reduction has shown to be highest in the postprandial state.[43] However, since it is possible that they may have lower VO_2 max and thus may need a gradually increasing training program with adequate rest periods. On the other hand for individuals treated with sulfonylureas or insulin, adequate measures should be taken to minimize the chances of hypoglycemia up to 24 hours after physical activity.[38]

Education of Self-management

The nutritional management of type 2 diabetes is a team effort with the person with diabetes in the center. The individual needs to be provided with the knowledge, skill, and motivation to incorporate self-management into their day to day life.

Conclusion

A single approach does not exist for MNT to diabetes and it involves a variety of interventions such as reduced energy/fat intake, healthy food choices, carbohydrate counting, exchange list, physical activity, and behavioral strategies. Nutrition education and counselling should be planned, keeping in mind the individual needs, preferences, economic status along with their willingness, and ability to change. The key goals of nutritional plan in diabetes is to achieve good glycemic control, maintain optimal body weight, serum lipids levels, and reduce risk of metabolic and microvascular complications. Additionally, follow-up visits should provide encouragement and ensure realistic expectations for the patient.

References

1. Sicree R, Shaw J, Zimmet P. Diabetes and impaired glucose tolerance. In Gan D (Ed). Diabetes Atlas. International Diabetes Federation. 3rd edition; Belgium. International Diabetes Federation; 2006. pp. 15-103.
2. Aucott L, Poobalan A, Smith WC, Avenell A, Jung R, Broom J, et al. Weight loss in obese diabetic and non-diabetic individuals and long-term diabetes outcomes—a systematic review. Diabetes Obes Metab. 2004;6(2):85-94.
3. Davies M, Tringham J, Peach F, Daly H. Prediction of the weight gain associated with insulin treatment. J Diabetes Nurs. 2003;7(3):94-8.
4. Balkau B, Picard P, Vol S, Fezeu L, Eschwege E, DESIR Study Group. Consequences of change in waist circumference on cardiometabolic risk factors over 9 years. Data from an Epidemiological Study on the Insulin Resistance Syndrome (DESIR). Diabetes Care. 2007;30(7):1901-3.
5. Vasquez G, Duval S, Jacobs DR, Silventoinen K. Comparison of Body Mass Index, waist circumference, and waist/hip ration in predicting incident diabetes: a meta-analysis. Epidemiol Rev. 2007;29:115-28.
6. Wing RR. Look AHEAD Research Group. Long-term effects of a lifestyle intervention on weight and cardiovascular risk factors in individuals with type 2 diabetes mellitus: four-year results of the Look AHEAD trial. Arch Intern Med. 2010;170(17):1566-75.
7. Kirk JK, Graves DE, Craven TE, Lipkin EW, Austin M, Margolis KL. Restricted-carbohydrate diets in patients with Type 2 diabetes: a meta-analysis. J Am Diet Assoc. 2008;108(1):91-100.
8. Dyson PA. A review of low and reduced carbohydrate diets in weight loss in type 2 diabetes. J Hum Nutr Diet. 2008;21(6):530-8.
9. Bravata DM, Sanders L, Huang J, Krumholz HM, Olkin I, Gardner CD, et al. Efficacy and safety of low-carbohydrate diets: a systematic review. JAMA. 2003;289(14):1837-50.
10. Hession, M, Rolland, C Kulkarni U, Wise A, Broom J. Systematic review of randomised controlled trials of low-carbohydrate vs. low-fat/low-calorie diets in the management of obesity and its comorbidities. Obes Rev. 2009; 10(1):36-50.
11. Nordmann AJ, Nordmann A, Briel M, Keller U, Yancy WS, Brehm BJ, et al. Effects of low-carbohydrate vs low-fat diets on weight loss and cardiovascular risk factors: a meta-analysis of randomized controlled trials. Arch Intern Med. 2006;166(3):285-93.
12. Norris SL, Zhang X, Avenell A, Gregg E, Brown TJ, Schmid CH, et al. Long-term non-pharmacologic weight loss interventions for adults with type 2 diabetes. Cochrane Database Syst Rev. 2005;(2):CD004095.
13. Heymsfield SB, van Mierlo CA, van der Knaap HC, Heo M, Frier HL. Weight management using a meal replacement strategy: meta and pooling analysis from six studies. Int J Obes Relat Metab Disord. 2003;27(5):537-49.

14. Boule NG, Haddad E, Kenny GP, Wells GA, Sigal RJ. Effects of exercise on glycemic control and body mass in Type 2 diabetes mellitus: a meta-analysis of controlled clinical trials. JAMA. 2001;286(10):1218-27.
15. Colberg SR, Albright AL, Blissmer BJ, Bruan B, Chasan-Tabler L, Fernhall B, et al. Exercise and type 2 diabetes: American College of Sports Medicine and the American Diabetes Association: joint position statement. Exercise and type 2 diabetes. Med Sci Sports Exerc. 2010;42(12):2282-303.
16. Shaw K, Gennat H, O'Rourke P, Del Marc. Exercise for overweight or obesity. Cochrane Database Syst Rev. 2006;(4):CD003817.
17. Thomas DE, Elliott EJ, Naughton GA. Exercise for type 2 diabetes mellitus. Cochrane Database Syst Rev. 2006;(3):CD002968.
18. API-I7CP Guidelines on Diabetes 2007. J Assoc Physicians India. 2007;55:1-50.
19. Opperman AM, Venter CS, Oosthuizen W, Thompson RL, Vorster HH. Meta-analysis of the health effects of using the glycaemic index in meal-planning. Br J Nutr. 2004;92(3):367-81.
20. Ma Y, Olendzki BC, Merriam PA, Chiriboga DE, Culver AL, Li W, et al. A randomized clinical trial comparing low-glycemic index versus ADA dietary education among individuals with type 2 diabetes. Nutrition. 2008;24(1):45-56.
21. Wolever TM, Gibbs AL, Mehling C, Chiasson JL, Connelly PW, Josse RG, et al. The Canadian Trial of Carbohydrates in Diabetes (CCD), a 1-y controlled trial of low-glycemic-index dietary carbohydrate in type 2 diabetes: no effect on glycated hemoglobin but reduction in C-reactive protein. Am J Clin Nutr. 2008;87(1):114-25.
22. Wolever T, Nguyen P-M, Chaisson J-L et al. Relationship between habitual diet and blood glucose and lipids in non-insulin dependent diabetes (NIDDM). Nutrition Research. 1995;15:843-57.
23. Jenkins DJ, Kendall CW, Augustin LS, Martini MC, Axelsen M, Faulkner D, et al. Effect of wheat bran on glycemic control and risk factors for cardiovascular disease in type 2 diabetes. Diabetes Care. 2002;25(9):1522-8.
24. Anderson JW, Randles KM, Kendall CW, Jenkins DJ. Carbohydrate and fiber recommendations for individuals with diabetes: a quantitative assessment and meta-analysis of the evidence. J Am Coll Nutr. 2004;23(1):5-17.
25. Malerbi DA, Paiva ES, Duarte AL, Wajchenberg BL. Metabolic effects of dietary sucrose and fructose in type II diabetic subjects. Diabetes Care. 1996;19(11):1249-56.
26. Nadeau J, Koski KG, Strychar I, Yale JF. Teaching subjects with type 2 diabetes how to incorporate sugar choices into their daily meal plan promotes dietary compliance and does not deteriorate metabolic profile. Diabetes Care. 2001;24(2):222-7.
27. Parker B, Noakes M, Luscombe N, Clifton P. Effect of a high-protein, high-monounsaturated fat weight loss diet on glycemic control and lipid levels in type 2 diabetes. Diabetes Care. 2002;25(3):425-30.
28. Brinkworth GD, Noakes M, Parker B, Foster P, Clifton PM. Long-term effects of advice to consume a high-protein, low-fat diet, rather than a conventional weight-loss diet, in obese adults with type 2 diabetes: one-year follow-up of a randomised trial. Diabetologia. 2004;47(10):1677-86.
29. Kodama S, Saito K, Tanaka S, Maki M, Yachi Y, Sato M, et al. Influence of fat and carbohydrate proportions on the metabolic profile in patients with type 2 diabetes: a meta-analysis. Diabetes Care. 2009;32(5):959-65.
30. Brehm B, Lattin B, Summer S, Boback JA, Gilchrist GM Jondeck RJ, et al. One-year comparison of a high-monounsaturated fat diet with a high-carbohydrate diet in type 2 diabetes. Diabetes Care. 2009;32(2):215-20.
31. Haimoto H, Iwata M, Wakai K, Umegaki H. Long-term effects of a diet loosely restricting carbohydrate on HbA1c levels, BMI and tapering of sulfonylureas in Type 2 diabetes: a 2-year follow up study. Diabetes Res Clin Pract. 2008;79(2):350-6.
32. Harding HA, Sargeant LA, Welch A, Oakes S, Luben RN, Bingham S, et al. Fat consumption and HbA(1c) levels: The EPIC-Norfolk study. Diabetes Care. 2001;24(11):1911-6.
33. Garg A. High-monounsaturated-fat diets for patients with diabetes mellitus: a meta-analysis. Am J Clin Nutr. 1998;67(3 Suppl):577S-582S.

34. Burr ML, Fehily AM, Gilbert JF, Rogers S, Holliday RM, Sweetnam PM, et al. Effects of changes in fat, fish, and fibre intakes on death and myocardial reinfarction: diet and reinfarction trial (DART). Lancet. 1989;2(8666):757-61.
35. Franz MJ, Bantle JP, Beebe CA, Brunzell JD, Chiasson JL, Garg A, et al. Evidence-based nutrition principles and recommendations for the treatment and prevention of diabetes and related complications. Diabetes Care. 2003;26 Suppl 1:S51-61.
36. Joe M. Chehade, Mae Sheikh-Ali, Arshag D. Mooradian. The Role of Micronutrients in Managing Diabetes. Diabetes Spectrum 2009;22:214-8.
37. Conn VS, Hafdahl AR, Mehr DR, LeMaster JW, Brown SA, Nielsen PJ. Metabolic effects of interventions to increase exercise in adults with type 2 diabetes. Diabetologia. 2007;50(5):913-21.
38. Nagi D, Gallen I. ABCD position statement on physical activity and exercise in diabetes. Pract Diab Int. 2010;27(4): 158-63a.
39. Castaneda C, Layne JE, Munoz-Orians L, Gordon PL, Walsmith J, Foldvari M, et al. A randomized controlled trial of resistance exercise training to improve glycemic control in older adults with type 2 diabetes. A randomized controlled trial of resistance exercise training to improve glycemic control in older adults with type 2 diabetes. Diabetes Care. 2002;25(12):2335-41.
40. Kelley GA, Kelley KS. Effects of aerobic exercise on lipids and lipoproteins in adults with type 2 diabetes; a meta-analysis of randomized-controlled trials. Public Health. 2007;121(9):643-55
41. Hills AP, Shultz SP, Soares MJ,Byrne NM, Hunter GR, King NA, et al. Resistance training for obese, type 2 diabetic adults: a review of the evidence. Obes Rev. 2010;11(10):740-9.
42. Gaudet-Savard T, Ferland A, Broderick TL, Garneau C, Tremblay A, Nadeau A, et al. Safety and magnitude of changes in blood glucose levels following exercise performed in the fasted and the postprandial state in men with type 2 diabetes. Eur J Cardiovasc Prev Rehabil. 2007;14(6):831-6.
43. Ferland A, Brassard P, Lemieux S, Bergeron J, Bogaty P, Bertrand F, et al. Impact of high-fat /low-carbohydrate, high-, low-glycaemic index or low-caloric meals on glucose regulation during aerobic exercise in Type 2 diabetes. Diabet Med. 2009;26(6):589-95.

CHAPTER 8

Gestational Diabetes Mellitus

> **Abstract**
>
> This chapter focuses on the nutritional management of gestational diabetes mellitus (GDM). Important aspects such as setting the nutritional goals, assessing the patient, planning a meal, and providing nutritional advice have been discussed in this chapter. The benefits of exercise and lifestyle management in GDM have also been highlighted.

Introduction

Gestational diabetes mellitus (GDM) is defined as any degree of glucose intolerance with onset or first recognition during pregnancy.[1] Most of the cases of GDM are diagnosed during the second or third trimester of pregnancy since there is an increase in insulin-antagonist hormone levels along with insulin resistance. The blood glucose levels return to normal in most women with GDM, but these women are at increased risk of developing type 2 diabetes. The prevalence of GDM in India varies from 3.8% to 21%, depending on the geographical locations and diagnostic methods used. GDM has been found to be more prevalent in urban areas than in rural areas.[2-5] The nutritional quality and quantity of the diet consumed by the mother has a large influence on the overall growth and development of the fetus and thus dietary intake is foundational to optimal pregnancy outcomes.

Risk Factors for Developing Gestational Diabetes Mellitus

Although genetic predisposition, age, and ethnicity play an important role in the development of GDM, maternal obesity has been consistently found to be a major modifiable risk factor.[6] Thus, it would be useful in counseling overweight/obese young nonpregnant women about their risk for GDM and encouraging them to reduce their weight, through lifestyle measures. A reduction of 1 kg/m^2 in body mass index (BMI) was associated with a reduction of almost 1% in the prevalence of GDM. Thus, a modest decrease in maternal prepregnancy BMI, could potentially result in a significant reduction in the incidence of GDM and adverse maternal and perinatal outcomes.

Principles of Nutritional Management of Gestational Diabetes Mellitus

A team approach is ideal for managing GDM with the team comprising of obstetrician, endocrinologist, diabetes educator, dietician, and pediatrician. Nutrition intervention for women with GDM has been recognized as the cornerstone of therapy. Nutritional quality and quantity affects the overall growth and development of the fetus and thus dietary intake is foundational to optimal pregnancy outcomes. Medical nutrition therapy (MNT) is most often the primary therapy for women diagnosed with GDM,[7,8] and the challenge for MNT for GDM is to balance the needs of a healthy pregnancy with the need to control glucose level. Patients diagnosed with GDM should receive individualized nutritional counseling by a qualified dietician. The goals of nutrition therapy are to provide the necessary nutrients for fetal development, maintenance of maternal health, maintaining normoglycemia, preventing ketosis, and achieving appropriate weight gain. The dietary prescriptions made need to be individualized, taking into consideration the pregnant woman's current weight, physical activity, and recommended weight gain. The nutritional management of GDM involves energy and nutrient restrictions, to normalize blood glucose levels. MNT for GDM is a "carbohydrate-controlled meal plan that promotes adequate nutrition with appropriate weight gain, normoglycemia, and the absence of ketosis".[9] Excessive energy restrictions should be avoided during pregnancy as it can lead to ketonemia and ketonuria, which can affect the fetus. The meal pattern should provide adequate calories and nutrients to meet the needs of pregnancy. Carbohydrate should be distributed into three moderate-sized meals and 2-3 snacks throughout the day. A minimum of 175 g of carbohydrates have to be provided daily.[10] In order to prevent ketosis at night, it is advisable to provide a late night snack. Since carbohydrates are not well tolerated at breakfast due to the increased levels of cortisol and growth hormones, the carbohydrate content of breakfast is limited and protein foods can be added to satisfy hunger.

Exercise can be used as an adjunct to nutrition therapy as it helps in overcoming peripheral resistance to insulin and controlling fasting and postprandial blood glucose levels. Moderate physical exercise has been shown to lower maternal glucose levels in women with GDM. Lifestyle intervention strategies using diet and exercise to reduce weight gain in pregnancy of obese women with GDM have shown to optimize pregnancy outcome and have significant impact on future behavior.[11]

Nutritional Goals for Gestational Diabetes Mellitus

The main nutrition goals for GDM are:
- To provide an individualized dietary plan that is appropriate for weight gain, normal blood glucose levels, and prevent ketone formation
- Optimal control of carbohydrate content at meals and snacks
- Promote well-balanced intake of micronutrients
- Distribute food intake into three small-to-moderate meals and 2–4 snacks
- Encourage physical activity, which improves glucose tolerance, and may avoid/delay the need for insulin
- Promote lifestyle intervention strategies postpartum to prevent recurrent GDM or type 2 diabetes.

Assessment of the Gestational Diabetes Mellitus Patient

A nutritional assessment needs to be carried out before arriving at the nutrient recommendations for the patient. These include:
- *Weight history*: History of total weight gain in previous pregnancies, significant weight fluctuations (gain or loss) during present pregnancy, weight fluctuations prior to pregnancy, history of any previous dieting, anorexia, and bulimia
- *Using prepregnancy weight, determine the BMI*: Assess the weight gain during pregnancy, if it has increased above recommended values, make sure to monitor that subsequent weight gain is slow, in order to avoid further excess weight gain
- *Physical activity assessment*: Assess the physical activity of the patient and if currently not active, assess the willingness to change. However, any advice on physical activity should be prescribed only after consulting the treating physician
- *Dietary assessment*: Details on the meal patterns, food preferences, and nutritional adequacy can be obtained using a 24-hour recall or food frequency questionnaire. Standard cups, bowls, and spoons of known weights can be used in order to obtain accurate amounts. Additional details on food allergies, intolerances, nausea, vomiting, snacking habits, need to be collected. A sample sheet for capturing the dietary intake is provided in table 1.

TABLE 1: Sample sheet for capturing the dietary intake

One day food record sheet				
Name: _____ Date: __/__/____				
Weekday/weekend: _____				
Meal	Time	Food item/drink	Amount	Additional comments
Early morning	7.00 am	Coffee	1 glass	Use artificial sweeteners
Breakfast				
Midmorning				
Lunch				
Evening				
Dinner				
Bedtime				

Weight Gain

The expected weight gain during pregnancy is 300–400 g/week, and total weight gain is 10–12 kg by term. The Indian pregnant woman gains about 8–12 kg throughout the pregnancy period. The additional energy requirements of Indian women during pregnancy have been estimated on the basis of weight gain between 10 kg and 12 kg. The recommended additional energy requirements for a normal pregnant woman is about 70–85 kcal/day in the first trimester; 230–280 kcal/day during the second trimester, and 390–470 kcal/day during the third trimester.[12] Thus, an average amount of 350 kcal/day can be recommended for Indian women of 55 kg body weight with expected weight gain of 10–12 kg.

The dietary plan should aim to provide sufficient calories to sustain adequate nutrition for the mother and fetus, while at the same time avoiding excess weight gain and postprandial hyperglycemia. The calorie requirement of a pregnant woman depends on age, activity, prepregnancy weight, and stage of pregnancy. Pregnancy is not the right time for weight reduction. Underweight subjects or those not gaining weight as expected, particularly in the third trimester, need to be followed up regularly to ensure adequate nutrition to prevent low-birth-weight infants. For obese women (BMI >30 kg/m^2), a 30–33% calorie restriction (up to 25 kcal/kg actual weight per day) has been shown to reduce hyperglycemia and plasma triglycerides with no increase in ketonuria.[13] Restriction of carbohydrates to 35–40% of calories has been shown to decrease maternal glucose levels and improve maternal and fetal outcomes.[14]

Calorie Counting

Severe energy restriction is not advisable as 50% energy restriction on short-term was found to be associated with ketonemia and ketonuria.[15] The American Diabetic Association (ADA) encourages obese women with BMI greater than or equal to 30 kg/m^2 to reduce their calorie intake by 30%.[16] Pregnant diabetic women are often advised to wisely distribute their calorie consumption, especially at breakfast, and this involves splitting the usual breakfast into two equal halves and consuming the portions with a 2-hour gap in between. This avoids sudden peak in plasma glucose levels, following the ingestion of the total quantity of breakfast at one time. For example, if 4 idlis/chapattis/slices of bread (applies to all types of breakfast menu) is consumed for breakfast at 8.00 am and 2 hours plasma glucose at 10.00 am is 140 mg/dL, the same quantity is divided into two equal portions, i.e., one portion at 8.00 am and remaining after 10.00 am, the 2 hours postprandial plasma glucose at 10.00 am could fall by 20–30 mg/dL.

Carbohydrate Intake

The key strategy in achieving optimal glycemic control is to monitor the total grams of carbohydrates, either by use of carbohydrate counting or exchanges.[9] Improved glycemic control in patients has been observed where there was a day-to-day consistency in the amount of carbohydrate eaten at meals and snacks. Low carbohydrate diets have been shown to be associated with lower number of macrosomic infants, Cesarean deliveries and pharmacotherapy.[14] On the other hand, it was observed that high carbohydrate diets were associated with lower macrosomic rates, but this was attributed to the diet being rich in complex carbohydrates and low glycemic foods.[17] The ADA recommends that the proportion of dietary carbohydrate should be limited to 40–45% of the total calorie consumption,[18] while other recommendations allow more carbohydrate consumption, if they are complex.[19] In patients who have to adjust their mealtime insulin dose, insulin doses have to be adjusted to match carbohydrate intake (insulin to carbohydrate ratios). In these patients, carbohydrate counting and exchange lists are useful in maintaining the blood glucose levels. Carbohydrate counting involves counting food portions of 15 g carbohydrates, regardless of the source; examples are provided in Appendix 2.

Glycemic index (GI) value of a food is the response of blood glucose to a particular food, compared with an equivalent amount of the standard glucose.[20] The consumption of carbohydrate foods typically results in a rise, peak and decline of blood glucose. Foods with low GI (whole grain cereals, whole grams, many fruits and vegetables) cause a gradual increase in blood glucose due to slow digestion and absorption, while high GI foods (potatoes, white bread) produce a rapid rise in blood glucose levels. Low GI diets have been shown to benefit those being treated for diabetes.[21]

Planning A Meal

The dietary plan should be culturally appropriate and individualized to take into account the patient's weight gain, age, and physical activity and modified as needed throughout pregnancy to achieve treatment goals. Adjusting the amount and type of carbohydrate to achieve the target for postprandial glucose concentrations is an important part of the treatment regimen. Nutrition interventions for GDM should emphasize overall healthy food choices, portion control, and cooking practices that can be continued postpartum and may potentially help prevent later diabetes, obesity, cardiovascular disease (CVD), and cancer.

Tips for Healthy Eating

Body weight and blood glucose levels can be controlled by a healthy diet, which includes all food groups. The following tips can be used for a healthy pregnancy (Table 2).

TABLE 2: Tips for healthy eating during pregnancy

Food	Tips
Fat: reduce fat intake	• Remove all skin and visible fat from chicken • Bake, boil, or grill meat instead of frying or adding extra fat • Use less oil in cooking and choose oil, such as ground nut, olive, rice bran, and soyabean oil • Choose low-fat milk, curds, cheese, and paneer
Fiber: increase fiber intake	• Include adequate amounts of whole grain foods, such as whole wheat chapattis, bread, whole grams (channa, rajma, green gram), brown rice, or bulgur • Choose fresh fruits over fruit juices • Choose dark green, red, or orange and yellow vegetables and fruits, such as *palak* (spinach), *methi* (fenugreek), carrots, orange, papaya, and pumpkin, which are good for pregnancy
Protein: ensure adequate protein intake	• Protein foods do not increase blood glucose levels • Use egg white, fish, and lean cuts of chicken • Nuts can also be used in moderation
Calcium	• Include 3–4 servings of low fat milk and dairy products daily
Low-calorie sweeteners	• Low-calorie sweeteners containing sucralose and aspartame are considered safe for use during pregnancy • Saccharin-based sweetener should be avoided
Caffeine	• Limit caffeine to <300 mg/day (2 cups coffee/day) • Since caffeine is also found in some soft drinks, tea, chocolate, and medications, it is important to read the labels
Mercury	• Mercury can damage the unborn baby's nervous system and high levels are found in mackerel and shark, while fish, such as salmon and sardines, have low levels

Reducing Fat Intake

Saturated fats, which are solid at room temperature, come from meat and animal products. They increase the maternal triglyceride levels, which are associated with bigger babies. Saturated fats should be limited to within 10% of the total calories. Unsaturated fats are liquids at room temperature, found in most vegetable oils such as sunflower, safflower, and groundnut should be used in moderation. But it should be remembered that any fat is a source of calorie and should not be used excessively.

Exercise and Lifestyle Modification

The use of nutrition and exercise interventions for patients with GDM has benefits not only for the current pregnancy, but also for reducing the risk for subsequent obesity and overt diabetes. Lifestyle interventions of weight maintenance or weight loss with nutritional guidance along with an exercise program during pregnancy for overweight and obese GDM patients could optimize pregnancy outcomes and have significant impact on future behaviors. Moderate exercise combined with either an isocaloric diet or hypocaloric diet for overweight and obese patients with GDM has shown to limit maternal weight gain during pregnancy.[11] Excess gestational weight gain can be associated with fetal macrosomia and unhealthy maternal postpartum weight retention. Planned physical activity of 30 min/day is recommended for all individuals, but no physical activity should be prescribed without consultation with the doctor. Regular aerobic exercise with proper warm-up and cool-down has been shown to lower fasting and postprandial glucose concentrations in several small studies of previously sedentary individuals with GDM.[1] The Diabetes Prevention Program showed that women with GDM, approximately a decade after their last pregnancy, were able to decrease their diabetes risk with a goal of weight reduction of 7% of their baseline weight.[22] The weight loss was achieved through increased physical activity and focus on caloric reduction and calorie quality.

Long-term Therapeutic Considerations

Providing dietary education and lifestyle advice that extends beyond the pregnancy period is extremely important, as this has the potential to lessen the future risk of GDM in women. Although in most women with GDM, the blood glucose levels return to normal postpartum, GDM is associated with high lifetime risk for diabetes. Glucose tolerance should be re-evaluated at 6 weeks after delivery. If glucose levels are normal postpartum, reassessment of glycemia should be undertaken at a minimum of 3-year interval. Women with impaired glucose tolerance in the postpartum period should be tested for diabetes annually. Patients should receive intensive MNT and should follow an individualized exercise program since they have high risk for development of diabetes. All patients with prior GDM should be educated regarding lifestyle modifications that reduce insulin resistance, including maintenance of normal body weight through MNT and physical activity. Women with prior GDM need to plan future pregnancies, and need preconception counseling on the risks of uncontrolled diabetes to the fetus and the mother. Regular evaluation of glucose tolerance should be done prior to conception and early in the pregnancy. It is important to train patients for subsequent lifestyle modifications aimed at losing weight and increasing physical activity are recommended.

Conclusion

The present nutrition recommendations for women with GDM are based on limited scientific evidence and future research is needed. Research areas for future studies include level of energy restriction, safety of ketone levels, and implementing strategies to manage weight gain during pregnancy. Regardless, MNT remains the cornerstone of treatment for GDM. Nutrition interventions for GDM should emphasize overall healthy food choices, portion control, and cooking practices that can be continued postpartum and may help prevent later diabetes, obesity, CVD, and cancer.

References

1. Metzger BE, Buchanan TA, Coustan DR, de Leiva A, Dunger DB, Hadden DR, et al. Summary and recommendations of the Fifth International Workshop-Conference on Gestational Diabetes Mellitus. Diabetes Care. 2007;30(Suppl 2):S251-60.
2. Seshiah V, Balaji V, Balaji MS, Panneerselvam A, Arthi T, Thamizharasi M, et al. Prevalence of gestational diabetes mellitus in South India (Tamil Nadu)—a community based study. J Assoc Physicians India. 2008;56:329-33.
3. Seshiah V, Balaji V, Balaji MS, Panneerselvam A, Kapur A. Pregnancy and diabetes scenario around the world: India. Int J Gynaecol Obstet. 2009;104(Suppl 1):S35-8.
4. Swami SR, Mehetre R, Shivane V, Bandgar TR, Menon PS, Shah NS. Prevalence of carbohydrate intolerance of varying degrees in pregnant females in western India (Maharashtra)—a hospital-based study. J Indian Med Assoc. 2008;106(11):712-4, 735.
5. Divakar H, Tyagi S, Hosmani P, Manyonda IT. Diagnostic criteria influence prevalence rates for gestational diabetes: implications for interventions in an Indian pregnant population. Perinatology. 2008;10:155-61.
6. Morisset AS, St-Yves A, Veillette J, Weisnagel SJ, Tchernof A, Robitaille J. Prevention of gestational diabetes mellitus: a review of studies on weight management. Diabetes Metab Res Rev. 2010;26(1):17-25.
7. Gunderson EP: Gestational diabetes and nutritional recommendations. Curr Diab Rep. 2004;4(5):377-86.
8. Kim C. Gestational diabetes: risks, management, and treatment options. Int J Womens Health. 2010;2:339-51.

9. American Diabetes Association. Standards of medical care in diabetes: Position statement. Diabetes Care. 2010; 33(Suppl 1):S11-S61.
10. Trumbo P, Schlicker S, Yates AA, Poos M; Food and Nutrition Board of the Institute of Medicine, The National Academies. Dietary reference intakes for energy, carbohydrate, fiber, fat, fatty acids, cholesterol, protein and amino acids. J Am Diet Assoc. 2002;102(11):1621-30.
11. Artal R, Catanzaro RB, Gavard JA, Mostello DJ, Friganza JC. A lifestyle intervention of weight-gain restriction: diet and exercise in obese women with gestational diabetes mellitus. Appl Physiol Nutr Metab. 2007;32(3):596-601.
12. National Institute of Nutrition, Indian Council of Medical Research. (2009). Nutrient Requirements and Recommended Dietary Allowances for Indians: A Report of the Expert Group of the Indian Council of Medical Research. [online] Available from: icmr.nic.in/final/RDA-2010.pdf. [Accessed August, 2014].
13. Franz MJ, Horton ES, Bantle JP, Beebe CA, Brunzell JD, Coulston AM, et al. Nutrition principles for the management of diabetes and related complications. Diabetes Care. 1994;17(5):490-518.
14. Major CA, Henry MJ, De Veciana M, Morgan MA. The effects of carbohydrate restriction in patients with diet-controlled gestational diabetes. Obstet Gynecol. 1998;91(4):600-4.
15. Magee MS, Knopp RH, Benedetti TJ. Metabolic effects of 1200-kcal diet in obese pregnant women with gestational diabetes. Diabetes. 1990;39(2):234-40.
16. American Diabetes Association. Gestational diabetes mellitus. Diabetes Care. 2004;27(Suppl 1):S88-90.
17. Romon M, Nuttens MC, Vambergue A, Vérier-Mine O, Biausque S, Lemaire C, et al. Higher carbohydrate intake is associated with decreased incidence of newborn macrosomia in women with gestational diabetes. J Am Diet Assoc. 2001;101(8):897-902.
18. Franz MJ, Bantle JP, Beebe CA, Brunzell JD, Chiasson JL, Garg A, et al. Evidence-based nutrition principles and recommendations for the treatment and prevention of diabetes and related complications. Diabetes Care. 2003;26(Suppl 1):S51-61.
19. Mazze R, Langer O. Medical nutrition therapy. In: Langer O (Ed). The Diabetes in Pregnancy Dilemma: Leading Change with Proven Solutions, 1st edition. Maryland, USA: University Press of America; 2006. pp. 251-63.
20. Foster-Powell K, Holt SH, Brand-Miller JC. International table of glycemic index and glycemic load values: 2002. Am J Clin Nutr. 2002;76(1):5-56.
21. Brand-Miller JC, Petocz P, Colagiuri S. Meta-analysis of low-glycemic index diets in the management of diabetes: response to Franz. Diabetes Care. 2003;26(12):3363-4.
22. Ratner RE, Christophi CA, Metzger BE, Dabelea D, Bennett PH, Pi-Sunyer X, et al. Prevention of diabetes in women with a history of gestational diabetes: effects of metformin and lifestyle interventions. J Clin Endocrinol Metab. 2008;93(12):4774-9.

CHAPTER 9

Nutrition in Complications of Diabetes

Abstract

The focus of this chapter is to emphasize the key role of medical nutrition therapy in preventing or delaying the complications of diabetes. The nutritional management of conditions such as diabetic nephropathy, diabetic neuropathy, and cardiovascular diseases has been discussed. Practical tips on restricting potassium, sodium, and fluid intake have been provided. The benefits and recommendations of physical activity in preventing complications of diabetes have also been outlined in this chapter.

Introduction

Medical nutrition therapy (MNT) plays a key role in preventing or delaying the complications of diabetes. The progression of complications of diabetes can be minimized by maintaining optimal blood glucose levels, body weight, lowering blood pressure, and following a moderate protein intake. The main complications of diabetes in which diet/nutrition plays a role can be broadly classified as acute and chronic.

Acute Complications

Hyperglycemia and Diabetic Ketoacidosis

Diabetic ketoacidosis (DKA) is seen mostly in type 1 diabetic patients, but also occurs sometimes in obese patients with type 2 diabetes mellitus (T2DM). Inadequate insulin for glucose utilization causes DKA, which causes the fat to be used as energy source. Build-up of ketone bodies in the blood occurs due to increased lipolysis (breakdown of lipids). DKA is characterized by high blood sugar levels and presence of ketones in urine and blood. DKA occurs when hyperglycemia is not treated properly. Treatment includes initial rehydration with subsequent potassium replacement and low-dose insulin therapy. The nutritional management of hyperglycemia includes a variety of interventions such as reduced energy/fat intake, healthy food choices, carbohydrate counting, exchange list, physical activity, and behavioral strategies. Guidance in making appropriate food choices to reduce risk, improve metabolic control, and quality of life should be provided. Preventive measures include patient education and instructions for the patient to contact the physician early during an illness.

Hypoglycemia

Low blood sugar levels often occur in the initial stages of insulin therapy either due to an overdose of insulin or insufficient carbohydrates in the meal. The immediate treatment includes providing either glucose or carbohydrate-rich foods. For patients not able to swallow, administration of glucose intravenously and in addition, subcutaneous or intramuscular glucagon needs to be provided. The long-term nutritional management focused towards preventing repeated episodes of hypoglycemia includes advising the patient to consume small frequent meals rather than three large meals with long periods of gap between them. Additionally, the intake of complex carbohydrates (whole grain cereals, legumes, fruits, and vegetables) with adequate fiber should be encouraged. Awareness by the patient regarding the symptoms of hypoglycemia and self-monitoring of blood glucose is essential, in order to prevent and treat hypoglycemia.

Chronic or Long-term Complications

Nutritional management is important in the long-term complications of diabetes. Long-term complications include disease of the larger vessels (macrovascular) and small vessels (microvascular).

Diabetic Nephropathy

Diabetes is one of the common causes of chronic kidney disease (CKD). Diabetic nephropathy is defined by the presence of proteinuria (>0.5 g/24 hours). Diet plays a significant role in the development of the disease and the nutritional recommendations depend on the degree of nephropathy and treatment such as dialysis and transplantation.

Nutritional Management

The goal of the treatment is to prevent the progression from microalbuminuria to macroalbuminuria, deterioration of renal function, and occurrence of cardiovascular events. Malnutrition is frequently present in patients with CKD and the nutritional assessment should be performed regularly.

Energy requirement: Energy requirement varies at different stages of CKD. The energy requirement of patients between stages 1 and 4 of CKD, not undergoing dialysis, is similar to that of healthy individuals. The energy demand increases with the progression of CKD. The aim should be to maintain a healthy body weight by consuming adequate calories and including daily physical activity. Obese patients require dietary and exercise recommendations for weight reduction.

Protein requirement: The amount and type of dietary protein have shown to be associated with diabetic nephropathy. A low-protein diet delays the decline of renal function and death in patients with type 1 diabetes with micro- and macroalbuminuria, while studies in type 2 diabetic patients are limited with short-term studies suggesting that low-protein diet decreases albuminuria. For patients with renal disease, the nutritional intervention should be planned to maintain a balance between an excessive protein energy intake-induced deterioration in glomerular filtration rate (GFR) and inadequate protein energy intake contributing to protein energy-malnutrition. In early stage of kidney disease, the protein intake should be between 0.8 g/kg and 1.0 g/kg body weight. Dietary protein restriction has been shown to delay the progression of diabetic nephropathy in patients with type 1 diabetes,[1] and a diet with a protein of 0.9 g/kg/day diet for type 1 diabetic patients with progressive nephropathy has been shown to reduce the risk of end-stage renal disease, or death by 76%, with no effect on GFR decline.[2] The data are still inconclusive about the potential benefit of plant protein in comparison to animal proteins in diabetic patients with microalbuminuria. Plant protein sources are associated with reduced GFR, lower protein, and phosphate intake and beneficial effects on blood pressure, body weight, and lipids. Improved lipid profile along with glomerular hemodynamics may be the mechanism by which a low-protein diet decreases the progression of diabetic nephropathy, but this needs to be confirmed. However, the use of low-protein diet for long periods is compromised by poor compliance and its long-term safety is not firmly established. A complementary source of protein (cereal and legume) can be recommended to ensure high-quality protein intake. Grains, such as rice, oats, wheat, corn, and *ragi* (finger millet) can act as complementary proteins for legumes such as lentils, since they contain the amino acids cysteine and methionine that lentils lack, while lentils provide the lysine that grains are deficient in.

In type 2 diabetic patients with microalbuminuria, the replacement of red meat with chicken in the diet reduced the urinary albumin excretion (UAE) by 46% along with reduction in total cholesterol, low-density lipoprotein (LDL) cholesterol, and apolipoprotein B.[3] The possible reason could have been the lower amount of saturated fat and higher level of polyunsaturated fatty acid in chicken meat, since the beneficial effect of polyunsaturated fats on endothelial function has shown to lower UAE.[4]

Lipid management: The serum lipid levels in patients with diabetic nephropathy are primarily evaluated to detect abnormalities that can increase the incidence of cardiovascular disease (CVD). Albumin excretion and the rate of progression of diabetic nephropathy may be influenced by dyslipidemia, and optimal lipid management has shown to delay the course of kidney disease progression,[5] suggesting that MNT designed to reduce the risk for CVD could have favorable effects on microvascular complications of diabetes. The lowering of lipid levels by drugs has shown to maintain GFR and reduce proteinuria in diabetic patients.[5] Advanced diabetic nephropathy with heavy proteinuria is associated with increased LDL cholesterol levels. The goal for a diabetic patient for LDL cholesterol is less than 100 mg/dL, while it is 70 mg/dL for a diabetic patient with CVD.[6] Nutritional therapy plays a key role in the management of lipid levels. Studies have shown that the replacement of saturated fats with carbohydrate in diabetic patients reduced LDL cholesterol with beneficial or no effects on serum triglycerides.[7] Supplementation with soy protein (0.5 g/kg) in a 8-week crossover trial of T2DM nephropathy patients showed an increase in high-density lipoprotein (HDL) cholesterol (4.5%) when compared to 0.5 g/kg casein supplementation.[8]

Sodium restriction: The restriction of sodium is important in achieving normal blood pressure levels and to achieve edema-free body weight in patients with diabetic nephropathy. The amount prescribed depends on the patient's CKD stage. Blood pressure should be regularly monitored, and the goal should be to maintain it below 130/80 mmHg. MNT for patients with elevated blood pressure includes reduction of sodium intake to 2,400 mg/day, weight reduction in obese patients, including adequate amounts of fruits, vegetables and whole grains, and regular exercise.

Potassium restriction: Hyperkalemia (elevated potassium levels) is a common feature of CKD. Dietary restriction of potassium depends on the presence or absence of hyperkalemia. Restriction of fruits, fruit juices, tender coconut water, vegetables rich in potassium, and high potassium containing cereals like *ragi* (finger millet), *bajra* (pearl millet), barley, and oats may be

TABLE 1: Potassium content of foods

Food group	High potassium foods (>100 mg/100 g)	Low potassium foods (<100 mg/100 g)
Cereals	*Ragi* (finger millet), *bajra* (pearl millet), barley, oats, broken wheat, whole wheat, corn	Rice, semolina (rava), vermicelli, noodles
Pulses	All whole grams and dals such as green gram, lima beans, masoor dal, cow pea, dry beans, chickpea flour (*besan*)	
Vegetables	Green leafy vegetables, carrot, onion, radish, pumpkin, French beans, cabbage, bitter gourd, brinjal, green plantain, drumstick, green papaya, mushroom, broccoli potato, sweet potato	*Methi* (fenugreek) leaves, ladies finger, peas, ridge gourd, field beans, green mango, *tinda* (round gourd), beetroot, *knol khol* (German turnip)
Fruits	Mango, pomegranate, sweet lime (*mosambi*), watermelon, muskmelon, banana, sapota (*chikoo*), peach, *amla* (Indian gooseberry), avocado, dried fruits, and orange	Pear, apple, pineapple, ripe papaya
Milk and its products	Cow's milk and it products like cheese, curds, cream, paneer, condensed milk, soya milk, tofu (bean curd)	Buffalo milk, buttermilk
Meat and its products	All fresh and processed meats like chicken, mutton, beef, fish, egg	

Note: Various resources use different milligram cut-off levels to determine what foods are higher and lower in potassium. Therefore, low potassium diet resources may vary.

necessary. In order to avoid unnecessary diet restriction, the counseling can be done in two stages:

1. *First stage*: Focus on consuming lower potassium, vegetables, fruits, and avoiding salt substitutes containing potassium chloride and sodium-reduced products that use potassium (Table 1).
2. *Second stage*: Move to this stage if potassium values are still above normal range.

Limit the intake of milk and milk products, *dals*, whole grams (*channa, rajma,* green gram), and meat.

Leaching of vegetables may prove useful to reduce its potassium content.

How to leach vegetables: Cut all vegetables into small pieces and cook in excess water. Discard the water after cooking and then consume the vegetables.

Phosphate restriction: Maintaining normal serum phosphate levels is important for preventing renal bone disease and calcification of the soft tissue in people with CKD. Increase in blood phosphate is usually seen in the later stages of CKD. Initially counseling is focused on sodium, potassium, and protein restriction which could indirectly reduce phosphorus in the diet. Dietary sources of phosphorus are bran of rice and oats, wheat germ, soyabean, processed meats, flaxseeds, sesame seeds, milk and milk products like curds, ice cream, cheese, and nuts like groundnuts, almonds and cashews. In the earlier stages of CKD, the use of fiber-rich grains and cereals can be encouraged to promote optimal blood glucose control. Beverages that contain phosphoric acid (regular and diet cola) or phosphates (beer, chocolates) should be discouraged.

Fluid intake: The fluid requirement of the individual will vary based on the urine output. The following tips can be employed to maintain fluid balance and quench thirst.

Tips
- Restrict the intake of salty and spicy foods
- Sip beverages to make them last longer
- Consume ice instead of beverages
- Rinse mouth with mouthwash or suck on lemon
- Maintain optimal blood glucose since thirst could be a side effect of high glucose levels.

Anemia

Patients with diabetic nephropathy often present with symptoms of anemia even with creatinine levels less than 1.8 mg/dL, and this is thought to be related to erythropoietin deficiency.[9] Anemia is associated with higher incidence of left ventricular hypertrophy,[10] recurrent cardiac failure, and increased cardiac-related hospitalizations.[11] Studies on whether anemia correction is beneficial to progression of diabetic nephropathy have shown conflicting results.[12-14] Further controlled studies are needed to clarify the prevalence and consequences of anemia in diabetic patients. The foods rich in iron, which can be advised in iron-deficiency anemia, are dried beans, green leafy vegetables, tofu (bean curd), dried fruits, meat, and organ meat (liver, kidney). The iron absorption from vegetarian sources can be enhanced by eating foods rich in vitamin C (orange, sweet lime, gooseberry, lemon, tomato, broccoli, and cabbage) along with an iron-rich meal. Foods containing tannins (tea, coffee, cola) should be avoided with an iron containing meal as they inhibit the absorption of iron.

Diabetic Neuropathy

Neuropathy is an adverse effect of hyperglycemia (high blood glucose levels). Gastroparesis or impaired gastric motility is a result of neuropathy of the nerves innervating the stomach leading to delayed gastric emptying due to irregular contractions of the stomach and can affect the digestion of food and slow glucose absorption. The disorders of the upper gastrointestinal motility seen in diabetes are referred to as gastropathy, which causes postprandial hyperglycemia. Early satiety, decreased appetite, bloating, abdominal discomfort, nausea, and vomiting are some of the symptoms which generally subside with improved blood glucose levels. MNT primarily involves effective glycemic controls through dietary and lifestyle modifications. Symptoms of gastroparesis can be relieved by minimizing abdominal stress. Small frequent meals low in fat and fiber and increased intake of liquid foods may help to accelerate gastric emptying. Occasionally, nutritional requirement may have to be met by nutritional and vitamin supplements. Regular self-monitoring of glucose is recommended to improve glycemic control.

Cardiovascular Disease

Cardiovascular disease is one of the most common complication of T2DM, and people with diabetes have threefold to fourfold increases for CVD. The risk factors for diabetes and CVD are similar. Risk assessment for CVD prevention should include family history, smoking habits, food and diet patterns, physical activity patterns, blood pressure, body mass index, waist circumference, blood glucose levels and lipid levels. Lifestyle modifications are associated with improved lipid levels, in diabetics. Type 2 diabetic patients are known to have smaller, dense LDL particle which increases atherogenicity. The primary goal is to lower LDL levels to 100 mg/dL or below.

Nutritional Management

The main nutritional interventions that have been successful in reducing the risk for cardiovascular events include reduction in the intake of dietary fat, saturated fat and cholesterol, interventions to improve blood pressure, maintain optimum body weight, and body composition. The primary goal for diabetic individuals with one or more risk factors of CVD such as low HDL cholesterol (<40 mg/dL), hypertension, cigarette smoking, or family history of premature coronary heart disease (CHD), is to maintain LDL cholesterol level less than 100 mg/dL. The reduction in the LDL cholesterol can be achieved by reduction of saturated fats intake (<7% of total energy), dietary cholesterol (<200 mg/dL), and trans fats (<1% of energy intake).[15] The diet can be substituted with monounsaturated fats or carbohydrates.[7] Patients with metabolic syndrome will benefit from better glycemic control, modest

TABLE 2: Types of dietary fat, its food sources, and effect on blood cholesterol

Type of fat	Effect on blood cholesterol	Sources
Saturated	Increases LDL and HDL	Butter, cheese, red meat, full-fat milk, yoghurt, lard, coconut and palm oil
Monounsaturated	Decreases LDL, increases HDL	Olive oil, peanut oil, mustard oil, gingelly oil, nuts (pistachio, almonds, hazelnuts, cashew, peanuts), avocados and their oils
Polyunsaturated	Decreases LDL, increases HDL	*Omega-6 polyunsaturated*: Sunflower seeds, safflower oil, wheat germ, sesame seeds, walnuts, soybean, corn and their oils *Omega-3 polyunsaturated*: Salmon, mackerel, herring, walnuts, soybean, flaxseed Plant sources include flax seed, oils (canola, soyabean and flaxseed), nuts and other seeds (walnut, sunflower seeds)
Trans-fatty acids	Increases LDL	Hydrogenated fats such as *vanaspathi* and *dalda*. Bakery products made from these fats such as biscuits, cakes and pastries

HDL, high-density lipoprotein; LDL, low-density lipoprotein.

weight loss, increased physical activity, and decreased intake of saturated fats. Consumption of fatty fish such as mackerel, sardine, tuna and salmon twice a week (~120 g) is recommended. The recommended fiber intake is 25–30 g/day with emphasis on 7–13 g of soluble fiber (fruits, vegetables, whole grains) to reduce LDL cholesterol. For individuals with very high serum triglycerides (>1,000 mg/dL), restriction of all fat intake except omega-3 fatty acids may be beneficial. Lipid lowering agents may be needed if levels are not controlled after dietary and lifestyle methods have not shown any improvement. Table 2 describes the types of fat, its food sources, and effect on blood cholesterol.

Glycemic control: It is important to maintain glycosylated hemoglobin (HbA1c) levels since every 1% increase in the HbA1c levels has been reported to increase the risk of developing CVD in type 2 diabetic patients by 18% and type 1 diabetics by 15%.[16] It is recommended to maintain the HbA1c levels less than 7% for diabetics in general, but targeting the HbA1c levels close to the normal range (<6%) without any hypoglycemic episodes.[17]

Hypertension

A common comorbidity of diabetes is hypertension, which should be treated immediately in order to prevent/reduce risk for macro- and microvascular diseases. Beneficial effects of reducing sodium intake have been demonstrated in both normo- and hypertensive patients. Reduction of sodium intake to 2,400 mg along with modest weight loss, balanced eating, regular physical activity, and diet low in fat and rich in fruits and vegetables have shown to help in lowering blood pressure. The Dietary Approaches to Stop Hypertension (DASH) diet which promotes the consumption of fruits vegetable, low fat dairy products, whole grains, poultry, fish, and nuts with reduction in red meats, fats, sweets, and sweetened beverages has shown to be helpful.[18] Additionally, regular physical activity (walking) has shown to decrease hypertension.[19,20] Consumption of high amounts of alcohol (>3 drinks/day) has been shown to increase blood pressure[7] and thus should be restricted.

Salt-free tips to flavor your food
*Use fresh or dried herbs and spices like oregano, thyme, basil, pepper, chilli flakes
*Flavor with lemon juice, vinegar or garlic.

Physical Activity

The benefits of physical activity for diabetic patients include management of body weight, blood glucose levels, blood pressure, and reduced risk for cardiovascular mortality. The type of physical activity will depend on the individual and can include walking, running, swimming, or any other exercise that increases exercise capacity endurance and skeletal muscle strength. The recommendation for physical activity to improve glycemic control, aid weight maintenance, and reduce the risk of CVD is to perform at least 150 minutes of moderate-intensity aerobic physical activity per week or at least 90 minutes of vigorous aerobic exercise per week. Diabetic patients should be encouraged to perform 30–60 minutes of moderate-intensity aerobic activity such as brisk walking on most days of the week (5-6 days/week). Additionally, they should be advised to reduce their sedentary time throughout the day. In case of patients requiring long-term maintenance of increased weight loss, at least 7 hours of moderate or vigorous aerobic physical activity per week may be needed.[15] The patient should, however, consult with the physician before starting any form of exercise.

Conclusion

Optimal nutritional management helps in the long-term health and quality of life of a diabetic individual. Achieving and maintaining healthy body weight, blood glucose, lipids, and blood pressure can help in preventing and reducing the risk of diabetes-related complications. Self-management education should be ongoing for the diabetic patient.

References

1. Pedrini MT, Levey AS, Lau J, Chalmers TC, Wang PH. The effect of dietary protein restriction on the progression of diabetic and nondiabetic renal diseases: a meta-analysis. Ann Intern Med. 1996;124(7):627-32.
2. Hansen HP, Tauber-Lassen E, Jensen BR, Parving HH. Effect of dietary protein restriction on prognosis in patients with diabetic nephropathy. Kidney Int. 2002;62(1):220-8.
3. Gross JL, Zelmanovitz T, Moulin CC, De Mello V, Perassolo M, Leitão C, et al. Effect of a chicken-based diet on renal function and lipid profile in patients with type 2 diabetes: a randomized crossover trial. Diabetes Care. 2002;25(4):645-51.
4. Ros E, Núñez I, Perez-Heras A, Serra M, Gilabert R, Casals E, et al. A walnut diet improves endothelial function in hypercholesterolemic subjects: a randomized crossover trial. Circulation. 2004;109(13): 1609-14.
5. Fried LF, Orchard TJ, Kasiske BL. Effect of lipid reduction on the progression of renal disease: a meta-analysis. Kidney Int. 2001;59(1):260-9.
6. Gross JL, de Azevedo MJ, Silveiro SP, Canani LH, Caramori ML, Zelmanovitz T. Diabetic nephropathy: diagnosis, prevention, and treatment. Diabetes Care. 2005;28(1):164-76.
7. American Diabetes Association. Position Statement: Evidence-based nutrition principles and recommendations for the treatment and prevention of diabetes and related complications. Diabetes Care. 2002;25(1):S50-60.
8. Teixeira SR, Tappenden KA, Carson L, Jones R, Prabhudesai M, Marshall WP, et al. Isolated soy protein consumption reduces urinary albumin excretion and improves the serum lipid profile in men with type 2 diabetes mellitus and nephropathy. J Nutr. 2004;134 (8):1874-80.
9. Bosman DR, Winkler AS, Marsden JT, Macdougall IC, Watkins PJ. Anemia with erythropoietin deficiency occurs early in diabetic nephropathy. Diabetes Care. 2001;24(3):495-910.
10. Levin A, Singer J, Thompson CR, Ross H, Lewis M. Prevalent left ventricular hypertrophy in the predialysis population: identifying opportunities for intervention. Am J Kidney Dis. 1996;27(3): 347-54.
11. Collins AJ, Li S, St Peter W, Ebben J, Roberts T, Ma JZ, et al. Death, hospitalization, and economic associations among incident hemodialysis patients with hematocrit values of 36 to 39%. J Am Soc Nephrol. 2001;12(11):2465-73.
12. Locatelli F, Aljama P, Barany P, Canaud B, Carrera F, Eckardt KU, et al. Revised European best practice guidelines for the management of anaemia in patients with chronic renal failure. Nephrol Dial Transplant. 2004;19(Suppl 2):ii1-47.
13. Kuriyama S, Tomonari H, Yoshida H, Hashimoto T, Kawaguchi Y, Sakai O. Reversal of anemia by erythropoietin therapy retards the progression of chronic renal failure, especially in nondiabetic patients. Nephron. 1997;77(2):176-85.
14. Silverberg DS, Wexler D, Blum M, Tchebiner JZ, Sheps D, Keren G, et al. The effect of correction of anaemia in diabetics and non-diabetics with severe resistant congestive heart failure and chronic renal failure by subcutaneous erythropoietin and intravenous iron. Nephrol Dial Transplant. 2003;18(1):141-6.
15. Buse JB, Ginsberg HN, Bakris GL, Clark NG, Costa F, Eckel R, et al. Primary prevention of cardiovascular diseases in people with diabetes mellitus: a scientific statement from the American Heart Association and the American Diabetes Association. Diabetes Care. 2007;30(1):162-72.
16. Selvin E, Mareinopoulos S, Berkinbilt G, Rami T, Brancoti FL, Powe NR, et al. Meta-analysis: glycosylated hemoglobin and cardiovascular disease in diabetes mellitus. Ann Intern Med. 2004;141(6):421-31.
17. American Diabetes Association. Standards of medical care in diabetes—2006. Diabetes Care. 2006;29(Suppl 1): S4-42.

18. National Heart, Lung, and Blood Institute, National Institutes of Health. National High Blood Pressure Education Program. Complete Report: The Seventh Report of the Joint National Committee on Prevention, Detection, Evaluation, and Treatment of High Blood Pressure. NIH Publication No. 04-5230. Bethesda, Maryland, USA: US Department of Health and Human Services; 2004.
19. Chobanian AV, Bakris GL, Black HR, Cushman WC, Green LA, Izzo JL, et al. Seventh report of the Joint National Committee on Prevention, Detection, Evaluation, and Treatment of High Blood Pressure. Hypertension. 2003;42(6):1206-52.
20. American Diabetes Association (2013). Diabetes: heart disease and stroke. [online] Available from: www.diabetes.org/diabetes-heart-disease-stroke.jsp [Accessed August, 2014].

CHAPTER 10

Complementary and Alternative Medicine Therapy for Obesity and Diabetes

Abstract

This chapter reviews the existing literature on some of the complementary and alternative therapies used for patients with obesity and diabetes. Some of the therapies discussed in this chapter include biologically based practices (dietary supplements and herbs), mind body medicine (Tai chi, yoga), manipulation and body-based practices (chiropractic therapy, osteopathic manipulation, and massage), energy medicine (reiki, acupuncture), and whole medical systems (Ayurveda, Homeopathy, Naturopathy, and Chinese medicine). The limited evidence on the effectiveness of these therapies has been explored.

Introduction

Complementary and alternative medicine (CAM) includes medical and health-care systems, products, and practices that are not considered as a part of contemporary medicine. Complementary medicine refers to therapies that are used along with conventional medicine, while "alternative" medicines are therapies that are used in place of conventional medicine. CAM is growing more popular among the consumer and professionals. The use of CAM in India is about 65%.[1] Although scientific evidence exists regarding some CAM therapies, more well-designed scientific studies are needed to assess if these therapies are safe or effective for the diseases or medical conditions for which they are used. CAM of proven quality, safety, and efficacy can contribute to the goal of ensuring that all people have access to care. The five domains of CAM are depicted in table 1.

TABLE 1: Domains of complementary and alternative medicine

CAM therapy	Description	Examples
Biologically-based practices	Use of substances found in nature with medical properties	Herbs and dietary supplements, such as vitamins and foods
Mind-body medicine	Practices that use the relationship of mind and body to achieve improved health or treat disease	Yoga, Tai Chi, and meditation
Manipulation and body-based practices	Involves manipulation or movement of specific body parts or the whole body	Chiropractic therapy, osteopathic manipulation, and massage
Energy therapies	Involves the use of energy fields. Two types of therapies are: • Biofield therapies • Bioelectromagnetic-based therapies involve the unconventional use of electromagnetic fields, such as pulsed field, magnetic fields, or alternating current	External Qi-gong, Reiki, and therapeutic touch
Whole medical systems	Complete medical systems that have evolved separately from or was earlier than conventional medicine	Homeopathy, naturopathy, ayurveda from India, and TCM

CAM, complementary and alternative medicine; TCM, traditional Chinese medicine.
Source: Adapted from National Center for Complementary and Medicine.

Biologically-based Practices

These practices involve the use of substances found in nature with medicinal properties and include dietary supplements and herbs. These products are consumed orally and contain vitamins, minerals, herbs, amino acids, and substances, such as enzymes, organ tissues, glandular substances, and metabolites. Supplements are often in the form of tablets, capsules, soft gels, liquids, or powders. Although dietary supplements are not treated as drugs by the Dietary Supplement Health and Education Act (DSHEA) of 1994, the manufacturers cannot make specific clinical claims that the supplement can treat or cure a specific disease.

TABLE 2: Common dietary supplements used for diabetes

Name	Possible effect and evidence
Chromium*	• Improvement in HbA1c levels, glucose tolerance, beneficial effects on insulin and cholesterol levels in subjects with T2DM[2] • Hypoglycemic effect in T2DM patients[3,4]
Alpha-lipoic acid	• Increase in glucose uptake, decrease of fasting insulin and improved insulin sensitivity in T2DM patients[5,6]
Vanadium	• Hypoglycemic effect in diabetes patients[7] • Decrease in fasting blood glucose, HbA1c, hepatic glucose production, increase in insulin-mediated glucose uptake and insulin sensitivity in T2DM patients[8-11]
Magnesium	• Improvement in glycemic control of T2DM patients[12,13] • Decrease in fasting blood glucose levels in T2DM patients[14] • Increase in glucose uptake, improved insulin sensitivity and glucose oxidation in T2DM patients[13,15,16] • Increase in the intake of dietary magnesium may reduce the risk of developing T2DM in normal individuals[17,18]
Vitamin E	• Improvement in glycemic control of insulin-dependent diabetes[19,20] and noninsulin-dependent diabetes[21-23] • Decrease in fasting blood glucose levels of T2DM patients[21,22]
Coenzyme Q10	• Improved glycemic control in T2DM patients[24-27]

HbA1c, glycosylated hemoglobin; T2DM, type 2 diabetes mellitus.
*The beneficial effects of chromium in individuals with diabetes were observed at levels higher than the upper limit of the estimated safe and adequate daily dietary intake.

Dietary Supplements and Type 2 Diabetes Mellitus

There is a lack of adequate scientific evidence to demonstrate that any dietary supplement can help manage or prevent type 2 diabetes mellitus (T2DM). There are some case reports linking some dietary supplement use to kidney disease, and thus it is important to monitor supplement use in patients who have or are at risk for kidney disease. Some of the common dietary supplements used for diabetes are summarized in table 2.

Herbs and Type 2 Diabetes Mellitus

Some of the botanical products used for diabetes treatment are mentioned in figure 1 and table 3 lists some of the common dietary and herbal supplements used for obesity.

Complementary and Alternative Medicine Therapy for Obesity and Diabetes

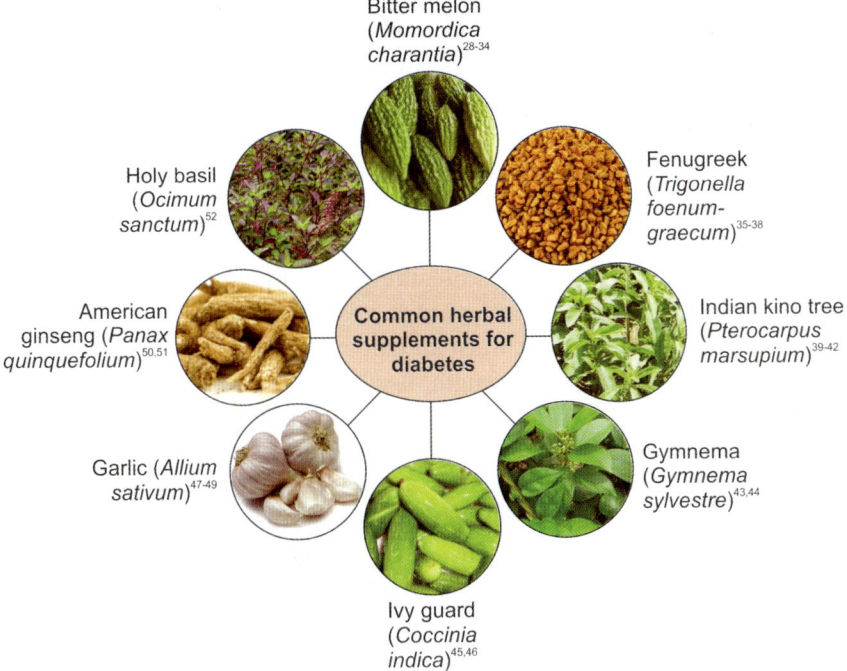

Figure 1 Common herbal supplements used for diabetes.
Note: The numbers in superscripts are the references for herbal supplement mentioned.

TABLE 3: Dietary and herbal supplements used for obesity

Chromium	Increase in lean body mass and decrease in the percentage of body fat, with associated weight loss[53]
Conjugated linoleic acid	Reduction in body fat mass[54-57]
Pyruvate	Decrease in body weight and fat loss[58,59]
Chitosan	Weight loss[60-62]
Glucomannan	Decrease in total cholesterol, LDL cholesterol, triglycerides, body weight and fasting blood glucose[63]
Green tea	Weight loss induced by dietary thermogenesis[64,65]
Caralluma fimbriata	Weight loss and reduction in body fat percentage suggested due to decreased energy intake caused by appetite suppression[66]

LDL, low-density lipoprotein.

Mind-body Medicine

This method uses specific techniques which are based on the concept that physical body and mind influence each other. Most of these therapies have been derived from yoga, tai chi and meditation. Yoga practices include techniques of movement, breathing, meditating, chanting, and lifestyle change, while tai chi has roots in martial arts and ancient healing traditions. Yoga interventions such as asana practice for 60 minutes or more (3–4 times a week for 3 months) along with breathing techniques and relaxing results in weight loss.[67-69] Beneficial effects of decreases in body mass index (BMI), fat mass, body fat percentage, waist and hip circumferences and increase in lean mass, improvement in strength, flexibility, and steadiness have been observed with yoga.[67,68,70-74] Yoga has shown to improve cardiovascular and aerobic capacity, enhance quality of life, improve self-esteem, self-efficiency, and reduce stress and anxiety.[68,74,75] Yoga was suggested to be a potentially successful intervention for weight maintenance and prevention of obesity.[76] The factors related to the effectiveness of yoga for weight loss include increased frequency of practice, longer intervention duration, yogic dietary component and residential component. A systematic review on the effects of yoga-based interventions on physiologic and anthropometric risk profiles and related clinical outcomes in adults with T2DM suggested that yoga could improve risk profiles in adults with T2DM and may help in the prevention and management of cardiovascular complications, however, only four out of 25 studies were randomized controlled trials.[77]

Clinical trial data on the effectiveness of tai chi for T2DM have not demonstrated convincing evidence that Tai Chi reduces fasting blood glucose levels or glycosylated hemoglobin (HbA1c) in patients with T2DM.[78] Tai chi when practiced over 6 months was found to reduce blood glucose, HbA1c levels, and improve quality of life;[79] however, these findings need to be further investigated. Although yoga and Tai chi are categorized as low-to-moderate intensity exercise, controlled clinical studies have not demonstrated long-term improvements in glycemic control.[80,81] Some studies have examined the therapeutic effect of incorporating tai chi exercises in weight management program;[82,83] however, the evidence is not strong.

While several reviews suggest positive effects of yoga, various methodical limitations, such as small sample size, heterogeneity of controls, and intervention, limit the generalization of these encouraging studies. However, since chronic diseases are often associated with diminished quality of life, anxiety, and depression, the mind and body therapies could help the patients improve mood and quality of life. Yoga and tai chi practices in diabetic patients have shown improvements in quality of life and stress levels.[84] Mind and body techniques when incorporated into cardiac rehabilitation programs, have demonstrated improvements in diet, exercise, and body weight.[85] Although the risks of practicing mind-body medicine are low, more extensive research with higher methodological quality and adequate control interventions are needed.

Manipulation and Body-based Practices

Manipulative and body-based practices include chiropractic and osteopathic manipulation, massage therapy, reexology, Rolfing, Bowen technique, and Trager approach. These treatment focuses on interactions among the brain, mind, body, and behavior and the ways in which emotional, mental, social, spiritual, and behavioral factors can directly affect health. Chiropractic care focuses on the relationship between body structure (spine) and body functions and on the effect of that relationship on health. Osteopathic manipulative medicine (OMM) or osteopathic manipulative treatment (OMT) is a technique of osteopathy based on the belief of the existence of a myofascial continuity—a tissue layer that interlinks all parts of the body. The practitioners diagnose and treat "somatic dysfunction" by manipulating the bones and muscles of a patient. Treatment with OMT has been suggested as an adjunct to the current methods of T2DM management with small studies observing that OMT may help in lowering glucose levels, increasing insulin secretion.[86] OMT could reduce diabetes-related complications, such as adhesive capsulitis.[87] However, osteopathic medical literature is still limited for evidence of OMT and management of T2DM. There is very limited or no literature available on the role of the other manipulation and body-based practices on obesity or diabetes.

Energy Medicine

Biofield therapies are "intended to affect energy fields that purportedly surround and penetrate the body". These therapies manipulate biofields by applying pressure or manipulating the body by placing the hands in or through these fields and include techniques such as acupuncture, Reiki, Chinese Qigong, and therapeutic touch. Some of these techniques have been used for weight management and weight loss. Reiki is believed to heal by charging affected parts of an individual's energy field with positive energy while removing the negative energy. The existing evidence is insufficient to suggest Reiki as an effective treatment for any condition.[88] Studies have suggested that training in energy healing techniques could help individuals in managing stress, controlling food cravings and in maintaining healthy lifestyle habits, even after the conclusion of the initial weight loss intervention.[89] Various experimental and clinical studies have demonstrated the beneficial effects of acupuncture in lowering serum glucose levels[90,91] and aiding in weight loss.[92] Application of ear acupuncture increased the feeling of fullness, while diet or physical exercise did not have an effect.[93] Obese women with electroacupuncture application demonstrated greater weight loss compared to the diet group, and the weight loss was postulated to be the result of increased satiety, which resulted in decreased food intake following acupuncture.[92] Although a pilot study on Tapas acupuncture technique (TAT) suggested more research is necessary on its weight loss maintenance ability,[94] the primary analysis of a randomized clinical trial testing the efficacy of TAT for weight loss maintenance showed no beneficial effects.[95] More research is necessary to elucidate the effectiveness and appropriate role for TAT interventions in long-term weight management. Qigong exercises consist of two aspects: a controlled synchronized breathing with slow body movements like aerobic exercise and relaxation. A small study observed that Qigong walking reduced plasma glucose levels in diabetic patients without a significant increase in pulse rate.[96] Qigong exercises were suggested to be a beneficial adjunctive treatment for T2DM patients with some benefits, such as improvement in glucose metabolism and insulin resistance.[97] The studies assessing the effectiveness of such interventions need to adhere to strict methodological guidelines of reproducibility, standardization of techniques, and practitioner training, length, and frequency of training.

Whole Medical Systems

These medical systems involve complete systems of theory and practice that have evolved independently or from parallel to conventional Western medicine. These include Ayurveda (traditional medicine form India), homeopathy, naturopathy, and traditional Chinese medicine (TCM).

Ayurveda which means "science of life" is derived from the *Sanskrit* words "Ayur" meaning *life* and "Veda" meaning *knowledge*. Ayurvedic treatment focuses on maintaining the three bodily humors (*doshas*) in a state of equilibrium, with the use of diet, meditation, herbs, and lifestyle management. Some of the herbs used to treat diabetes include *shilajit*, turmeric, *neem*, *Coccinia indica*, *amalaki*, *triphala*, bitter gourd, rose apple, leaves of *bilva* (stone apple), cinnamon, *gymnema*, fenugreek, bay leaf, and aloe vera.[98,99] Few probable mechanisms of actions suggested are delayed gastric emptying and carbohydrate absorption, inhibition of glucose transport, increased glycogen synthesis, and peripheral glucose utilization.[98]

Ayurvedic treatments/medicines (using several herbal medicinal plants) have shown improvement in the levels of HbA1c, fasting glucose, postprandial blood glucose, total cholesterol, and low-density lipoprotein (LDL).[43,44,100-104] Beneficial effect of promoting weight loss, decrease in BMI, hip and waist circumference, serum cholesterol, and triglyceride levels[105-109] have also been observed with ayurvedic treatment. Although some studies with ayurvedic herbal mixtures have shown significant improvement in diabetes control and body weight, the existing evidence is insufficient to recommend the use of these interventions. Further research is warranted in this area.

Homeopathy is a system of alternative medicine created by the German physician Christian Friedrich Samuel Hahnemann. Homeopathy uses minute doses of a substance that causes symptoms to stimulate body's self-healing response and selects substances by matching a patient's symptoms with symptoms produced by these substances in healthy individuals. Homeopathic and conventional therapies in patients with diabetic polyneuropathy showed improvement in diabetic neuropathy symptom, quality of life, slight decrease in the fasting blood glucose, and HbA1c.[110]

Naturopathy, which was originated from Europe, works on the principle of the body's ability to heal itself naturally. It uses a combination of practices like dietary and lifestyle changes, homeopathy, herbal medicines, hydrotherapy, spinal and soft-tissue manipulation, physical therapies using electric currents, mud therapy, and light therapy. Naturopathic care in T2DM patients has shown improvement in glycemic control, self-management of glucose levels, mood, and self-efficacy.[111,112] Naturopathy as an adjunct to conventional primary care was observed to have benefits beyond primary care alone.[113] However, the evidence is limited and requires future research to confirm these benefits.

Traditional Chinese medicine is a system of healing that originated thousands of years ago and has now evolved into a well-developed, coherent system of medicine that uses several methods in the treatment and prevention of illness. The most commonly used therapeutic methods in TCM include acupuncture, moxibustion, Chinese herbal medicine, *Tui Na* (Chinese therapeutic massage), dietary therapy, mind-body exercises such as Qigong and tai chi.[114] Acupuncture and moxibustion (burning an herb above the skin to apply heat to acupuncture points) traditionally have been used in the management of diabetes to reduce blood glucose levels and normalize the endocrine function. The role of acupuncture in T2DM and weight loss has been described earlier in the chapter. *Tui Na* is a traditional form of Chinese massage that is used to stimulate acupuncture points and other parts of the body to create balance and harmony in the system by using techniques, such as pulling, kneading, pushing, and grasping, but there is no evidence for its role in obesity or T2DM. Herbal medicine is an integral part of TCM, and the prescriptions are formulated or prescribed based on the patient's predominant symptoms. Some of the herbal substances used for the management of diabetes are *Momordica charantia abreviata* (balsam pear), *Lagenaria siceraria* (bottle gourd), and *Psidium guajava* (guava).

These herbal substances do not appear to increase insulin levels, but rather enhance carbohydrate utilization.[115]

A systemic review on the use of Chinese medicine in overweight and obese patients showed reduction in body weight and BMI.[116] TCM does not offer a cure for diabetes, but instead aims at optimizing the normal functioning of the body. There is still a great need for more controlled studies research on the efficacy and safety of these therapies.

Reasons for using Complementary Alternative Medicine

Patients opt for CAM for various reasons. Certain patients with T2DM might feel that their needs are not being met by allopathic medicine and hence seek alternative treatments.[117] A person with poorer diabetes control has shown to be more likely to visit a CAM doctor, and there is a need to further evaluate the role of CAM in controlling symptoms and improving quality of life. Regardless of the reasons for the use of CAM, it is important to know which forms of CAM are safe and effective for the treatment of DM. Although CAM is more often used for improving general well-being than for diabetes-related symptoms and complications, the potential benefits of CAM in prevention and management of chronic diseases and in achieving integrative care for diabetics need to be studied further.

Conclusion

The increasing prevalence of obesity and T2DM and the simultaneous increase in interest of CAM gives adequate reason for the need to study the various CAM, use behaviors and the potential role of CAM in the treatment and management of obesity and diabetes. The treating physician should update his/her knowledge of the existing therapeutic options available to their patients (both allopathic and CAM) along with knowledge of the services being used by the individuals in order to provide evidence-based information on the safety and appropriateness of the CAM used.

The evidence supporting the effectiveness of CAM as a treatment option for obesity and diabetes is scarce. While reviewing and examining the efficacy of CAM, it is important to consider many factors. The lack of regulation of some of the common practices will increase heterogeneity, thus making treatment effect difficult to measure. Double blinding or concealing the allocation of treatment is difficult for therapies, such as acupuncture. Finally, it has been demonstrated that individuals who practice general positive health behaviors are more likely to use CAM than those who exhibit more risk factors, independent of their health status, health access, and sociodemographic factors.

References

1. World Health Organization (WHO). (2002). Traditional Medicine Strategy 2002-2005. [online] Available from: www.wpro.who.int/health_technology/book_who_traditional_medicine_strategy_2002_2005.pdf. [Accessed August, 2014].
2. Anderson RA, Cheng N, Bryden NA, Polansky MM, Cheng N, Chi J, et al. Elevated intakes of supplemental chromium improve glucose and insulin variables in individuals with type 2 diabetes. Diabetes. 1997;46(11):1786-91.
3. Bahijiri SM, Mira SA, Mufti AM, Ajabnoor MA. The effects of inorganic chromium and brewer's yeast supplementation on glucose tolerance, serum lipids and drug dosage in individuals with type 2 diabetes. Saudi Med J. 2000;21(9):831-7.
4. Cheng N, Zhu X, Shi H, Wu W, Chi J, Cheng J, et al. Follow-up survey of people in China with type 2 diabetes mellitus consuming supplemental chromium. J Trace Elem Exp Med. 1999;12:55-60.
5. Konrad T, Vicini P, Kusterer K, Höflich A, Assadkhani A, Böhles HJ, et al. alpha-Lipoic acid treatment decreases serum lactate and pyruvate concentrations and improves glucose effectiveness in lean and obese patients with type 2 diabetes. Diabetes Care. 1999;22(2):280-7.
6. Jacob S, Ruus P, Hermann R, Tritschler HJ, Maerker E, Renn W, et al. Oral administration of RAC-alpha-lipoic acid modulates insulin sensitivity in patients with type-2 diabetes mellitus: a placebo-controlled pilot trial. Free Radic Biol Med. 1999;27(3-4):309-14.
7. Cam MC, Brownsey RW, McNeill JH. Mechanisms of vanadium action: insulin-mimetic or insulin-enhancing agent? Can J Physiol Pharmacol. 2000;78(10):829-47.
8. Cohen N, Halberstam M, Shlimovich P, Chang CJ, Shamoon H, Rossetti L. Oral vanadyl sulfate improves hepatic and peripheral insulin sensitivity in patients with non-insulin dependent diabetes mellitus. J Clin Invest. 1995;95(6):2501-9.
9. Halberstam M, Cohen N, Shlimovich P, Rossetti L, Shamoon H. Oral vanadyl sulfate improves insulin sensitivity in NIDDM but not in obese nondiabetic subjects. Diabetes. 1996;45(5):659-66.
10. Boden G, Chen X, Ruiz J, van Rossum GD, Turco S. Effects of vanadyl sulfate on carbohydrate and lipid metabolism in patients with non-insulin-dependent diabetes mellitus. Metabolism. 1996;45(9):1130-5.
11. Goldfine A, Simonson D, Folli F, Patti ME, Kahn R. Metabolic effects of sodium metavanadate in humans with insulin-dependent and non-insulin dependent diabetes mellitus in vivo and in vitro studies. J Clin Endocrinol Metab. 1995;80(11):3311-20.
12. Lima DLM, Cruz T, Pousada JC, Rodrigues LE, Barbarosa K, Cangucu V. The effect of magnesium supplementation in increasing doses on the control of type 2 diabetes. Diabetes Care. 1998;21(5):682-6.
13. Paolisso G, Sgambato S, Pizza G, Passariello N, Varricchio M, D'Onofrio F: Improved insulin response and action by chronic magnesium administration in aged NIDDM subjects. Diabetes Care. 1989;12(4):265-9.
14. Paolisso G, Sgambato S, Gambardella A, Pizza G, Tesauro P, Varricchio M, et al. Daily magnesium supplements improve glucose handling in elderly subjects. Am J Clin Nutr. 1992;55(6):1161-7.
15. de Valk HW. Magnesium in diabetes mellitus. Neth J Med. 1999;54(4):139-46.
16. Paolisso G, Scheen A, Cozzolino D, Di Maro G, Varricchio M, D'Onofrio F, et al. Changes in glucose turnover parameters and improvement of glucose oxidation after 4-week magnesium administration in elderly noninsulin-dependent (type II) diabetic patients. J Clin Endocrinol Metab. 1994;78(6):1510-4.
17. Larsson SC, Wolk A. Magnesium intake and risk of type 2 diabetes: a meta-analysis. J Intern Med. 2007;262(2):208-14.
18. Schulze MB, Schulz M, Heidemann C, Schienkiewitz A, Hoffmann K, Boeing H. Fiber and magnesium intake and incidence of type 2 diabetes: a prospective study and meta-analysis. Arch Intern Med. 2007;167(9):956-65.
19. Pozzolli P, Vissali N, Cavallo MG, Signore A, Baroni MG, Buzzetti R, et al. Vitamin E and nicotinamide have similar effects in maintaining residual â cell function in recent onset insulin-dependent diabetes (The IMDIAB IV study). Eur J Endocrinol. 1997;137(3):234-9.

20. Jain SK, McVie R, Jaramillo JJ, Palmer M, Smith T. Effect of modest vitamin E supplementation on blood glycated hemoglobin and triglyceride levels and red cell indices in type 1 diabetic patients. J Am Coll Nutr. 1996;15(5): 458-61.
21. Paolisso G, D'Amore A, Giugliano D, Cereillo A, Varricchio M, D'Onofrio F. Pharmacological doses of vitamin E improve insulin action in healthy subjects and non-insulin dependent diabetic patients. Am J Clin Nutr. 1993;57(5):650-6.
22. Paolisso G, D'Amore A, Galzerano D, Balbi V, Giugliano D, Varriccho M, et al. Daily vitamin E supplements improve metabolic control but not insulin secretion in elderly type 2 diabetic patients. Diabetes Care. 1993;16(11):1433-7.
23. Cerillo A, Giugliano D, Quataro A, Donzella C, Dipalo G, Lefebrve PJ. Vitamin E reduction of protein glycosylation in diabetes. New prospect for prevention of diabetic complications? Diabetes Care. 1991;14(1):68-72.
24. Hodgson JM, Watts GF, Playford DA, Burke V, Croft KD. Coenzyme Q10 improves blood pressure and glycaemic control: a controlled trial in subjects with type 2 diabetes. Eur J Clin Nutr. 2002;56(11): 1137-42.
25. Kolahdouz Mohammadi R, Hosseinzadeh-Attar MJ, Eshraghian MR, Nakhjavani M, Khorami E, Esteghamati A. The effect of coenzyme Q10 supplementation on metabolic status of type 2 diabetic patients. Minerva Gastroenterol Dietol. 2013;59(2):231-6.
26. Mezawa M, Takemoto M, Onishi S, Ishibashi R, Ishikawa T, Yamaga M, et al. The reduced form of coenzyme Q10 improves glycemic control in patients with type 2 diabetes: an open label pilot study. Biofactors. 2012;38(6):416-21.
27. Dzugkoev SG, Kaloeva MB, Dzugkoeva FS. Effect of combination therapy with coenzyme Q10 on functional and metabolic parameters in patients with type 1 diabetes mellitus. Bull Exp Biol Med. 2012;152(3):364-6.
28. Ahmad N, Hassan MR, Halder H, Bennoor KS. Effect of Momordica charantia (Karolla) extracts on fasting and postprandial serum glucose levels in NIDDM patients. Bangladesh Med Res Counc Bull. 1999;25(1):11-3.
29. Tongia A, Tongia SK, Dave M. Phytochemical determination and extraction of Momordica charantia fruit and its hypoglycemic potentiation of oral hypoglycemic drugs in diabetes mellitus (NIDDM). Indian J Physiol Pharmacol. 2004;48(2):241-4.
30. Srivastava Y, Venkatakrishna-Bhatt H, Verma Y, Venkaiah K, Raval B. Antidiabetic and adaptogenic properties of Momordica charantia extract: an experimental and clinical evaluation. Phytother Res. 1993;7(4),285-9.
31. Welihinda J, Karunanayake EH, Sheriff MH, Jayasinghe KS. Effect of Momordica charantia on the glucose tolerance in maturity onset diabetes. J Ethnopharmacol. 1986;17(3):277-82.
32. Akhtar MS. Trial of Momordica charantia Linn (Karela) powder in patients with maturity-onset diabetes. J Pak Med Assoc. 1982;32(4):106-7.
33. Bever BO. Oral hypoglycemic plants in West Africa. J Ethnopharmacol. 1980;2(2):119-27.
34. Nadkarni KM. Indian Materia Medica, 3rd revised and enlarged edition. Mumbai, India: Popular Prakashan (P) Limited; 1976.
35. Raju J, Gupta D, Rao AR, Yadava PK, Baquer NZ. Trigonellafoenum graecum (fenugreek) seed powder improves glucose homeostasis in alloxan diabetic rat tissues by reversing the altered glycolytic, gluconeogenic and lipogenic enzymes. Mol Cell Biochem. 2001;224(1-2):45-51.
36. Gupta A, Gupta R, Lal B. Effect of Trigonella foenum graecum (fenugreek) seeds on glycemic control and insulin resistance in type 2 diabetes mellitus: A double blind controlled study. J Assoc Physicians India. 2001;49:1057-61.
37. Anderson JW, Chen WJ. Plant fiber. Carbohydrate and lipid metabolism. Am J Clin Nutr. 1979;32(2): 346-63.
38. Raghuram TC, Sivakumar RD, Shivkumar B, Sahay BK. Effect of *Trigonella foenum-graecum* (Fenugreek) seeds on intravenous glucose disposition in NIDDM patients. Phytother Res. 1994; 8:83-6.

39. Kedar P, Chakrabarti CH. Blood sugar, blood urea and serum lipid as influenced by Gurmar preparation. *Pterocarpus marsupium* and *Tamarindus indica* in diabetes mellitus. Maharashtra Med J. 1981;28:165.
40. Flexible dose open trial of Vijayasar in cases of newly-diagnosed non-insulin-dependent diabetes mellitus. Indian Council of Medical Research (ICMR), Collaborating Centres, New Delhi. Indian J Med Res. 1998;108:24-9.
41. Ahmad F, Khalid P, Khan M.M, Rastogi AK, Kidwai JR. Insulin like activity in (-) epicatechin. Acta Diabetol Lat. 1989;26(4):291-300.
42. Chakravarthy BK, Gupta S, Gambhir SS, Gode KD. Pancreatic beta-cell regeneration in rats by (-)-epicatechin. Lancet. 1981;2(8249):759-60.
43. Baskaran K, Kizar Ahamath B, Radha Shanmugasundaram K, Shanmugasundaram ER. Antidiabetic effect of a leaf extract from Gymnema sylvestra in non-insulin-dependent diabetes mellitus patients. J Ethnopharmacol. 1990;30(3):295-300.
44. Shanmugasundaram ER, Rajeswari G, Baskaran K, Rajesh Kumar BR, Radha Shanmugasundaram K, Kizar Ahmath B. Use of Gymnema sylvestre leaf extract in the control of blood glucose in insulin-dependent diabetes mellitus. J Ethnopharmacol. 1990;30(3):281-94.
45. Kuriyan R, Rajendran R, Bantwal G, Kurpad AV. Effect of supplementation of Coccinia cordifolia extract on newly detected diabetic patients. Diabetes Care. 2008;31(2):216-20.
46. Azad Khan AK, Akhtar S, Mahtab H. Coccinia indica in the treatment of patients with diabetes mellitus. Bangladesh Med Res Counc Bull. 1979;5(2):60-6.
47. Sheela CG, Augusti KT. Antidiabetic effects of S-allyl cysteine sulphoxide isolated from garlic Allium sativum Linn. Indian J Exp Biol. 1992;30(6):523-6.
48. Keisewetter H, Jung F, Pindur G, Jung EM, Mrowietz C, Wenzel E. Effect of garlic on thrombocyte aggregation, microcirculation, and other risk factors. Int J Clin Pharmacol Ther Toxicol. 1991;29(4):151-5.
49. Isaacsohn JL, Moser M, Stein EA, Dudley K, Davey JA, Liskov E, et al. Garlic powder and plasma lipids and lipoproteins: a multicenter, randomized, placebo-controlled trial. Arch Intern Med. 1998;158(11):1189-94.
50. Sotaniemi EA, Haapakoski E, Rautio A: Ginsing therapy in non-insulin dependent diabetic patients. Diabetes Care. 1995;18(10):1373-5.
51. Vuksan V, Sievenpiper JL, Xu Z, Wong EY, Jenkins AL, Beljan-Zdravkovic U, et al. Konjacmannan and American ginsing: emerging alternative therapies for type 2 diabetes mellitus. J Am Coll Nutr. 2001;20(5 Suppl):370S-380S.
52. Agrawal P, Rai V, Singh RB, Azad Khan AK, Akhtar S, Mahtab H. Randomized placebo-controlled single-blind trial of holy basil leaves in patients with noninsulin-dependent diabetes mellitus: *Coccinia indica* in the treatment of patients with diabetes mellitus. Int J Clin Pharmacol Ther. 1996;34:406-9.
53. Anderson RA. Effects of chromium on body composition and weight loss. Nutr Rev. 1998;56(9):266-70.
54. Blankson H, Stakkestad JA, Fagertun H, Thom E, Wadstein J, Gudmundsen O. Conjugated linoleic acid reduces body fat mass in overweight and obese humans. J Nutr. 2000;130(12):2943-8.
55. Gaullier JM, Halse J, Høye K, Kristiansen K, Fagertun H, Vik H, et al. Conjugated linoleic acid supplementation for 1 y reduces body fat mass in healthy overweight humans. Am J Clin Nutr. 2004;79(6):1118-25.
56. Gaullier JM, Halse J, Høye K, Kristiansen K, Fagertun H, Vik H, et al. Supplementation with conjugated linoleic acid for 24 months is well tolerated by and reduces body fat mass in healthy, overweight humans. J Nutr. 2005;135(4):778-84.
57. Smedman A, Vessby B. Conjugated linoleic acid supplementation in humans—metabolic effects. Lipids. 2001;36(8):773-81.
58. Kalman D, Colker CM, Wilets I, Roufs JB, Antonio J. The effects of pyruvate supplementation on body composition in overweight individuals. Nutrition. 1999;15(5):337-40.
59. Kalman D, Colker CM, Stark R, Minsch A, Wilets I, Antonio J. Effect of pyruvate supplementation on body composition and mood. *Current Therapeutic Research*. 1998;59(11):793-802.

60. Kaats GR, Michalek JE, Preuss HG. Evaluating efficacy of a chitosan product using a double-blinded, placebo-controlled protocol. J Am Coll Nutr. 2006;25(5):389-94.
61. Jull AB, Ni Mhurchu C, Bennett DA, Dunshea-Mooij CA, Rodgers A. Chitosan for overweight or obesity. Cochrane Database Syst Rev. 2008;(3):CD003892.
62. Ni Mhurchu C, Dunshea-Mooij CA, Bennett D, Rodgers A. Chitosan for overweight or obesity. Cochrane Database Syst Rev. 2005;(3):CD003892.
63. Sood N, Baker WL, Coleman CI. Effect of glucomannan on plasma lipid and glucose concentrations, body weight, and blood pressure: systematic review and meta-analysis. Am J Clin Nutr. 2008;88(4):1167-75.
64. Shixian Q, VanCrey B, Shi J, Kakuda Y, Jiang Y. Green tea extract thermogenesis-induced weight loss by epigallocatechin gallate inhibition of catechol-O-methyltransferase. J Med Food. 2006;9(4):451-8.
65. Westerterp-Plantenga M, Diepvens K, Joosen AM, Berube-Parent S, Tremblay A. Metabolic effects of spices, teas, and caffeine. Physiol Behav. 2006;89(1):85-91
66. Kuriyan R, Raj T, Srinivas SK, Vaz M, Rajendran R, Kurpad AV. Effect of Caralluma fimbriata extract on appetite, food intake and anthropometry in adult Indian men and women. Appetite. 2007;48(3):338-44.
67. Thomley BS, Ray SH, Cha SS, Bauer BA. Effects of a brief, comprehensive, yoga-based program on quality of life and biometric measures in an employee population: a pilot study. Explore (NY). 2011;7(1):27-9.
68. Benavides S, Caballero J. Ashtanga yoga for children and adolescents for weight management and psychological well being: an uncontrolled open pilot study. Complement Ther Clin Pract. 2009;15(2):110-4.
69. Satyanarayana M, Rajeswari KR, Rani NJ, Krishna CS, Rao PV. Effect of Santhi Kriya on certain psychophysiological parameters: a preliminary study. Indian J Physiol Pharmacol. 1992;36(2):88-92.
70. Telles S, Naveen VK, Balkrishna A, Kumar S. Short term health impact of a yoga and diet change program on obesity. Med Sci Monit. 2010;16(1):CR35-40.
71. Bera TK, Rajapurkar MV. Body composition, cardiovascular endurance and anaerobic power of yogic practitioner. Indian J Physiol Pharmacol. 1993;37(3):225-8.
72. Littman AJ, Bertram LC, Ceballos R, Ulrich CM, Ramaprasad J, McGregor B, et al. Randomized controlled pilot trial of yoga in overweight and obese breast cancer survivors: effects on quality of life and anthropometric measures. Support Care Cancer. 2012;20(2):267-77.
73. Raju PS, Prasad KV, Venkata RY, Murthy KJ, Reddy MV. Influence of intensive yoga training on physiological changes in 6 adult women: a case report. J Altern Complement Med. 1997;3(3):291-5.
74. Tran MD, Holly RG, Lashbrook J, Amsterdam EA. Effects of Hatha Yoga Practice on the Health-Related Aspects of Physical Fitness. Prev Cardiol. 2001;4(4):165-170.
75. McCaffrey R, Ruknui P, Hatthakit U, Kasetsomboon P. The effects of yoga on hypertensive persons in Thailand. Holist Nurs Pract. 2005;19(4):173-80.
76. Rioux JG, Ritenbaugh C. Narrative review of yoga intervention clinical trials including weight-related outcomes. Altern Ther Health Med. 2013;19(3):32-46.
77. Innes KE, Vincent HK. The influence of yoga-based programs on risk profiles in adults with type 2 diabetes mellitus: a systematic review. Evid Based Complement Alternat Med. 2007;4(4):469-86
78. Lee MS, Pittler MH, Kim MS, Ernst E. Tai chi for Type 2 diabetes: a systematic review. Diabet Med. 2008;25(2):240-1.
79. Song R, Ahn S, Roberts BL, Lee EO, Ahn YH. Adhering to a t'ai chi program to improve glucose control and quality of life for individuals with type 2 diabetes. J Altern Complement Med. 2009;15(6):627-32.
80. Aljasir B, Bryson M, Al-Shehri B. Yoga Practice for the Management of Type II Diabetes Mellitus in Adults: A systematic review. Evid Based Complement Alternat Med. 2010;7(4):399-408.
81. Zhang Y, Fu FH. Effects of 14-week Tai Ji Quan exercise on metabolic control in women with type 2 diabetes. Am J Chin Med. 2008;36(4):647-54.
82. Dechamps A, Gatta B, Bourdel-Marchasson I, Tabarin A, Roger P. Pilot study of a 10-week multidisciplinary Tai Chi intervention in sedentary obese women. Clin J Sport Med. 2009;19(1):49-53.

83. Beebe N, Magnanti S, Katkowski L, Benson M, Xu F, Delmonico MJ, et al. Effects of the addition of t'ai chi to a dietary weight loss program on lipoprotein atherogenicity in obese older women. J Altern Complement Med. 2013;19(9):759-66.
84. Kosuri M, Sridhar GR. Yoga practice in diabetes improves physical and psychological outcomes. Metab Syndr Relat Disord. 2009;7(6):515-7.
85. Astin JA, Shapiro SL, Eisenberg DM, Forys KL. Mind-body medicine: state of the science, implications for practice. J Am Board Fam Pract. 2003;16(2):131-47.
86. Licciardone JC. Rediscovering the classic osteopathic literature to advance contemporary patient-oriented research: A new look at diabetes mellitus. Osteopath Med Prim Care. 2008;2:9.
87. Heinking KP. Upper extremities. In: Chila AG (Ed). Foundations of Osteopathic Medicine, 3rd edition. Baltimore, MD: Lippincott Williams & Wilkins; 2010. p. 658.
88. Lee MS, Pittler MH, Ernst E. Effects of reiki in clinical practice: a systematic review of randomised clinical trials. Int J Clin Pract. 2008;62(6):947-54.
89. Pittler MH, Ernst E. Complementary therapies for reducing body weight: a systematic review. Int J Obes (Lond). 2005;29(9):1030-8.
90. Chen DC, Gong DQ, Zhai Y: Clinical and experimental studies in treating diabetes mellitus by acupuncture. J Tradit Chin Med. 1994;14(3):163-6.
91. Mao-liang Q. The treatment of diabetes by acupuncture. J Chinese Med. 1984;15:3-5.
92. Carbioglu MT, Ergene N, Tan U. The treatment of obesity by acupuncture. Int J Neurosci. 2006;116(2):165-75.
93. Asamoto S, Takeshige C. Activation of the satiety center by auricular acupuncture point stimulation. Brain Res Bull. 1992;29(2):157-64.
94. Elder C, Ritenbaugh C, Mist S, Aickin M, Schneider J, Zwickey H, et al. Randomized trial of two mind-body interventions for weight-loss maintenance. J Altern Complement Med. 2007;13(1):67-78.
95. Elder CR, Gullion CM, Debar LL, Funk KL, Lindberg NM, Ritenbaugh C, et al. Randomized trial of Tapas Acupressure Technique for weight loss maintenance. BMC Complement Altern Med. 2012;12:19.
96. Iwao M, Kajiyama S, Mori H, Oogaki K. Effects of qigong walking on diabetic patients: a pilot study. J Altern Complement Med. 1999;5(4):353-8.
97. Tsujiuchi T, Kumano H, Yoshiuchi K, He D, Tsujiuchi Y, Kuboki T, et al. The effect of Qi-gong relaxation exercise on the control of type 2 diabetes mellitus: a randomized controlled trial. Diabetes Care. 2002;25(1):241-2.
98. McWhorter LS. Biological Complementary Therapies: A Focus on Botanical Products in Diabetes. Diabetes Spectrum. 2001;14:199-208.
99. Saxena A, Vikram NK. Role of selected Indian plants in management of type 2 diabetes: a review. J Altern Complement Med. 2004;10(2):369-78.
100. Sharma RD, Raghuram TC, Rao NS. Effect of fenugreek seeds on blood glucose and serum lipids in type 1 diabetes. Eur J Clin Nutr. 1990;44(4):301-6.
101. Sharma RD, Sarkar A, Hazra DK, Miehra B, Singh JB, Sharma SK, et al. Use of fenugreek seed powder in the management of non-insulin-dependent diabetes mellitus. Nutr Res. 1996;16:1331-9.6
102. Khanna P, Jain SC, Panagariya A, Dixit VP. Hypoglycemic activity of polypeptide-p from a plant source. J Nat Prod. 1981;44(6):648-55.
103. Dhanabal SP, Kokate CK, Ramanathan M, Kumar EP, Suresh B, et al. Hypoglycaemic activity of Pterocarpus marsupium Roxb. Phytother Res. 2006;20(1):4-8.
104. Mohan V. Evaluation of Diabecon (D-400) as an antidiabetic agent—A double-blind placebo-controlled trial in NIDDM patients with secondary failure to oral drugs. Indian Journal of Clinical Practice. 1998;8(9):18.
105. Sharma S, Puri S, Agarwal T, Sharma V. Diets based on Ayurvedic constitution—potential for weight management. Altern Ther Health Med. 2009;15(1):44-7.
106. Paranjpe P, Patki P, Patwardhan B. Ayurvedic treatment of obesity: a randomised double-blind, placebo-controlled clinical trial. J Ethnopharmacol. 1990;29(1):1-11.

107. Vasudeva N, Yadav N, Sharma SK. Natural products: a safest approach for obesity. Chin J Integr Med. 2012; 18(6):473-80.
108. Pattonder RK, Chandola HM, Vyas SN. Clinical efficacy of Shilajatu (Asphaltum) processed with Agnimantha (Clerodendrum phlomidis Linn.) in Sthaulya (obesity). Ayu. 2011;32(4):526-31.
109. Goyal R, Kaur M, Chandola HM. A clinical study on the role of Agnimanthadi compound in the management of Sthaulya (obesity). Ayu. 2011;32(2):241-9.
110. Pomposelli R, Piasere V, Andreoni C, Costini G, Tonini E, Spalluzzi A, et al. Observational study of homeopathic and conventional therapies in patients with diabetic polyneuropathy. Homeopathy. 2009;98(1):17-25.
111. Oberg EB, Bradley RD, Allen J, McCrory MA. CAM: naturopathic nutrition program for type 2 diabetes. Complement Ther Clin Pract. 2011;17(3):157-61.
112. Bradley R, Sherman KJ, Catz S, Calabrese C, Oberg EB, Jordan L, et al. Adjunctive naturopathic care for type 2 diabetes: patient-reported and clinical outcomes after one year. BMC Complement Altern Med. 2012;12:44.
113. Oberg EB, Bradley R, Hsu C, Sherman KJ, Catz S, Calabrese C, et al. Patient-reported experiences with first-time naturopathic care for type 2 diabetes. PLoS One. 2012;7(11):e48549.
114. Lao L. Traditional Chinese Medicine. In: Jonas WB, Levin JS (Eds). Essentials of Complementary and Alternative Medicine. Baltimore, MD, USA: Lippincott Williams & Wilkins; 1999. pp. 216-32.
115. Keji C. Understanding and treatment of diabetes mellitus by traditional Chinese medicine. Am J Chin Med. 1981;9(1):93-4.
116. Sui Y, Zhao HL, Wong VC, Brown N, Li XL, Kwan AK, et al. A systematic review on use of Chinese medicine and acupuncture for treatment of obesity. Obes Rev. 2012;13(5):409-30.
117 Ernst E, Pittler MH, Wider B, Boddy K. The Desktop Guide to Complementary and Alternative Medicine, 2nd edition. Edinburgh, United Kingdom: Elsevier Mosby; 2006.

APPENDIX 1

Nutritive Value of Common Indian Cooked Foods

A. Nutritive Value (Macronutrients and Fats for 100 g of the Food Items)

S No	Food items	Macronutrients					Fats			
		Energy (kcals)	Protein (g)	Fat (g)	CHO (g)	Dietary fiber (g)	SFA (g)	PUFA (g)	MUFA (g)	Cholesterol (mg)
Cereals										
1	Idli	113.4	4.3	0.3	23.4	0.2	0.1	0.1	0	0
2	Vegetable upma	152.4	4.5	2.6	27.7	1.6	0.3	0.6	1.7	0
3	Upma	157.1	4	3.9	26.4	0.2	0.6	1.3	1.7	0
4	Vermicelli upma	137.9	3.6	2.3	25.7	4.1	0.2	0.6	1.5	0
5	Poha (flattened rice)	174.8	3.3	2.2	35.4	0.2	0.1	0.4	1.1	0
6	Idiyappam (Nooputt or string hoppers)	214.3	4.2	0.3	48.6	2.7	0.1	0.1	0.1	0
7	Poori	434.8	8	24.3	46	1.3	4.1	7.9	10.9	0
8	Dalia (broken/cracked wheat) with milk	193.6	6.9	2.8	35.2	0.8	1.4	0.5	0	8.3
9	Puttu (rice pudding)	269	5.1	6.7	47	4.3	5.8	0.7	0.2	0
10	Adai (multigrain)	249.9	6.7	11.1	30.8	3	1	2.8	7.1	0
11	Wheat dosa	163.3	5.3	3	28.8	3.1	0.4	0.7	1.8	0
12	Onion dosa	167	5.1	1.1	34.2	2.5	0.2	0.3	0.6	0
13	Onion wheat dosa	163.3	5.3	3	28.8	3.1	0.4	0.7	1.8	0
14	Plain dosa	209.5	5.3	5.4	34.8	0.2	1	1.7	2.4	0

Continued

Continued

S No	Food items	Macronutrients					Fats			
		Energy (kcals)	Protein (g)	Fat (g)	CHO (g)	Dietary fiber (g)	SFA (g)	PUFA (g)	MUFA (g)	Cholesterol (mg)
15	Masala dosa	200.5	4.7	6.5	30.8	0.8	1.1	2.1	2.9	0
16	Pesarattu (green gram dosa)	186.7	10	5.1	25.2	0.6	0.9	1.6	2.2	0
17	Avalakki (beaten rice)	197.6	3.8	3.1	38.6	0.4	0.6	1	1.3	0
18	Ragi chapatti	255.8	4.9	5.3	47.3	2.4	0.9	1.7	2.4	0
19	Channa (gram) chapatti	236	10.9	2.4	42.7	5.8	0.3	0.7	1.4	0
20	Jowar (sorghum chapatti)	232.7	6.9	1.3	48.4	6.4	0.4	0.4	0.7	0
21	Bajra (millet chapatti)	257.5	8.3	3.6	48.1	2.9	1.1	1.8	0.8	0
22	Rice chapatti (roti)	263.9	4.6	4.5	51.1	0.4	0.8	1.4	2	0
23	Tandoori chapatti	198.8	7.1	1	40.5	4.1	0.3	0.5	0.5	0
24	Phulka (chapatti)	198.8	7.1	1	40.5	1.1	0.2	0.4	0.1	0
25	Stuffed paratha	240.6	6.9	3.5	45.5	1.2	0.6	1.2	1.3	0
26	Mix-vegetable methi (fenugreek) paratha	230.2	7.3	5.1	38.8	4.2	1	1.6	2.5	0.3
27	Methi (fenugreek) chapatti	210.3	6.5	4.5	36.1	3.9	0.6	1.1	2.9	0
28	Tomato chapatti	263.1	8.6	4.2	47.8	5.2	0.6	1.1	2.4	0
29	Plain chapatti	297.2	8.3	8.1	47.9	4.8	1	2.1	5.2	0
30	Puliyogare (tamarind rice)	265.9	5.8	12.9	31.7	2.2	2.3	2.2	5.3	0
31	Peas pulao	183	4.8	3.1	33.9	2.2	0.4	0.8	1.8	0
32	Mushroom cauliflower pulao	119	2.8	2.2	21.9	1.6	0.3	0.6	1.3	0
33	Pongal (rice dish)	169.7	5.2	6.7	22.1	0.4	2.6	1.2	2.5	8.3
34	Curd rice	138.1	3.8	6.4	16.2	1.1	2	1.7	2.8	6.6
35	Chinese veg fried rice	152.2	2.6	3.6	27.3	0.5	0.8	1.3	1.4	0
36	Tomato rice	127.9	2.6	2.6	23.4	1.7	0.3	0.7	1.6	0
37	Masala bhath	169.2	4.56	2.97	32.6	0.9	0.5	0.8	0.9	0
38	Sprouted green gram garlic rice	86.4	1.8	1.4	16.5	1.2	0.2	0.4	0.9	0
39	Lemon rice	176	3.6	4.3	30.6	0.5	1.7	0.9	1.3	0

Continued

Nutritive Value of Common Indian Cooked Foods

Continued

S No	Food items	Macronutrients					Fats			
		Energy (kcals)	Protein (g)	Fat (g)	CHO (g)	Dietary fiber (g)	SFA (g)	PUFA (g)	MUFA (g)	Cholesterol (mg)
40	Methi (fenugreek) pulao	129.3	2.4	3.0	23	0.6	0.7	1.0	1.2	0
41	Vegetable biryani	149.4	2.8	4.3	24.8	1.8	0.5	1.1	2.7	0
42	Vegetable pulao	127.4	2.2	3	22.9	0.3	0.5	0.9	1.3	0
43	Plain rice	99.7	2.2	0.3	22.1	1.3	0.1	0.1	0.1	0
44	Coconut rice	191.2	3.5	9	24	2.6	4.8	2.6	1.6	0
45	Sweet pongal	258.1	4.5	9.7	38.1	1.3	5.8	3.1	0.8	20.6
46	Chicken biryani	182.3	10	7.0	19.8	0.4	3.3	1.2	2.1	25.2
47	Mutton biryani	165.8	6.2	7.0	19.4	0.5	3.4	0.9	2.2	16.6
48	Bisibele bhath (hot lentil sour rice)	197.6	4.9	9.7	22.4	3.3	7.3	0.6	1.8	7.9
49	Vegetable khichdi	122.1	5.1	2.1	20.8	1.1	0.4	0.7	0.8	0
50	Bread	245.0	7.8	0.7	51.9	7	0.2	0.2	0.3	0
51	Brown bread	244.0	8.8	1.4	49	12.4	0.4	0.4	0.6	0
52	Plain ragi ball	110.7	2.5	0.4	24.3	1.2	0.1	0.2	0.2	0
53	Ragi and rice ball	107.0	2.4	0.4	23.6	1.1	0.1	0.1	0.1	0
54	Ragi porridge	46.5	1	0.2	10.2	0.5	0	0.1	0.1	0
55	Vada	267.3	9.5	14.5	24.6	0.5	2.5	4.7	6.5	0
56	Corn flakes	357.0	7.5	0.4	84.1	3.3	0.1	0.2	0.1	0
57	Pizza/burger	271	11.9	10.8	31.2	1.8	5.0	1.8	2.9	24
58	Vegetable noodles	111.7	1.4	0.2	25.2	0.8	0.1	0.1	0.1	0
59	Macaroni and cheese	149	5.6	6.41	17.28	1.1	2.61	1.36	1.43	10
60	Bagel	275	10.5	1.6	53.4	2.3	0.22	0.7	0.13	0
61	French toast	229	7.7	10.8	25	-	2.72	2.59	4.52	116
62	Pancake	227	6.4	9.7	28.3	-	2.12	4.45	2.47	59
63	Waffle	291	7.9	14.1	32.9	-	2.87	6.79	3.52	69
64	Tortilla	237	7.28	0.95	49.94	2.4	0.3	0.39	0.19	-
65	Soba noodles, plain boiled (Japanese)	99	5.06	0.1	21.44	-	0.02	0.03	0.03	0
66	Somen, plain boiled (noodles, Japanese)	131	4	0.18	27.54	-	0.03	0.07	0.02	0
67	Noodles, chowmein	459	10.58	17.64	67.02	2.7	1.76	10.58	5.29	0

Continued

Continued

S No	Food items	Macronutrients					Fats			
		Energy (kcals)	Protein (g)	Fat (g)	CHO (g)	Dietary fiber (g)	SFA (g)	PUFA (g)	MUFA (g)	Cholesterol (mg)
68	Rice noodles, cooked	109	0.91	0.2	24.9	1	0.02	0.02	0.03	0
69	Tofu pad Thai	94.7	3.1	4.2	11.7	1.3	0.6	0.6	2.7	0
70	Vegetable soba noodles	138.2	4.1	9.2	11.5	2.4	1.2	1.5	5.4	0
71	Burrito (with beans and cheese)	205	7.35	6.05	31.23	4.2	2.31	2.23	1.26	5
72	Spaghetti and meatballs	97	4.46	4	10.89	-	1.44	0.49	1.61	7
73	Spaghetti in tomato and cheese sauce	80	2.7	0.6	15.8	1.2	0.2	-	-	2
74	Ravioli (cheese filled)	77	2.48	1.45	13.64	1.3	0.72	0.18	0.42	3
75	Lasagna, cheese	130	6.54	5.33	13.84	1.7	2.11	1.02	1.57	13
76	Black bean tortilla casserole	124.6	4.9	2.5	21.6	3.8	0.6	0.5	1.08	2.3
77	Pasta in tomato sauce (plain)	70	2.2	0.4	14.2	0.9	0.1	0.08	0.2	0.1
78	Vegetable congee	122.1	5.1	2.1	20.8	1.1	0.4	0.7	0.8	0
Dals/curries										
79	Plain sambhar	72.5	2.9	3	8.6	0.7	0.5	1	1.3	0
80	Tur dal sambhar with vegetables	72.7	3.1	2.6	9.3	0.7	0.4	0.8	1.1	0
81	Whole (gram) channa curry	87.2	2.9	3.1	11.8	1.3	1.6	0.6	0.6	0
82	Green leafy vegetable curry	67.3	3.6	3.1	6.2	1.2	0.5	1	1.4	0
83	Paneer gravy	125.9	5	8.5	7.6	0.7	4.4	0.9	2.7	11
84	Rasam (SI soup)	45.4	0.6	3	4	0.5	0.5	1	1.4	0
85	Kadhi (curd sambhar) (NI)	55.2	1.7	3.8	3.6	0.5	1	1	1.6	2.4
86	Mosaru huli (curd sambar) (SI)	88.2	2.7	6.6	4.7	0.4	3.5	0.9	1.8	7.3
87	Bengal gram curry	141.9	6.6	4.1	19.7	0.7	0.6	1.5	1.5	0
88	Black gram dal curry	135.6	7.7	2.9	19.8	0.7	0.5	1	1.2	0

Continued

Continued

S No	Food items	Macronutrients					Fats			
		Energy (kcals)	Protein (g)	Fat (g)	CHO (g)	Dietary fiber (g)	SFA (g)	PUFA (g)	MUFA (g)	Cholesterol (mg)
Vegetable dishes										
89	Baked vegetable	122.1	5.5	5.1	14.2	3.6	0.4	1	2.6	0
90	Aloo gobi sabzi (cauliflower potato vegetables)	99	3.2	2.6	15.7	2.5	0.3	0.6	1.7	0
91	Vegetable saagu	78.9	2.8	3.4	9.3	1.6	1.4	0.6	1.4	0
92	Methi paneer (Fenugreek)	140.6	7.5	9.1	7.2	2.6	4.5	2.4	2.2	16.1
93	Dahi bhindi (Curd lady finger)	137.2	6.1	6.1	14.7	5.7	0.7	1.4	3.8	0
94	Palak (Corn spinach)	82.1	2.8	2.8	11.8	3.2	0.4	0.6	1.7	0
95	Paneer matar (peas) masala	261.8	17.1	13.4	18	2.0	3.4	4.9	3.4	19.6
96	Mushroom with baby corn	194.1	5.7	10	21	3.7	0.9	2.3	6	0
97	Green leafy vegetable (SI)	77.9	3.2	4.8	5.5	1	0.7	1.5	2	0
98	Green leafy vegetable (NI)	104.4	2.8	7.6	6.1	1.1	0.9	4.8	1.3	0
99	Potato (SI)	127.4	2.3	4	20.8	0.7	0.7	1.3	1.7	0
100	Potato (NI)	154.9	1.9	6.2	23	0.6	0.7	4	1.2	0
101	Carrot (SI)	147.5	1.4	10.2	12.4	1.3	1.7	3.2	4.7	0
102	Carrot (NI)	123.8	1.3	6.8	14.6	1.7	0.7	4.3	1.3	0
103	Radish (SI)	62.6	1.9	2.3	8.6	1.4	0.3	0.7	1.1	0
104	Radish (NI)	101.8	1.2	8.5	5.2	1.1	0.9	5.5	1.6	0
105	Cabbage (SI)	107.8	3	6.6	9	1.4	1.1	2.1	2.9	0
106	Cabbage (NI)	81	1.8	5.4	6.2	1.2	0.6	3.5	1	0
107	Beans (SI)	89.5	2.1	6.3	6.2	1.8	1.1	2	2.8	0
108	Beans (NI)	106.2	1.8	7.4	8.1	1.6	0.8	4.8	1.4	0
109	Lady's finger (sabji) (SI)	108.9	2.1	8.2	6.6	1.7	1.4	2.6	3.7	0
110	Lady's finger (sabji) (NI)	148.1	2.5	11.6	8.4	1.6	1.3	7.4	2.2	0
111	Cauliflower (SI)	75.2	2.7	1.7	12.3	1.3	0.3	0.6	0.6	0
112	Cauliflower (NI)	82.7	2.7	5	6.8	1.4	0.5	3.2	1	0
113	Brinjal (SI)	141.6	2.9	10.3	9.4	2.3	1.8	3.4	4.5	0

Continued

Continued

S No	Food items	Macronutrients					Fats			
		Energy (kcals)	Protein (g)	Fat (g)	CHO (g)	Dietary fiber (g)	SFA (g)	PUFA (g)	MUFA (g)	Cholesterol (mg)
114	Brinjal (NI)	105.1	1.6	7.3	8.3	1.1	0.8	4.7	1.4	0
115	Mushroom (SI)	86.5	2.6	4.5	8.2	1.3	0.8	1.5	1.8	0
116	Mushroom (NI)	109.9	2.7	8.3	5	0.9	0.9	5.2	1.5	0
117	Fresh peas (SI)	108.0	6.8	10.3	22.0	4.2	1.8	3.3	4.7	0
118	Fresh peas (NI)	189.6	8.5	7.5	22.2	4.8	0.8	4.8	1.4	0
119	Pumpkin (SI)	93	1.9	2.5	15.6	1.3	1	0.6	0.8	0
120	Pumpkin (NI)	101.4	2.2	6.8	7.7	1.3	0.8	4.3	1.4	0
121	Pointed gourd (parwal) (SI)	171.4	4.5	11.6	12.4	2	3.4	3.3	4.1	0
122	Stuffed pointed gourd (parwal) (NI)	178.5	2.5	14.7	9	4.2	1.5	8.9	3.5	0
123	Capsicum (SI)	92.2	2.4	4.9	9.8	1.8	0.8	1.6	2.2	0
124	Capsicum (NI)	97.2	1.3	7	7.5	0.9	0.7	4.5	1.3	0
125	Drumstick (SI)	135	2.5	9.5	9.9	3.3	1.6	3.1	4.3	0
126	Drumstick (NI)	109.2	2.1	8.3	6.5	3.5	0.9	5.4	1.6	0
127	Colocasia (SI)	94.7	2.3	3.5	13.4	1.5	1.8	0.6	0.8	0
128	Colocasia (NI)	124.7	2.4	5.6	16.1	1.3	0.6	3.6	1.2	0
129	Yam palya (SI)	91	1.5	2.3	16.2	1.4	1.1	0.4	0.6	0
130	Yam palya (NI)	193	2.1	9.3	25.2	2.1	1	5.7	2	0
131	Bottle gourd	75.4	0.7	5.6	5.5	1.3	0.7	3.5	1.2	0
132	Ridge gourd	95.8	0.7	8.6	3.9	1	1.4	2.7	3.9	0
133	Jackfruit tender	92.9	1.5	5.2	10.3	1.4	0.9	1.7	2.3	0
134	Chow chow marrow	54	0.8	2.9	6.2	0.6	0.5	0.9	1.3	0
135	Raw banana palya	83.8	1.7	4.2	9.8	1.7	1.7	1	1.2	0
136	Bittergourd	129.8	3.6	4.4	18.8	3	0.5	0.9	1.3	0
137	Lotus stem	186.7	2.7	7.3	27.7	12.3	1.4	2	2.9	0
138	Tinda	166.1	2.4	14.5	6.6	2.8	2.4	4.6	6.5	0
139	Aviyal (SI)	127.1	2.6	8.2	12.6	1.7	6.8	0.2	0.6	2.5
140	Asparagus, boiled	22	2.4	0.22	4.11	2	0.05	0.11	0	0
141	Broccoli, boiled	35	2.38	0.41	7.18	3.3	0.08	0.17	0.04	0
142	Brussels sprouts, boiled	36	2.55	0.5	7.1	2.6	0.1	0.26	0.04	0
143	Celery, boiled	18	0.83	0.16	4	1.6	0.04	0.08	0.03	0
144	Sweet corn, boiled	96	3.41	1.5	20.98	2.4	0.2	0.6	0.37	0

Continued

Continued

S No	Food items	Macronutrients					Fats			
		Energy (kcals)	Protein (g)	Fat (g)	CHO (g)	Dietary fiber (g)	SFA (g)	PUFA (g)	MUFA (g)	Cholesterol (mg)
145	Mushroom, stir fried	26	3.58	0.33	4.04	1.8	0.04	0.16	0	0
146	Mashed potatoes	83	1.91	0.57	17.57	1.5	0.3	0.07	0.12	2
147	Hash brown potato	327	2.61	21.65	32.2	2.7	4.95	3.8	11.55	0
148	Chinese cabbage (bok choy, boiled)	12	1.56	0.16	1.78	1	0.02	0.08	0.01	0
149	Bamboo shoot, boiled	11	1.53	0.22	1.52	1	0.05	0.1	0.01	0
150	Wax gourd (tung qwa), cooked	14	0.4	0.2	3.04	1	0.02	0.09	0.04	0
Fruits										
151	Amla (gooseberry)	58	0.5	0.1	13.7	3.4	0	0	0	0
152	Apple	59	0.2	0.5	13.4	1	0.1	0.1	0	0
153	Banana	116	1.2	0.3	27.2	0.4	0.1	0.1	0	0
154	Custard apple	104	1.6	0.4	23.5	3.1	0.2	0	0	0
155	Dates (dry)	317	2.5	0.4	75.8	3.9	0	0	0	0
156	Grapes	58	0.6	0.4	13.1	2.8	0.1	0.1	0	0
157	Guava, country	51	0.9	0.3	11.2	5.2	0.1	0.1	0	0
158	Jackfruit	88	1.9	0.1	19.8	1.1	0	0	0	0
159	Jamoon (Jambu)	62	0.7	0.3	14	0.9	0	0	0	0
160	Kiwi	61	1.1	0.5	14.7	3	0	0.3	0	0
161	Sweet lime (mosambi)	43	0.8	0.3	9.3	0.5	0	0.1	0	0
162	Litchis	61	1.1	0.2	13.6	0.5	0	0.1	0.1	0
163	Mango	74	0.6	0.4	16.9	0.7	0.1	0.1	0.1	0
164	Muskmelon	17	0.3	0.2	3.5	0.4	0.1	0.1	0	0
165	Orange	48	0.7	0.2	10.9	0.3	0	0	0	0
166	Palmyra (tar/thati pandu)	87	0.7	0.2	20.7	0.5	0.1	0.1	0.1	0
167	Papaya	32	0.6	0.1	7.2	0.8	0	0	0	0
168	Passion fruit	54	0.9	0.1	12.4	9.6	0	0	0	0
169	Peach	50	1.2	0.3	10.5	1.2	0	0.1	0.1	0
170	Pears	52	0.6	0.2	11.9	1	0	0	0	0
171	Pineapple	46	0.4	0.1	10.8	0.5	0	0	0	0
172	Plums	52	0.7	0.5	11.1	0.4	0	0.1	0.2	0

Continued

Continued

S No	Food items	Macronutrients					Fats			
		Energy (kcals)	Protein (g)	Fat (g)	CHO (g)	Dietary fiber (g)	SFA (g)	PUFA (g)	MUFA (g)	Cholesterol (mg)
173	Pomegranate	65	1.6	0.1	14.5	5.1	0	0	0	0
174	Sapota	98	0.7	1.1	21.4	2.6	0	0	0	0
175	Strawberry	44.0	0.7	0.2	9.8	1.1	0	0	0	0
176	Sugarcane	398	0.1	0	99.4	0	0	0	0	0
177	Watermelon	16	0.2	0.2	3.3	0.2	0	0.1	0	0
178	Ziziphus (elantha pazham)	74	0.8	0.3	17	0	0	0	0	0
179	Fruit custard with milk	155.2	2.8	3.2	29	1.1	1.8	0.2	0.9	9.4
180	Persimmons (kaki, raw)	70	0.58	0.19	18.59	3.6	0.02	0.043	0.037	0
181	Persimmons (kaki, dried)	274	1.38	0.59	73.43	14.5	-	-	-	0
Dry fruits and nuts										
182	Almond (badam)	655	20.8	58.9	10.5	1.7	4.5	14.2	37.4	0
183	Apricot	306	1.6	0.7	73.4	2.1	0	0	0	0
184	Cashew nut	596	21.2	46.9	22.3	1.3	9.3	7.9	27.6	0
185	Dates (dry)	317	2.5	0.4	75.8	3.9	0	0	0	0
186	Figs	37	1.3	0.2	7.6	2.2	0	0	0	0
187	Groundnut (peanut)	567	25.3	40.1	26.1	3.1	5.6	12.7	19.9	0
188	Pistachio nut	656	19	59.1	12.1	3.8	7.2	17.9	31	0
189	Raisins	308	1.8	0.3	74.6	1.1	0.1	0.1	0	0
190	Walnut	687	15.6	64.5	11	2.6	-	-	-	-
191	Ginkgo nuts (raw)	182	4.32	1.68	37.6	-	0.319	0.618	0.619	0
Nonvegetarian										
192	Methi (fenugreek) chicken	163.8	19	7	4.8	0.8	0.4	2.9	1.1	58.3
193	Chicken dry	212.6	20.9	11	6.1	0.1	0.2	5.3	2.0	65.6
194	Chicken gravy	137.6	13.4	6.9	4.4	0.4	0.5	3.3	1.3	41.3
195	Pepper chicken	113.7	12.6	4.8	4.1	1.3	0.3	2.1	0.7	37.4
196	Grilled chicken	165	31.0	3.5	0	0	1	0.8	1.2	85.0
197	Chicken kabab	130.9	24.5	3	1.8	0.4	1.6	0.3	0.8	70.9
198	Chicken curry	104	12.3	5.1	2.2	0.8	4.2	0.1	0.4	31.3
199	Chicken fry	209.1	28.6	6.7	8.9	0.6	1.2	2.1	2.9	74.1
200	Mutton curry	157.3	10.9	11.5	2.4	0.6	5.2	1.4	4.2	40.5

Continued

Continued

S No	Food items	Macronutrients					Fats			
		Energy (kcals)	Protein (g)	Fat (g)	CHO (g)	Dietary fiber (g)	SFA (g)	PUFA (g)	MUFA (g)	Cholesterol (mg)
201	Mutton fry	235.8	19.3	16.4	2.6	0.3	6.4	2	6.9	73.2
202	Fish curry	287.9	7.3	25.1	8.5	0.7	15	3.4	5.3	20.1
203	Fish fry	302.4	28.4	19.9	2.4	0.5	3.5	6.2	9	103.9
204	Liver fry	174.3	18.8	8.8	6.6	0.7	2.1	2.4	3.3	334.6
205	Prawn	233.5	24.1	12.2	6.9	0.6	2.1	4	5.2	186.3
206	Boiled egg	155	12.6	10.6	1.1	0	3.3	1.4	4.1	373
207	Scrambled eggs	149	9.99	10.98	1.61	0	3.33	2.43	4.44	277
208	Baked egg white with mushroom	19.2	3.8	0.1	0.7	0	0	0	0	0
209	Salami (fermented and air-dried meat)	262	15	20.7	2.8	0	9	1	9.4	65
210	Chicken pot pie	198	4.82	11.45	18.99	1	4.18	2.75	3.93	17
211	Lemon chicken	226	10.7	11.7	19.1	1.1	1.9	5.7	2.5	32
212	Steamed fish (halibut)	111	22.5	1.61	0	0	0.4	0.4	0.6	60
Snacks										
213	Masala murmure (puffed rice)	413.8	11.9	11.1	66.5	4.8	0.4	0.9	2.2	0
214	Sundal (white chickpeas)	215.9	8.3	7.5	28.8	6.7	3.7	1.2	2.5	0
215	Cutlet	177.9	7.4	4.4	28.1	7.8	0.4	1	2.6	0
216	Peanut masala	442.5	19.6	30.5	22.4	3.7	0	0	0	0
217	Paneer toast	380.2	14.3	12.8	52	13	4.7	3.3	4.6	14.8
218	Egg sandwich	190.3	9.1	6.4	24.1	3.3	2.3	1.7	2.4	7.3
219	Grilled chicken sandwich	272	15.1	10.9	27.7	3.8	4.2	2.6	2.4	50.5
220	Mixture	685.2	12.6	59.6	25.8	4.5	9.7	19.3	27.2	0
221	Potato chips	513.3	4.2	29.7	57.7	1.2	5	9.5	13.6	0
222	Banana chips	491.4	4.5	36.6	35.6	0	8.2	19.2	9.3	0
223	Potato bajji (pakora)	276.5	7.9	14.8	29	3.8	2.1	5	6.3	0
224	Bajji	290.4	3.2	20.1	24.1	2.6	4.4	10.5	5.3	0
225	Mysore bonda	457.1	15.3	26.9	38.3	5.7	9.3	11.8	5.8	0
226	Potato bonda	287.4	7.7	12.5	36	4.2	2.5	5.8	4.2	0
227	Pakoda	437.8	13.5	23.5	43.1	7.3	4.8	11.5	7.2	0
228	Maddur vada	485.8	7.4	31.6	42.9	4	14.1	12.4	5	40.9

Continued

Continued

S No	Food items	Macronutrients					Fats			
		Energy (kcals)	Protein (g)	Fat (g)	CHO (g)	Dietary fiber (g)	SFA (g)	PUFA (g)	MUFA (g)	Cholesterol (mg)
229	Urad vada (SI)	233.1	10.5	9.6	26.2	3.1	2.1	4.9	2.5	0
230	Kachori	355	10.3	15.5	43.5	3.4	3.4	8	4.1	0
231	Thair vada (curd vada)	148.5	5.9	8.8	11.5	1	3	3.9	1.8	7.2
232	Karasev	375.6	16.5	8.6	58.1	8.3	3.5	2.2	2.8	11.8
233	Murukku	467.9	9.4	17.9	67.2	4.3	4.7	9	4.3	3.9
234	Vegetable puff	423	6.2	27.4	38.4	1.8	25.2	0.2	0.1	25.7
235	Sweet cookies	500.7	5.6	25.5	62.2	1.5	17.6	6.9	1	0
236	Biscuits (salted)	448.3	13.2	4.4	89	0.4	2.4	0.6	0.9	9.3
237	Biscuits (sweet/creamed)	452.9	8	10.3	82.3	0.2	6.4	0.6	2.4	26.9
238	Bhelpuri	447.4	11.9	23.2	47.7	2.3	3.6	7.5	10.9	0
239	Dhokla	283.7	11.1	12.1	33.7	4.1	2.8	3.6	4.6	6.1
240	Pavbhaji	133.7	4.1	8.1	11.7	1.8	2.5	2	3.2	1.6
241	Healthy green kebab	167.6	4.3	3.2	30	3.9	0.3	0.7	2	0
242	Corn chat	38.7	1.4	0.4	7.8	4.6	0	0	0	0
243	Popcorn	500	9	28.1	57.2	10	4.89	13.4	8.17	0
244	Hot dog	247	10.6	14.84	18.4	-	5.21	1.74	6.99	45
245	Croissant (butter)	406	8.2	21	45.8	2.6	11.6	1.09	5.53	67
246	Croissant (cheese)	414	9.2	20.9	47	2.6	10.6	2.38	6.51	57
247	Doughnut (plain)	418	5.87	23.55	45.63	1.6	7.13	2.66	12.73	9
248	Egg roll	250	8.3	11.9	24.3	2.6	2.1	5.6	3.0	16
249	Cheese burger	263	12.97	11.79	27.81	1.1	4.44	0.36	3.63	35
250	Popcorn chicken	351	17.67	21.74	21.18	1	3.95	10.1	5.66	40
251	Fried chicken, drumstick	239	22.3	14.22	5.39	-	3.24	4.29	5.12	117
252	Nachos, with cheese	306	8.05	16.77	32.15	-	6.89	1.98	7.07	16
253	Taco (with beef and cheese)	226	8.86	12.7	19.85	3.9	4.38	3.04	4.41	28
254	Thai lettuce roll	61.7	2.9	2.6	8.5	1.6	0.38	0.4	1.6	0
255	Dim sum (steamed wanton)	255.5	6.5	3.8	48	2.3	0.5	0.59	2.3	0
256	Green gram sprouts, steamed	19	2.03	0.09	3.6	0.8	0.02	0.03	0.01	0

Continued

Continued

S No	Food items	Macronutrients					Fats			
		Energy (kcals)	Protein (g)	Fat (g)	CHO (g)	Dietary fiber (g)	SFA (g)	PUFA (g)	MUFA (g)	Cholesterol (mg)
257	Wo tou (steamed corn bun)	266	6.7	7.1	43.5	-	1.5	3.2	1.8	40
258	Garlic bread	350	8.36	16.61	41.72	2.5	5.2	5.4	4.6	0
259	Spinach corn and cheese sandwich	276	6.2	14.5	30.2	1.9	5.1	0.3	2.1	0.02
260	Mixed-vegetable sandwich	276	6.3	13.9	31.3	1.9	5.6	0.7	2.6	0.02
Sweets										
261	Cake/sweet pastry	469.4	7.1	27.1	50	0.1	15.6	1.5	8.1	179.6
262	Payasam, kheer	165	3.8	5.9	24.2	0.1	3.4	0.3	1.9	16
263	Bread pudding	171.2	4.7	5.2	26.4	0.1	2.4	0.5	2	10.8
264	Ice cream	201	3.1	11	23.6	0	6.8	0.4	3.2	44
265	Mysore pak	434.3	6.3	27.2	42	3	16.7	1.7	6.5	70.8
266	Peda	332.5	6.6	9.7	47.1	0.6	6.4	0.3	2.5	27.7
267	Badusha (Balushahi)	527.3	5.5	12.6	97.9	0.1	6	1.8	3.9	22.3
268	Kesari bhath	230.3	2.2	12	28.4	0.1	6.5	0.8	3.7	0
269	Kaju katli	439.5	9	29.3	34.9	0.6	10.1	3.7	14	26.2
270	Shrikhand	162.2	2.3	2.7	32.2	0.4	1.7	0.1	0.7	8.5
271	Chocolate	553	7.2	32.8	57.9	1.9	0	0	0	22
272	Besan ladoo	491.6	8.4	26.6	54.6	3.6	16.8	7.6	2.2	63.4
273	Boondi ladoo	387.6	4.4	10.8	68.2	1.7	2.3	5.6	2.9	0
274	Gajar (carrot) halwa	417.8	5.8	15.7	63.3	0.5	10.2	4.8	0.8	45.2
275	Coconut burfi	425.2	5.6	22.5	50	4.3	18.7	3.2	0.6	16.8
276	Jalebi	452.2	3.5	14.8	76.1	0.9	3.3	7.8	3.8	0.3
277	Kalakand	504.4	11.2	26.5	55.2	0	17.7	7.7	1.1	82.2
278	Rasgulla	249.1	14.3	15.7	12.8	0.1	10.9	4.2	0.5	42
279	Narayal doodh mithai (coconut milk sweet)	601.4	5.3	38.1	59.3	9.7	32.9	4.2	0.9	16.2
280	Caramel custard (flan)	145	4.53	4.03	22.78	0	1.8	0.39	1.27	90
281	Egg custard, baked	104	5.02	4.58	11	0	2.16	0.41	1.38	84
282	Chocolate mousse	225	4.14	16	16.07	0.6	9.15	0.88	5.03	140
283	Apple pie	265	2.4	12.5	37.1	1.6	3.05	3.34	5.39	0
284	Brownie	405	4.57	16.84	64.95	2.8	5.22	4.4	6.38	16

Continued

Continued

S No	Food items	Macronutrients					Fats			
		Energy (kcals)	Protein (g)	Fat (g)	CHO (g)	Dietary fiber (g)	SFA (g)	PUFA (g)	MUFA (g)	Cholesterol (mg)
Chutney and raita										
285	Green tomato chutney	67.3	2.9	2.5	8.2	1.4	0.2	0.6	1.5	0
286	Red capsicum chutney	87.9	3.6	3.1	11.5	2.6	0.3	0.7	2	0
287	Cabbage chutney	199.1	6.9	13	13.6	2.7	0.8	2.1	5.6	0
288	Green peas chutney	49.4	3.6	0.1	8.5	0.9	0	0	0.1	0
289	Ridge gourd chutney	130.4	1.2	11.6	5.2	2.3	1.1	2.9	7.7	0
290	Gherkin chutney	95.5	2.3	7	5.8	0	0.7	1.7	4.4	0
291	Tomato chutney	128.1	3.4	6.8	13.4	2.6	0.7	1.6	4.5	0
292	Mint chutney	57.7	1.9	0.5	11.5	2	0	0.1	0.1	0
293	Coconut chutney	92.8	1	8.3	3.5	0.9	7.4	0.1	0.4	0
294	Groundnut chutney	301.5	13.2	18	23	4	4.3	5.1	7.5	0
295	Chili chutney	134.9	2.6	10	8.6	3.3	1.7	3.2	4.5	0
296	Tamarind chutney	293.4	2.7	13.9	39.4	2.3	6.2	2.5	4.4	0
297	Mango chutney	159.3	2	14	6.3	1.9	12.3	0.2	0.6	0
298	Brinjal chutney	175.6	2.5	14	9.8	2.5	2.3	4.5	6.4	0
299	Urad dal chutney	152.3	9.1	3	22.2	0.5	0.7	0.9	1.1	0.8
300	Chutney powder	481.8	23.1	25	41	3.2	3.5	8.5	11.6	0
301	Onion raita	111	2.5	8.6	6	0.6	2.3	2.2	4.1	7.5
302	Vegetable raita	38.1	1.6	1.4	4.8	1	0.9	0.4	0.1	3.8
Salad										
303	Salad with green gram	114.7	6.4	2.8	16	2.7	0.5	1.2	1	0
304	Salad with macaroni	127.9	2.4	5.4	17.4	3.7	4	0.8	0.6	0
305	Crunchy salad	100.6	2	0.4	22.8	1.4	0.1	0.1	0.1	0
306	Vegetable salad	37.9	0.9	0.2	7.9	0.9	0	0.1	0	0
307	Caesar salad	44	3.18	2.05	4.28	1.6	1.18	0.14	0.46	5
308	Moong dal and green mango salad	114	6.3	2.7	15.9	2.7	0.5	1	1.1	0
309	Sprouts salad	30	3	0.1	5.9	1.8	0.04	0.05	0.02	0

Continued

Continued

S No	Food items	Macronutrients					Fats			
		Energy (kcals)	Protein (g)	Fat (g)	CHO (g)	Dietary fiber (g)	SFA (g)	PUFA (g)	MUFA (g)	Cholesterol (mg)
310	Asparagus salad	22	2.4	0.22	4.1	2	0.05	0.1	0	0
311	Greek salad	20	1	2.1	4.3	1.6	0.02	0.1	0	0
312	Tossed salad	16	1.2	0.07	3.2	2	0.01	0.03	0	0
Soup										
313	Creamy broccoli soup	48.4	1.8	1.6	28.9	7.8	1	0.4	0.1	4.4
314	Carrot and coriander soup	95.8	1.7	2.8	16	2.9	1.8	0.7	0.3	6.5
315	Garlic-vegetable soup	77.5	3.1	3.4	8.6	1.1	1.7	0.9	0.8	9.1
316	Noodle soup, chicken	39	3.09	1.16	4	0.8	0.41	0.11	0.19	5
317	Wonton soup, Chinese	32	2.08	0.26	5.25	0.2	0.06	0.07	0.08	4
318	Drumstick soup	52.3	2.6	2.4	5.2	0.8	1.5	0.6	0.2	7.9
319	Button mushroom soup	103.8	4.8	2.8	178.9	28	1.8	0.7	0.1	8.9
320	Vegetable manchow soup	49.2	1	1.7	7.6	0.9	0.2	0.4	1	0
321	Spinach soup	89.2	3.2	5.2	7.4	0.5	3.6	1.4	0.2	18.1
322	Chicken herb soup	58.6	5.3	3.1	2.3	0.3	1.3	1.4	0.5	3.8
323	Tomato soup	35.6	0.9	1.8	4	0.7	1.2	0.5	0.1	4.4
324	Tomato soup with cream	55.5	1.6	2.2	7.5	1.5	1.4	0.5	0.2	5.1
325	Tomato mint soup	45.6	0.8	3.2	3.3	0.5	1	0.4	0.1	9.7
326	Vegetable soup	81.4	2.6	3.1	10.9	1.4	0.7	0.3	0.1	9.3
327	Miso soup	91	4.8	1.3	15.4	6.8	0.3	0.4	0.5	0
328	Tom yum soup	51	1.4	1.5	7.9	0.5	0.2	0.6	0.6	0
Beverages										
329	Tea with sugar	64.5	2	2.3	9	0	1.5	0.1	0.7	7.8
330	Coffee with sugar	81.6	3	3.8	8.9	0	2.4	0.1	1.1	12.6
331	Plain milk with sugar	83.6	3.2	4.1	8.5	0	2.6	0.2	1.2	13.6
332	Horlicks	93.1	3.7	4.2	10.5	0	2.5	0.1	1.2	13.2
333	Curd	66.7	3.2	4.1	4.4	0	2.5	0.2	1.2	13.5
334	Buttermilk	19.2	0.7	1.4	0.8	0.1	0.6	0.2	0.5	2.5

Continued

Continued

S No	Food items	Macronutrients					Fats			
		Energy (kcals)	Protein (g)	Fat (g)	CHO (g)	Dietary fiber (g)	SFA (g)	PUFA (g)	MUFA (g)	Cholesterol (mg)
335	Fresh fruit juice	113.4	1.4	0.5	25.9	0.9	0.1	0.2	0	0
336	Soft drinks	41	0	0	10.4	0	0	0	0	0
337	Beer	41	0.3	0	3.7	0.2	0	0	0	0
338	Wine	70	0.2	0	1.4	0	0	0	0	0
339	Spirits (whisky/gin/rum, etc.)	231	0	0	0	0	0	0	0	0
340	Local arrack/toddy	38	0.1	0.3	1.8	0	0	0	0	0
341	Raw green mango squash (aam ka panna)	14.3	0.3	0.1	3.1	0.4	0	0	0	0
Miscellaneous										
342	Butter/cream	729	0.9	81	0.1	0	50.4	3	23.4	218.9
343	Ghee	900	0	100	0	0	66	3.4	24.1	280
344	Jam	278	0.4	0.1	68.9	1.1	0	0	0	0
345	Sugar	398	0.1	0	99.4	0	0	0	0	0
346	Honey	319	0.3	0	79.5	0.2	0	0	0	0
347	Jaggery	383	0.4	0.1	95	0	0	0	0	0
348	Cheese	348	24.1	25.1	6.3	0	15.8	0.7	7.4	55.2
349	Ketchup, tomato sauce	30	1.3	0.2	7.2	1.4	0	0.1	0	0
350	Mango pickle	150.3	1.1	13	7.2	1.2	2.1	4.1	6.1	0
351	Papad (papadum)	676.3	30.8	27	77.8	2	4.8	8.7	11.9	0
352	Maple syrup	260	0.04	0.06	67.04	0	0.01	0.02	0.01	0

CHO, carbohydrates; SFA, saturated fatty acids; PUFA, polyunsaturated fatty acid; SI, South Indian; NI, North Indian.

B. Nutritive Value (Vitamins for 100 g of Food Items)

S No	Food items	β-carotene (µg)	Thiamin (mg)	Riboflavin (mg)	Niacin (mg)	Vitamin B6 (mg)	Folate (µg)	Vitamin C (mg)
Cereals								
1	Idli	4.6	0.1	0	0.6	0.1	17.7	0
2	Vegetable upma	300	0.1	0	0.7	0	6	9.9
3	Upma	50.7	0.1	0	0.6	0.1	28	2
4	Vermicelli upma	214.3	0.1	0	0.7	0	9.4	6.2
5	Poha (flattened rice)	158.9	0.1	0	1.8	0	1.2	5.5
6	Idiyappam (Nooputt or string hoppers)	0	0	0	1.2	0	0	0
7	Poori	19.2	0.3	0.1	2.9	0.2	23.7	0
8	Dalia (broken/cracked wheat)	28.4	0.4	0.2	2.5	0.3	16.3	1
9	Puttu (rice pudding)	1.2	0.1	0.1	2.4	0	1.8	0.1
10	Adai (multigrain)	30.6	0.2	0.1	1.5	0.1	29.3	0.2
11	Wheat dosa	366.9	0.2	0.1	1.8	0	15.1	10.9
12	Onion dosa	127.6	0.1	0.1	1.6	0	16.6	2.9
13	Onion wheat dosa	366.9	0.2	0.1	1.8	0	15.1	10.9
14	Plain dosa	4.6	0.1	0	0.9	0.1	18.5	0
15	Masala dosa	18.6	0.1	0	1	0.2	21.1	6.4
16	Pesarattu (green gram dosa)	175.3	0.2	0.1	1	0.2	57	6.7
17	Avalakki (beaten rice)	54.6	0.1	0	2	0	9.6	1.5
18	Ragi chapatti	120.6	0.3	0.1	0.8	0.3	13.1	5.4
19	Channa (gram) chapatti	52.1	0.3	0.1	2.2	0	60.4	0.3
20	Jowar (sorghum chapatti)	31.3	0.2	0.1	2.1	0.1	13.3	0
21	Bajra (millet chapatti)	94.2	0.2	0.2	1.6	0	32.5	0
22	Rice chapatti (roti)	194.6	0.1	0	1.3	0.1	7	7.7
23	Tandoori chapatti	16.9	0.3	0.1	2.5	0	20.9	0
24	Phulka (chapatti)	16.9	0.3	0.1	2.5	0.2	20.9	0
25	Stuffed paratha	37.7	0.3	0.1	2.7	0.3	21.6	7.8

Continued

Continued

S No	Food items	β-carotene (μg)	Thiamin (mg)	Riboflavin (mg)	Niacin (mg)	Vitamin B6 (mg)	Folate (μg)	Vitamin C (mg)
26	Mix-vegetable methi (fenugreek) paratha	400.6	0.3	0.1	2.4	0	23.8	13
27	Methi (fenugreek) chapatti	235.3	0.3	0.1	2.3	0	60.4	9.9
28	Tomato chapatti	225	0.4	0.1	3.1	0	40.8	16.8
29	Plain chapatti	20	0.3	0.1	3	0	24.7	0
30	Puliyogare (tamarind rice)	53.2	0.2	0.1	2.9	0	1.5	1.1
31	Peas pulao	174.8	0.1	0.1	1.7	0	1.7	5.6
32	Mushroom cauliflower pulao	93.3	0.1	0.1	1.8	0	0.5	10.4
33	Pongal (rice dish)	35.3	0.1	0	0.7	0.1	23.4	0.2
34	Curd rice	213.6	0.1	0.1	0.8	0	11.8	5.9
35	Chinese fried rice	158	0.1	0.1	1.4	0	6	11
36	Tomato rice	120.7	0.1	0.1	1.3	0	0.2	10
37	Masala bhath	218.6	0.1	0.1	1.7	0	0.6	11.8
38	Sprouted green gram garlic rice	70.7	0.1	0	0.9	0	2.7	10.5
39	Lemon rice	55.5	0.05	0	1.0	0.08	8.4	6.4
40	Methi (fenugreek) pulao	429	0.0	0.0	0.7	0.1	12.2	11.2
41	Vegetable biryani	173.1	0.1	0.1	1.3	0	7	6.1
42	Vegetable pulao	251.9	0	0	0.6	0.1	6.9	3.5
43	Plain rice	0.6	0.1	0	1.1	0	0	0
44	Coconut rice	500.7	0.1	0.1	1.3	0	4.6	6.9
45	Sweet pongal	182.4	0.1	0.1	0.8	0	14.1	0.1
46	Chicken biryani	40	0	0.1	3	0.2	6.2	3..2
47	Mutton biryani	61.9	0.1	0.1	2	0.1	7	3.5
48	Bisibele bhath (hot lentil sour rice)	28	0.1	0	0.5	0.1	11.5	0.7
49	Vegetable khichdi	93.5	0.1	0.1	0.9	0.2	34.4	13.5
50	Bread	0	0.1	0	0.7	0	0	0
51	Brown bread	0	0.2	0	2.5	0	0	0
52	Plain ragi ball	14.2	0.1	0.1	0.4	0.2	6.2	0
53	Ragi with rice ball	12.2	0.1	0.1	0.4	0.2	5.6	0
54	Ragi porridge	5.9	0.1	0	0.2	0.1	2.6	0

Continued

Nutritive Value of Common Indian Cooked Foods

Continued

S No	Food items	β-carotene (µg)	Thiamin (mg)	Riboflavin (mg)	Niacin (mg)	Vitamin B6 (mg)	Folate (µg)	Vitamin C (mg)
55	Vada	123.7	0.2	0.1	0.8	0.1	52.3	4.3
56	Corn flakes	83	1.3	1.5	18	1.8	357	21
57	Pizza	116	0.3	0.3	3.3	0.1	-	0
58	Vegetable noodles	170.7	0	0	0.2	0	11.2	16.2
59	Macaroni and cheese	20	0.05	0.06	0.74	0.04	7	0
60	Bagel	-	0.54	0.32	4.56	0.05	88	0
61	French toast	66	0.2	0.32	1.63	0.07	43	0.3
62	Pancake	-	0.2	0.28	1.57	0.05	38	0.3
63	Waffle	-	0.26	0.35	2.07	0.06	46	0.4
64	Tortilla	-	0.37	0.11	4.13	0.06	98	0
65	Soba noodles, plain boiled (Japanese)	-	0.09	0.03	0.51	0.04	7	0
66	Somen, plain boiled (noodles, Japanese)	-	0.02	0.03	0.1	0.01	2	0
67	Noodles, chowmein	0	0.58	0.42	5.95	0.11	109	0
68	Rice noodles, cooked	-	0.02	0	0.07	0.01	3	0
69	Tofu pad Thai	1,422.2	0.04	0.07	0.4	0.07	18.5	7.4
70	Vegetable soba noodles	97.6	0.08	0.11	1.4	0.1	65	8.8
71	Burrito (with beans and cheese)	24	0.19	0.1	2.02	0.1	104	0.4
72	Spaghetti and meatballs	147	0.1	0.09	2.23	0.07	-	2.2
73	Spaghetti in tomato and cheese sauce	-	0.06	0.06	1.2	-	32	0
74	Ravioli (cheese filled)	124	0.07	0.08	1.06	0.1	20	0
75	Lasagna, cheese	-	0.11	0.15	1.36	0.07	21	17.1
76	Black bean tortilla casserole	94.8	0.12	0.07	0.7	0.16	43.5	5.6
77	Pasta in tomato sauce (plain)	407	0.05	0.05	1.3	0.05	31	0
78	Vegetable congee	93.5	0.1	0.1	0.9	0.2	34	13.5

Continued

Continued

S No	Food items	β-carotene (μg)	Thiamin (mg)	Riboflavin (mg)	Niacin (mg)	Vitamin B6 (mg)	Folate (μg)	Vitamin C (mg)
Dals/curries								
79	Plain sambhar	102.5	0.1	0	0.5	0.1	18.6	7.1
80	Tur dal sambhar with vegetables	44.1	0.1	0	0.5	0.1	21.4	4.2
81	Whole (gram) channa curry	92.4	0.1	0	0.6	0.1	31.3	5.6
82	Green leafy vegetable curry	4,019.3	0	0.2	1.1	0.2	110.4	72
83	Paneer gravy	336.5	0.1	0.1	0.4	0.1	23	20.8
84	Rasam (SI soup)	173	0	0	0.2	0	2.6	4.7
85	Kadhi (curd sambhar) (NI)	12.2	0	0	0.1	0	22.2	0.3
86	Mosaru huli (curd sambar) (SI)	50.9	0.1	0.1	0.2	0	12.5	1.4
87	Bengal gram curry	82.6	0.2	0.1	0.8	0.2	49.3	4.4
88	Black gram dal curry	56.6	0.2	0.1	0.7	0.1	44.6	4.1
Vegetable dishes								
89	Baked vegetable	985.2	0.4	0.1	1.1	0	3,398	91.7
90	Aloo gobi sabzi (cauliflower potato vegetables)	235.3	0.1	0.1	1.2	0	130.2	39.5
91	Vegetable saagu	570.9	0.1	0.1	0.5	0	15.2	20
92	Methi paneer (Fenugreek)	675.6	0.5	0.1	0.4	0	20.9	122.3
93	Dahi bhindi (Curd lady finger)	150.7	0.1	0.3	1	0	115.6	15.3
94	Palak (Corn spinach)	2,450.6	0.1	0.2	0.7	0	70.5	33.8
95	Paneer matar (peas) masala	567.6	0.3	0.3	1	0.1	32.9	34.9
96	Mushroom with baby corn	24.7	0.2	0.5	4.6	0	1.7	9.2
97	Green leafy vegetable (SI)	7,073.1	0.1	0.3	0.8	0.3	157.4	37
98	Green leafy vegetable (NI)	6,618.9	0.1	0.3	0.7	0.3	150.9	40.5
99	Potato (SI)	203.1	0.1	0	1.1	0.2	17.8	23.1
100	Potato (NI)	137.4	0.1	0	1.2	0.3	8.1	19.9
101	Carrot (SI)	1,766	0.1	0	0.7	0.2	16.6	6.1

Continued

Continued

S No	Food items	β-carotene (μg)	Thiamin (mg)	Riboflavin (mg)	Niacin (mg)	Vitamin B6 (mg)	Folate (μg)	Vitamin C (mg)
102	Carrot (NI)	2,264.6	0.1	0	0.8	0.2	19	5.6
103	Radish (SI)	75.3	0.1	0	0.8	0.1	27.3	15.9
104	Radish (NI)	7.3	0.1	0	0.6	0.1	32.6	18.9
105	Cabbage (SI)	155.8	0.1	0.1	0.6	0.2	33.5	157.2
106	Cabbage (NI)	139	0.1	0.1	0.5	0.1	23.3	104
107	Beans (SI)	127.4	0.1	0.1	0.4	0.1	45.9	24.7
108	Beans (NI)	94.7	0.1	0.1	0.4	0.1	34.5	21.5
109	Lady's finger (sabji) (SI)	55.3	0.1	0.1	0.7	0.2	94	12.3
110	Lady finger (sabji) (NI)	60.1	0.1	0.1	0.7	0.3	112	16.1
111	Cauliflower (SI)	161.4	0.1	0.1	1.2	0.3	47.7	49.7
112	Cauliflower (NI)	31.9	0.1	0.1	1	0.2	49.5	49.4
113	Brinjal (SI)	110	0.1	0.2	1.5	0.2	52.7	18.1
114	Brinjal (NI)	92.2	0.1	0.1	0.9	0.1	27.1	13.5
115	Mushroom (SI)	174.1	0.1	0.3	2.6	0.2	23.8	17.7
116	Mushroom (NI)	59.5	0.1	0.3	3.2	0.1	10.3	2.9
117	Fresh peas (SI)	127.0	0.2	0.0	1.3	0.3	59.9	17.9
118	Fresh peas (NI)	153.9	0.3	0	1.1	0.3	78.2	19.4
119	Pumpkin (SI)	171.7	0.1	0	0.5	0.6	17.9	25
120	Pumpkin (NI)	64.2	0.1	0.1	0.7	0.1	16.6	2.9
121	Pointed gourd (parwal) (SI)	166.7	0.2	0.1	1.2	0.2	79.3	15.5
122	Stuffed pointed gourd (parwal) (NI)	159.9	0.1	0.1	0.8	0.2	39.4	12
123	Capsicum (SI)	533.3	0.7	0.1	0.4	0.4	29.9	156.3
124	Capsicum (NI)	243.8	0.3	0	0.2	0.2	14.9	81
125	Drumstick (SI)	319.1	0.2	0.1	0.8	0.2	28.2	70.6
126	Drumstick (NI)	73.1	0.1	0.1	0.3	0	1.69	72.4
127	Colocasia (SI)	104.4	0.1	0	0.6	0.1	36.8	7.7
128	Colocasia (NI)	21.3	0.1	0	0.4	0	39.3	0.5
129	Yam palya (SI)	335.9	0.1	0.1	0.7	0.3	23.6	8.1
130	Yam palya (NI)	93.4	0.1	0	0.8	0.1	17.6	1
131	Bottle gourd	9.9	0.1	0	0.4	0.1	10.7	0.9
132	Ridge gourd	117.3	0	0.1	0.3	0.1	13	6
133	Jackfruit tender	113.4	0.1	0	0.5	0.1	14.8	17.6

Continued

Continued

S No	Food items	β-carotene (μg)	Thiamin (mg)	Riboflavin (mg)	Niacin (mg)	Vitamin B6 (mg)	Folate (μg)	Vitamin C (mg)
134	Chow chow marrow	39.4	0	0	0.3	0.1	47.7	7
135	Raw banana palya	88	0.1	0	0.5	0.1	7	7.4
136	Bittergourd	199.3	0.1	0.1	0.7	0.1	112.7	153.3
137	Lotus stem	78	0.4	0.6	1.2	0.1	8.3	10
138	Tinda	126.5	0.1	0.2	0.6	0.2	19.1	48.9
139	Aviyal (SI)	108.9	0.1	0.1	0.5	0.1	35.4	16.6
140	Asparagus, boiled	604	0.16	0.14	1.08	0.08	149	7.7
141	Broccoli, boiled	929	0.06	0.12	0.55	0.2	108	64.9
142	Brussels sprouts, boiled	465	0.11	0.08	0.61	0.18	60	62
143	Celery, boiled	313	0.02	0.07	0.37	0.09	33	6.1
144	Sweet corn, boiled	66	0.09	0.06	1.68	0.14	23	5.5
145	Mushroom, stir fried	0	0.1	0.46	3.99	0.04	20	0
146	Mashed potatoes	2	0.09	0.04	1.12	0.23	8	6.2
147	Hash brown potato	0	0.14	0.08	1.67	0.22	20	2.9
148	Chinese cabbage (bok choy, boiled)	2,549	0.03	0.06	0.43	0.17	41	26
149	Bamboo shoot, boiled	-	0.02	0.05	0.3	0.1	2	0
150	Wax gourd (tung qwa), cooked	0	0.03	0	0.38	0.03	4	10.5
Fruits								
151	Amla (gooseberry)	110	0	0	0.3	0	8	0
152	Apple	0	0	0	0	0	2.8	1
153	Banana	78	0.1	0.1	0.5	0.6	19.1	7
154	Custard apple	0	0.1	0.1	0.5	0.2	0	19.2
155	Dates (dry)	89	0.1	0	1.6	0.2	15	0
156	Grapes	3	0	0	0.2	0.1	3.9	1
157	Guava, country	0	0	0	0.4	0.1	14	212
158	Jackfruit	175	0	0.1	0.4	0.1	14	7
159	Jamoon (Jambu)	17	0.1	0	0.2	0.1	2	3
160	Kiwi	52	0	0	0.3	0.1	25	92.7
161	Sweet lime (mosambi)	0	0	0	0	0.1	10.6	50

Continued

Continued

S No	Food items	β-carotene (μg)	Thiamin (mg)	Riboflavin (mg)	Niacin (mg)	Vitamin B6 (mg)	Folate (μg)	Vitamin C (mg)
162	Litchis	0	0	0.1	0.6	0.1	14	71.5
163	Mango	2,743	0.1	0.1	0.9	0.1	14	16
164	Muskmelon	169	0.1	0.1	0.3	0.1	21	39
165	Orange	1,104	0.1	0	0.3	0.1	30.3	30
166	Palmyra (tar/thati pandu)	0	0	0.7	0.6	0.1	14	71.5
167	Papaya	666	0	0.3	0.2	0	38	57
168	Passion fruit	54	0.1	0.1	1.6	-	-	25
169	Peach	162	0	0.3	0.8	0	4	6.6
170	Pears	0	0	0	0.2	0	8	3.8
171	Pineapple	18	0.2	0.1	0.1	0.1	10.6	39
172	Plums	190	0	0.3	0.4	0	5	9.5
173	Pomegranate	0	0.1	0.1	0.3	0.1	6	16
174	Sapota	97	0	0	0.2	0	0	6
175	Strawberry	18	0	0	0.2	-	-	52
176	Sugarcane	0	0	0	0	0	0	0
177	Watermelon	0	0	0	0.1	0.1	2.2	1
178	Ziziphus (elantha pazham)	0	0	0	0.9	0.8	0	69
179	Fruit custard	229.1	0.1	0.2	0.3	0.2	15.3	7.7
180	Persimmons (kaki, raw)	253	0.03	0.02	0.1	0.1	8	7.5
181	Persimmons (kaki, dried)	374	-	0.029	0.18	-	-	0
Dry fruits and nuts								
182	Almond (badam)	3	0.2	0.8	3.9	0.1	29	0
183	Apricot	58	0.2	-	2.3	-	-	2
184	Cashew nut	60	0.6	0.2	1.2	0.3	69.2	0
185	Dates (dry)	26	0	0	0.9	-	-	3
186	Figs	162	0.1	0.1	0.6	-	-	5
187	Groundnut (peanut)	37	0.9	0.1	19.9	0.3	20	0
188	Pistachio nut	332	0.9	0.2	1.3	1.7	51	5
189	Raisins	2.4	0.1	0.2	0.7	0.2	3.3	1
190	Walnut	6	0.5	0.4	1	-	-	0
191	Ginkgo nuts (raw)	-	0.22	0.09	6	0.33	54	15

Continued

Continued

S No	Food items	β-carotene (μg)	Thiamin (mg)	Riboflavin (mg)	Niacin (mg)	Vitamin B6 (mg)	Folate (μg)	Vitamin C (mg)
Nonvegetarian								
192	Methi (fenugreek) chicken	279.4	0.1	0.1	7.2	0.3	16.0	20.4
193	Chicken dry	125.6	0.1	0.1	7.9	0.3	2.8	10.4
194	Chicken gravy	49.3	0.09	0.09	5	0.2	2.1	5.9
195	Pepper chicken	496	0.2	0.1	4.6	0.2	17.5	55.4
196	Grilled chicken	139.1	0.2	0.3	11.1	0	0.7	7.2
197	Chicken kabab	119.1	0.1	0.1	7.7	0.4	8.6	3.6
198	Chicken curry	42.5	0	0.1	3.8	0.2	5.2	2.6
199	Chicken fry	16.8	0.1	0.2	9.5	0.6	21.8	8.8
200	Mutton curry	118.9	0.1	0.1	4	0.1	9.2	7.1
201	Mutton fry	125.8	0.2	0.2	7.1	0.2	13.3	8.3
202	Fish curry	136.1	0.1	0.1	3.1	0.2	20.3	14.3
203	Fish fry	6	0.3	0.5	13.7	0.7	3.8	1.4
204	Liver fry	167.5	0.4	3.3	14.8	0.9	169.6	14.3
205	Prawn	77.3	0.1	0.1	6.1	0.2	7.9	7.1
206	Boiled egg	493	0.1	0.5	0.1	0.2	91.9	0
207	Scrambled eggs	26	0.04	0.38	0.08	0.13	36	0
208	Baked egg white with mushroom	3.9	0	0.1	0.6	0	0	0.4
209	Salami (fermented and air-dried meat)	0	0.1	0.2	3.2	0.2	2	0
210	Chicken pot pie	352	0.07	0.02	1.48	0.08	35	1
211	Lemon chicken	1	0.05	0.06	3.6	0.2	11	2.5
212	Steamed fish (halibut)	0	0.05	0.04	7.9	0.6	14	0
Snacks								
213	Masala murmure (puffed rice)	491.9	0.3	0.1	7.9	0	0	2.4
214	Sundal (white chickpeas)	605.5	0.1	0.1	1.4	0	8.2	13.5
215	Cutlet	405.3	0.2	0.1	1.3	0	108.3	10.6
216	Peanut masala	240.3	0.7	0.1	15.2	0	15.2	9
217	Paneer toast	5,438.6	0.5	0.1	2.4	0	114.2	105.7
218	Egg sandwich	474.8	0	0.1	0.4	0	132.4	5

Continued

Continued

S No	Food items	β-carotene (µg)	Thiamin (mg)	Riboflavin (mg)	Niacin (mg)	Vitamin B6 (mg)	Folate (µg)	Vitamin C (mg)
219	Grilled chicken sandwich	261.8	0.1	0.1	4.5	0.2	0	17.1
220	Mixture	187.7	0.3	0.1	4.2	0.2	161.3	0.1
221	Potato chips	63.6	0.3	0	3.1	0.7	18.5	43.6
222	Banana chips	96.1	0.1	1.4	0	0	0	0
223	Potato bajji (pakora)	54.1	0.2	0	1.2	0.3	141.4	8.3
224	Bajji	322.2	0	1.4	0	0	0.2	69.4
225	Mysore bonda	243.2	0.2	1.4	0	0.1	0	123.6
226	Potato bonda	55.3	0.1	1.6	0	0	1	35.2
227	Pakoda	426.8	0.1	1.7	0	0.1	0	0
228	Maddur vada	594.8	0.1	1.4	0	0	1.3	0
229	Urad vada (Sl)	267.9	0.1	0.9	0	0.1	0	88.3
230	Kachori	350	0.1	1.7	0	0	0	15.5
231	Thair vada (curd vada)	109.3	0.1	0.4	0	0	0.1	30.7
232	Karasev	268.5	0.1	2.1	0	0.1	1.4	8.3
233	Murukku	69.5	0.1	1.7	0	0	5.7	48.2
234	Vegetable puff	33.3	0.1	0	1.5	0.2	25.5	8.8
235	Sweet cookies	637.5	0	1.2	0	0	0	11.6
236	Biscuits (salted)	50	0.1	0.1	2.9	0.1	31.2	0
237	Biscuits (sweet/creamed)	75.7	0.1	0.1	1.7	0	18.8	0
238	BhelPoori	41.3	0.3	0.1	6	0.3	32.3	2.7
239	Dhokla	63.9	0.2	0.1	0.9	0.2	178.9	0.5
240	Pavbhaji (pakora)	405.3	0.2	0.1	0.6	0.2	27.7	51.7
241	Healthy green kebab	3.7	0.18	0.08	1.6	0	0.5	33.6
242	Corn chat	0.1	0.1	0.03	0.5	0.01	7.5	28.2
243	Popcorn	-	0.13	0.14	1.55	0.21	17	0.3
244	Hot dog	-	0.24	0.28	3.72	0.05	49	0.1
245	Croissant (butter)	38	0.39	0.24	2.19	0.06	88	0.2
246	Croissant (cheese)	89	0.52	0.33	2.16	0.07	74	0.2
247	Doughnut (plain)	1	0.24	0.15	1.97	0.03	80	1.3
248	Egg roll	-	0.16	0.07	2.7	0.16	-	0
249	Cheese burger	-	0.22	0.26	4.03	-	59	0.6
250	Popcorn chicken	-	0.18	0.13	8.11	0.5	-	-

Continued

Continued

S No	Food items	β-carotene (µg)	Thiamin (mg)	Riboflavin (mg)	Niacin (mg)	Vitamin B6 (mg)	Folate (µg)	Vitamin C (mg)
251	Fried chicken, drumstick	-	0.04	0.21	4.99	0.22	-	-
252	Nachos, with cheese	-	0.17	0.33	1.36	0.18	9	1.1
253	Taco (with beef and cheese)	46	0.05	0.06	1.65	0.09	19	0.4
254	Thai lettuce roll	1,508.6	0.07	0.09	0.8	0.1	59.3	10.4
255	Dim sum (momo)	8.02	0.47	0.3	3.5	0.07	117.2	7.2
256	Green gram sprouts, steamed	1	0.05	0.1	0.8	0.05	29	11.4
257	Wo tou (steamed corn bun)	-	0.3	0.3	2.2	0.1	77	0.3
258	Garlic bread	0	0.5	0.2	4.1	0.08	186	0.2
259	Spinach corn and cheese sandwich	0.8	0.02	0.07	0.14	0	0.01	4.3
260	Mixed-vegetable sandwich	0.8	0.06	0.09	0.9	0	0.01	4.1
Sweets								
261	Cake/sweet pastry	397.1	0.1	0.1	0.7	0.1	29.8	0
262	Payasam, kheer	55.2	0.1	0.2	0.3	0.1	9.8	1.7
263	Bread pudding	44.4	0.1	0.2	0.2	0	34.7	1.6
264	Ice cream	195	0	0.2	0.1	0	5	0.6
265	Mysore pak	187.8	0.1	0	0.5	0.1	121.9	0
266	Peda	70.1	0.1	0.2	0.2	0	9.9	1.5
267	Badusha (Balushahi)	60.1	0.1	0.1	1.2	0	13.3	0.1
268	Kesari bhath	86.4	0	0	0.3	0	14.6	0
269	Kaju katli	81.7	0.3	0.1	0.5	0.1	29.4	0
270	Shrikhand	22	0	0.1	0.1	0	8.1	0.7
271	Chocolate	0	0	0	0	0	0	0
272	Besan ladoo	510.7	0.1	0.9	0	0.1	0	22.1
273	Boondi ladoo	23.1	0	0.5	0	0	0	18.6
274	Gajar (carrot) halwa	876.6	0.3	0.4	0	0	0.1	74.6
275	Coconut burfi	124.4	0.2	0.4	0	0	0	7.4
276	Jalebi	8.5	0	0.7	0	0	0	0
277	Kalakand	1,118.6	0.6	0.4	0	0	0	27.2
278	Rasgulla	274.5	0	0.1	0	0	0	23.3

Continued

Continued

S No	Food items	β-carotene (µg)	Thiamin (mg)	Riboflavin (mg)	Niacin (mg)	Vitamin B6 (mg)	Folate (µg)	Vitamin C (mg)
279	Narayal doodh mithai (coconut milk sweet)	120	0.1	1.1	0	0	1.7	25.8
280	Caramel custard (flan)	5	0.03	0.21	0.08	0.04	9	0
281	Egg custard, baked	6	0.04	0.24	0.11	0.05	10	0
282	Chocolate mousse	27	0.05	0.21	0.15	0.06	15	0.1
283	Apple pie	-	0.15	0.11	1.23	0.03	24	1.7
284	Brownie	-	0.12	0.21	0.97	0.04	29	5.3
Chutney and raita								
285	Green tomato chutney	361.3	0.1	0	0.5	0	5.1	36.1
286	Red capsicum chutney	186.8	0.1	0.1	0.6	0	27.2	16.6
287	Cabbage chutney	85.2	0.2	0.1	2.8	0	224.7	69.5
288	Green peas chutney	258.5	0.1	0	0.4	0	0.5	12.3
289	Ridge gourd chutney	212.6	0.1	0	0.4	0	12.6	18.4
290	Gherkin chutney	38.5	0.1	0.1	0.5	0	0.4	20.8
291	Tomato chutney	848.5	0.3	0.2	1.5	0	70.8	71.4
292	Mint chutney	1,788.4	0.7	0	0.5	0	4.3	46.1
293	Coconut chutney	4.8	0	0	0.2	0	3.3	2.8
294	Groundnut chutney	209.1	0.4	0.1	8.1	0.3	30.6	6.7
295	Chili chutney	75.8	0.1	0.2	0.5	0.3	14.1	45.7
296	Tamarind chutney	24.7	0.1	0.1	0.7	0.1	10.4	5.6
297	Mango chutney	486.5	0	0.1	0.4	0.1	8.7	17.2
298	Brinjal chutney	292.6	0.1	0.2	1	0.2	44.7	35.4
299	Urad dal chutney	21.2	0.2	0.1	0.8	0.1	50.2	3.3
300	Chutney powder	288.2	0.7	0.2	11.1	0.5	73.5	6.1
301	Onion raita	137.6	0.1	0.1	0.2	0	10.2	7.7
302	Vegetable raita	317	0.1	0.1	0.3	0	17.6	12.5
Salad								
303	Salad with green gram	342.7	0.2	0.1	0.8	0	42.8	14.3
304	Salad with macaroni	198	0.1	0	0.6	0	6.4	10.1

Continued

Continued

S No	Food items	β-carotene (µg)	Thiamin (mg)	Riboflavin (mg)	Niacin (mg)	Vitamin B6 (mg)	Folate (µg)	Vitamin C (mg)
305	Crunchy salad	1,496.2	0.4	0.5	4.3	0.6	127.8	17.7
306	Vegetable salad	583.7	0.1	0	0.4	0.1	18.3	15.8
307	Caesar salad	-	0.04	0.03	0.2	-	54	14.1
308	Moong dal and green mango salad	0.3	0.15	0.7	0.8	0	0.04	14.2
309	Sprouts salad	6	0.08	0.1	0.7	0.08	0	13.2
310	Asparagus salad	604	0.1	0.1	1	0.07	149	7.7
311	Greek salad	-	0.04	0.04	0.2	-	57	15.7
312	Tossed salad	-	0.03	0.05	0.5	0.08	0	23.2
Soup								
313	Creamy broccoli soup	74.1	0.1	0	0.3	0	160.5	11.6
314	Carrot and coriander soup	3,048.3	0.1	0	0.9	0	10.9	19.8
315	Garlic-vegetable soup	268.6	0.3	0.1	0.3	0	8.8	9.9
316	Noodle soup, chicken	593	0.02	0.02	1.2	0.05	9	0.4
317	Wonton soup, Chinese	6	0.02	0.02	0.58	0.08	13	0.7
318	Drumstick soup	1,094.6	0.2	0.1	0.2	0	218.3	25.6
319	Button mushroom soup	149.1	0.2	0.2	1.1	0	163.7	2.2
320	Vegetable manchow soup	1,845.5	0.1	0	0.3	0	39.2	12.1
321	Spinach soup	759.5	0.4	0.2	0.3	0	21.1	5.7
322	Chicken herb soup	496.6	0	0.1	2	0	8.7	4.4
323	Tomato soup	364.7	0	0	0.2	0	10	12.4
324	Tomato soup with cream	1,602.2	0.2	0.1	0.5	0	26.9	35
325	Tomato mint soup	333.4	0	0	0.1	0	7.1	8.9
326	Vegetable soup	421.8	0.1	0	0.4	0	13.1	5.5
327	Miso soup	219	0.04	0.04	0.4	0.07	66	0.2
328	Tom yum soup	1,198	0.03	0.03	0.5	0.08	7	2.5

Continued

Nutritive Value of Common Indian Cooked Foods

Continued

S No	Food items	β-carotene (µg)	Thiamin (mg)	Riboflavin (mg)	Niacin (mg)	Vitamin B6 (mg)	Folate (µg)	Vitamin C (mg)
Beverages								
329	Tea with sugar	30.2	0	0.1	0.2	0	6	1.1
330	Coffee with sugar	49.1	0	0.2	0.3	0	7.9	1.9
331	Plain milk with sugar	53	0.1	0.2	0.1	0	8.5	2
332	Horlicks	51.5	0.1	0.2	0.8	0	8.3	1.9
333	Curd	52.7	0	0.2	0.1	0	8.5	2
334	Buttermilk	17.2	0	0	0	0	2.8	0.5
335	Fresh fruit juice	0	0.1	0	0	0.1	18.2	85.6
336	Soft drinks	0	0	0	0	0	0	0
337	Beer	0	0	0	0.5	0.1	6	0
338	Wine	0	0	0	0.1	0	1.1	0
339	Spirits (whisky/gin/rum, etc.)	0	0	0	0	0	0	0
340	Local arrack/toddy	0	0	0	0	0	0	0
341	Raw green mango squash (aam ka panna)	29.3	0	0	0.1	0	4.2	0.9
Miscellaneous								
342	Butter/cream	3.2	0	0	0	0	0	0
343	Ghee	600	0	0	0	0	0	0
344	Jam	0	0	0	0	0	33	8.8
345	Sugar	0	0	0	0	0	0	0
346	Honey	0	0	0	0.1	0	2	0.5
347	Jaggery	0	0	0	0	0	0	0
348	Cheese	82	0	0.4	0.1	0.1	7	0
349	Ketchup, tomato sauce	1,070	0.1	0.1	1.1	0.2	9.4	13.1
350	Mango pickle	113.8	0	0	0.3	0.1	11.4	2.3
351	Papad (papadum)	81.4	0.6	0.3	2.8	0.4	173	0.7
352	Maple syrup	0	0.07	1.27	0.08	0	0	0

NI, North Indian; SI, South Indian.

C. Nutritive Value (Minerals for 100 g of Food Items)

S No	Food items	Calcium (mg)	Phosphorus (mg)	Iron (mg)	Sodium (mg)	Potassium (mg)	Magnesium (mg)	Zinc (mg)
Cereals								
1	Idli	21	79.8	0.6	318.9	115	29	0.6
2	Vegetable upma	32.4	100.1	1	251	74.9	19.8	0.2
3	Upma	14.3	47.1	0.7	193.3	60.4	22	0.4
4	Vermicelli upma	32.8	84.4	1	330.4	89.1	25.7	0.2
5	Poha (flattened rice)	30.5	116.1	9.1	512.3	89.5	53.8	0.1
6	Idiyappam (hoppers) nooputt or string	7.8	99.4	0.4	240.7	0	60.9	0.9
7	Poori	31.9	235.4	3.3	83.5	208.9	87.5	1.5
8	Dalia (broken/cracked wheat)	80	201.8	2.3	43.3	194.7	61.3	1.2
9	Puttu (rice pudding)	9.2	147.1	2.1	286	81.6	92.4	1.1
10	Adai (multigrain)	21.8	117.9	1.7	442.4	212.8	60.8	0.6
11	Wheat dosa	75.3	149.6	2.2	449.8	147	62.1	1
12	Onion dosa	30.9	124.7	1.3	136.5	105.4	58.7	0.8
13	Onion wheat dosa	75.3	149.6	2.2	449.8	147	62.1	1
14	Plain dosa	22.3	102.7	0.7	600.7	125.8	38.2	0.8
15	Masala dosa	31.5	97.6	1	920.9	178.4	44.6	0.8
16	Pesarattu (green gram dosa)	40.9	171.3	1.8	430.5	486.4	62.6	1.2
17	Avalakki (beaten rice)	17.3	124.6	9.5	192.3	102.8	52.2	0.6
18	Ragi chapatti	227.1	188.5	2.6	877.6	288.8	91.4	1.5
19	Channa (gram) chapatti	34.3	226.2	3.4	30.7	341.2	86.4	1.3
20	Jowar (sorghum) chapatti	16.7	148	2.7	4.9	87.3	114	1.1
21	Bajra (millet) chapatti	30	211.1	5.7	7.8	219	97.7	2.2
22	Rice chapatti	22.5	113.3	0.7	541.5	93.4	47.9	0.9
23	Tandoori chapatti	28	207	2.9	11.7	183.7	77	1.3
24	Phulka (chapatti)	28	207	2.9	11.7	183.7	77	1.3
25	Stuffed paratha	30	200	2.7	703.2	271.8	81.1	1.4
26	Mix-vegetable methi (fenugreek) paratha	94.7	252.9	3.2	658.5	207.8	83.8	1.3
27	Methi (fenugreek) chapatti	76.4	186.5	3	468.3	186.2	72.5	1.2
28	Tomato chapatti	64.5	246.8	4	582.3	294	87.1	1.7

Continued

Continued

S No	Food items	Calcium (mg)	Phos-phorus (mg)	Iron (mg)	Sodium (mg)	Potassium (mg)	Magne-sium (mg)	Zinc (mg)
29	Plain chapatti	36.4	244.8	3.4	515	217.3	91	1.5
30	Puliyogare (tamarind rice)	76.8	118.3	2.6	593.2	63.5	53.2	0.9
31	Peas pulao	19.3	111.7	2.2	298.8	27.7	73.7	0.6
32	Mushroom cauliflower pulao	16.4	75.9	1.3	307.6	73.7	46	0.5
33	Pongal (rice dish)	26.2	95.6	1	570.6	211.8	39.4	0.7
34	Curd rice	96.6	98.7	0.9	445.7	103.3	40.3	0.4
35	Chinese fried rice	17.7	98.8	1.7	28.7	29.4	62.2	0.7
36	Tomato rice	32.7	67.1	1.5	162	57.5	50.4	0.6
37	Masala bhath	48.4	146.4	2.1	391.1	91.6	70.4	0.7
38	Sprouted green gram garlic rice	13	56.8	0.9	263.7	26.2	36	0.4
39	Lemon rice	21.9	85.4	0.6	185.8	97.1	34	0.6
40	Methi (fenugreek) pulao	44.7	60.8	0.7	243.7	93.6	29.9	0.6
41	Vegetable biryani	25.1	105.9	1.4	331	38.9	58.7	0.6
42	Vegetable pulao	14.7	74.5	0.4	397.3	47.7	26	0.5
43	Plain rice	2.9	54.8	0.9	0	0	45.2	0.4
44	Coconut rice	49.6	96.5	2.1	624.7	87.6	47.7	0.7
45	Sweet pongal	61.2	96.4	2.5	4.2	126.5	51.4	0.7
46	Chicken biryani	16.2	131.9	0.8	325.5	131.7	36	0.9
47	Mutton biryani	52.9	93	1.1	356.5	131.2	29	1.2
48	Bisibele bhath (hot lentil sour rice)	67.8	98.8	1.8	348.6	243.5	41.2	0.6
49	Vegetable khichdi	33.7	94.6	1.5	245.8	227	32.1	0.6
50	Bread	11	0	1.1	530	91	0	0
51	Brown bread	16	75	1.6	500	0	0	0
52	Plain ragi ball	116.2	95.5	1.3	243	137.7	46.2	0.8
53	Ragi with rice ball	100.1	87.6	1.2	3.2	121.3	41.9	0.7
54	Ragi porridge	49	40.1	0.6	504.4	57.9	19.4	0.3
55	Vada	68.7	157.2	1.6	467.6	334.8	58	1.2
56	Corn flakes	86.2	72.1	7	287.9	118.9	12.1	0.4
57	Pizza	209	249	1.95	685	173	22	1.65
58	Vegetable noodles	18.4	80.3	1	267.3	57.7	17.6	0.5
59	Macaroni and cheese	114	119	0.57	290	95	0.216	0.8

Continued

Continued

S No	Food items	Calcium (mg)	Phosphorus (mg)	Iron (mg)	Sodium (mg)	Potassium (mg)	Magnesium (mg)	Zinc (mg)
60	Bagel	18	96	3.56	534	101	0.54	0.88
61	French toast	100	117	1.67	479	134	0.188	0.67
62	Pancake	219	159	1.8	439	132	0.2	0.56
63	Waffle	255	190	2.31	511	159	0.27	0.68
64	Tortilla	70	146	3.81	482	105	0.27	0.32
65	Soba noodles, plain boiled (Japanese)	4	25	0.48	60	35	0.37	0.12
66	Somen, plain boiled (noodles, Japanese)	8	27	0.52	161	29	0.25	0.22
67	Noodles, chowmein	20	161	4.73	847	120	-	1.4
68	Rice noodles, cooked	4	20	0.14	19	4	0.11	0.25
69	Tofu pad (Thai)	55.1	44.7	0.7	224.1	154.9	15.4	0.32
70	Vegetable soba noodles	66.4	86.8	1.7	362.4	236.3	36.3	0.76
71	Burrito (with beans and cheese)	124	163	2.37	563	261	0.46	0.86
72	Spaghetti and meatballs	36	62	1.22	315	201	0.15	0.55
73	Spaghetti in tomato and cheese sauce	8	-	0.3	377	-	-	-
74	Ravioli (cheese filled)	33	50	0.74	306	232	0.18	0.36
75	Lasagna, cheese	111	107	1.27	284	182	0.2	0.91
76	Black bean tortilla casserole	45.7	126.1	1.1	126	219.2	41.2	0.8
77	Pasta in tomato sauce (plain)	13	39	0.9	272	192	14	0.38
78	Vegetable congee	33.7	94.6	1.5	245.8	227	32.1	0.6
Dals/curries								
79	Plain sambhar	27.7	47.4	0.6	331.3	169.2	16.7	0.3
80	Tur dal sambhar with vegetables	28.7	49.6	1	247.7	199.4	17.6	0.2
81	Whole channa (gram) curry	48.3	65.9	1.2	262.6	186.3	30.5	0.6
82	Green leafy vegetable curry	295.1	74.6	2.8	442.2	280.9	93.6	0.2
83	Paneer gravy	97.7	66.5	0.6	220.2	164.9	14.4	0.5
84	Rasam (Sl soup)	23	17.5	0.7	450.8	55.9	7.3	0.1
85	Kadhi (curd sambar) NI	32.4	36.3	0.4	481.2	71.4	11.5	0.3

Continued

Continued

S No	Food items	Calcium (mg)	Phos-phorus (mg)	Iron (mg)	Sodium (mg)	Potassium (mg)	Magne-sium (mg)	Zinc (mg)
86	Mosaru huli (curd sambar) (SI)	108.2	79.3	0.5	769.1	121.6	14.8	0.5
87	Bengal gram curry	29.1	109.2	2	256	257.7	45	0.6
88	Black gram dal curry	63	127.6	1.6	246.2	285.7	46.7	1
Vegetable dishes								
89	Baked vegetable	181	171.1	3.3	369.7	301.1	31.5	0.9
90	Cauliflower potato vegetables (aloo sabji)	39.7	72.1	1.3	442.2	201.7	35.1	0.5
91	Vegetable saagu	66	91	2.1	421.9	116.8	29.9	0.4
92	Methi (fenugreek) paneer	125.4	86.8	1.2	327	117.9	18.4	0.4
93	Curd lady finger (dahi bhindi)	270.1	199.9	1.5	620.6	348.9	75.5	0.7
94	Corn spinach (palak)	79.1	61	1.3	553.7	243.1	43.9	0.8
95	Paneer matar (peas) masala	212	294.3	2.2	998	346	41.9	0.9
96	Mushroom with baby corn	33.6	177	2.2	1115.7	396.9	27.1	0.9
97	Green leafy vegetable (SI)	116.1	49.5	1.8	566.8	297.2	94.4	0.5
98	Green leafy vegetable (NI)	101.2	38.4	2.7	718	325.8	88.3	0.5
99	Potato (SI)	32.7	53.3	0.8	155.2	259.7	34.9	0.6
100	Potato (NI)	16	46.5	1.3	479.1	276	36.5	0.6
101	Carrot (SI)	94.5	495.1	1.2	405.6	136	25	0.5
102	Carrot (NI)	104.9	643.2	1.9	425.8	170.3	29.4	0.5
103	Radish (SI)	60.3	54.4	0.7	694.6	177.1	20.7	0.5
104	Radish (NI)	44.4	33.5	1.3	596.4	196.8	18.6	0.4
105	Cabbage (SI)	56.2	71.6	2.1	509.7	370.9	50.1	0.5
106	Cabbage (NI)	44.7	48.1	1.5	479.1	256.4	31.7	0.4
107	Beans (SI)	54.7	37.2	0.7	532.4	139.7	41.3	0.5
108	Beans (NI)	54.1	45.3	1.4	436.9	158.2	38.1	0.5
109	Lady finger vegetable (sabji) (SI)	68.1	60	0.6	249.5	114.1	53.4	0.4
110	Lady finger vegetable (sabji) (NI)	74.7	70	1.6	731.3	161	67.5	0.6
111	Cauliflower (SI)	53.6	64.7	1.3	242.3	226.4	27	0.6
112	Cauliflower (NI)	46.2	65.3	1.7	324.5	167.2	23.7	0.5

Continued

Continued

S No	Food items	Calcium (mg)	Phosphorus (mg)	Iron (mg)	Sodium (mg)	Potassium (mg)	Magnesium (mg)	Zinc (mg)
113	Brinjal (SI)	34.6	86.5	1.7	538.1	346.1	31.6	0.5
114	Brinjal (NI)	22.8	46.8	1.4	564.5	226.6	21.2	0.4
115	Mushroom (SI)	46.9	87.1	2	748.8	336.5	19.9	0.7
116	Mushroom (NI)	18	94.2	1.8	468.2	330.1	15.5	0.6
117	Fresh peas (SI)	36.0	142.0	2.0	1387.0	202	50.1	1.3
118	Fresh peas (NI)	46.4	174.4	3.2	885.5	196.9	53	1.6
119	Pumpkin (SI)	30.2	46.8	5.9	911.7	215.9	18.9	0.2
120	Pumpkin (NI)	24.4	52.4	2	631.4	225.3	54.5	0.4
121	Pointed gourd (parwal) (SI)	101.2	104.4	1.5	1436.9	177.5	65.2	1
122	Stuffed pointed gourd (parwal) (NI)	84	71.9	3	709	193.4	52.6	0.6
123	Capsicum (SI)	39.9	63.6	1.4	1619.1	271	25.8	0.4
124	Capsicum (NI)	27.6	39.5	1.2	501.4	175.1	17.3	0.3
125	Drumstick (SI)	73.2	86.6	0.9	468.9	276.9	29.8	0.6
126	Drumstick (NI)	35.8	92.7	1.3	765.3	248.2	30.7	0.3
127	Colocasia (SI)	39	96.2	0.5	566	343.3	22.6	0.4
128	Colocasia (NI)	45.6	105.3	1.4	629.7	406.7	24.5	0.3
129	Yam palya (SI)	39.2	61.1	1	465.4	650	27.2	0.4
130	Yam palya (NI)	60	42.3	2.6	473.3	276.4	31.6	0.6
131	Bottle gourd	52.5	28.2	1.7	310	189.3	56.1	0.5
132	Ridge gourd	27.4	26.3	1.5	18.3	64.2	40.2	0.4
133	Jackfruit tender	40.9	35	1.4	465.1	212.5	30	0.4
134	Chow chow marrow	84.7	32.6	0.9	923	115.7	16.1	0.5
135	Raw banana palya	32.3	42.2	1.2	595.8	254.4	51.1	0.5
136	Bittergourd	46.6	72.1	3.5	445.3	307.2	64	0.8
137	Lotus stem	219.1	84.7	28.6	760.4	1473.1	98.4	0.4
138	Tinda	43.4	59.5	2.3	638.7	174.9	98	0.9
139	Aviyal (SI)	77	82.6	2.2	548.4	206	33.3	0.5
140	Asparagus, boiled	23	54	0.91	14	224	0.15	0.6
141	Broccoli, boiled	40	67	0.67	41	293	0.19	0.45
142	Brussels sprouts, boiled	36	56	1.2	21	317	0.23	0.33
143	Celery, boiled	42	25	0.42	91	284	0.11	0.14
144	Sweet corn, boiled	3	77	0.45	1	218	0.17	0.62
145	Mushroom, stir fried	4	105	0.25	12	396	0.05	0.57

Continued

Continued

S No	Food items	Calcium (mg)	Phosphorus (mg)	Iron (mg)	Sodium (mg)	Potassium (mg)	Magnesium (mg)	Zinc (mg)
146	Mashed potatoes	24	46	0.27	302	296	0.12	0.28
147	Hash brown	16	110	0.67	518	356	0.15	0.34
148	Chinese cabbage (bok choy, boiled)	93	29	1.04	34	371	0.14	0.17
149	Bamboo shoot, boiled	12	20	0.24	240	533	0.11	0.47
150	Wax gourd (tung qwa), cooked	18	17	0.38	107	5	0.06	0.59
Fruits								
151	Amla (gooseberry)	50	20	1.2	5	225	7	0.1
152	Apple	10	14	0.7	28	75	7	0.1
153	Banana	17	36	0.4	36.6	88	41	0.2
154	Custard apple	30	21	0	4	382	84	0.8
155	Dates (dry)	120	50	7.3	1	696	54	0.4
156	Grapes	20	23	0.5	2	185	82	0.1
157	Guava, country	10	28	0.3	5.5	91	24	0.2
158	Jackfruit	20	41	0.6	3	303	24	0.1
159	Jamoon (jambu)	15	15	0.4	2	210	7	0.1
160	Kiwi	34	34	0.3	3	312	17	0.1
161	Sweet lime (mosambi)	40	30	0.7	138	490	16	0
162	Litchis	5	31	0.3	124.9	171	10	0.1
163	Mango	14	16	1.3	26	205	270	0.3
164	Muskmelon	32	14	1.4	104	341	31	0.2
165	Orange	26	20	0.3	4.5	93	9	0.1
166	Palmyra (tar/thati pandu)	9	33	0.7	124.9	159	10	0.1
167	Papaya	17	13	0.5	6	69	11	0
168	Passion fruit	10	60	2	28	348	29	0.1
169	Peach	15	41	2.4	2	453	21	0.2
170	Pears	8	15	0.5	6.1	96	7	0
171	Pineapple	20	9	2.4	34.7	37	33	0.1
172	Plums	10	12	0.6	0.8	247	147	0.1
173	Pomegranate	10	70	1.8	0.9	133	44	0.8
174	Sapota	28	27	1.3	5.9	269	25	0.2
175	Strawberry	30.0	30.0	1.8	-	-	-	-
176	Sugarcane	12	1	0.2	0	0	0	0

Continued

Continued

S No	Food items	Calcium (mg)	Phos-phorus (mg)	Iron (mg)	Sodium (mg)	Potassium (mg)	Magne-sium (mg)	Zinc (mg)
177	Water melon	11	12	7.9	27.3	160	13	0
178	Ziziphus (elantha pazham)	4	9	0.5	3	250	13	0.1
179	Fruit custard	97.5	83	0.5	62.9	180.2	34.7	0.4
180	Persimmons (kaki, raw)	8	17	0.15	1	161	0.355	0.11
181	Persimmons (kaki, dried)	25	81	0.74	2	802	1.39	0.42
Dry fruits and nuts								
182	Almond (badam)	230	490	5.1	1	728	373	3.6
183	Apricot	110	70	4.6	-	-	-	-
184	Cashew nut	50	450	5.8	16	565	349	6
185	Dates (dry)	120	50	7.3	-	-	-	-
186	Figs	80	30	1	-	-	-	-
187	Groundnut (peanut)	90	350	2.5	18	705	168	3.9
188	Pistachio nut	279	528	8.5	1	1025	121	2.2
189	Raisins	87	80	7.7	12	751	33	0.3
190	Walnut	100	380	2.6	-	-	302	2.3
191	Ginkgo nuts (raw)	2	124	1	7	510	0.113	0.34
Nonvegetarian								
192	Methi (fenugreek) chicken	71.7	174.0	1.7	398.6	296.8	31.6	1.6
193	Chicken dry	65	191	1.7	1286	274	42	1.7
194	Chicken gravy	52.3	129.7	1.09	1155	197	29	1.1
195	Pepper chicken	55.9	116.7	1.2	817	212.8	26.1	1.1
196	Grilled chicken	120.9	341.6	2.9	587.6	113.8	17.1	0.1
197	Chicken kabab	41.5	238.1	1.1	575.3	244.1	35.4	1.5
198	Chicken curry	21.8	144.3	0.7	384.4	162.6	21.3	0.9
199	Chicken fry	40.6	289.3	2.5	1225.1	315.1	41.9	1.9
200	Mutton curry	102.8	104.2	2	372.5	215.5	23.5	2.1
201	Mutton fry	170.9	167.7	3	352.4	334.8	33.4	3.6
202	Fish curry	159	158.4	2.5	342.4	280.4	45.5	0.7
203	Fish fry	642.4	463.1	7.8	1384.7	515.5	120	1
204	Liver fry	48.2	277.8	7.5	528	251.7	35.7	4.5
205	Prawn	427.8	366.2	7.2	463.5	397.4	62.5	1.6
206	Boiled egg	70.4	258.3	2.5	147.9	142	11.7	1.3
207	Scrambled eggs	66	165	1.31	145	132	0.02	1.04

Continued

Nutritive Value of Common Indian Cooked Foods

Continued

S No	Food items	Calcium (mg)	Phos-phorus (mg)	Iron (mg)	Sodium (mg)	Potassium (mg)	Magne-sium (mg)	Zinc (mg)
208	Baked egg white with mushroom	4.7	17.3	0.2	141.3	79.9	0.6	0
209	Salami (fermented and air-dried meat)	9	113	2.2	1176	224	14	2.2
210	Chicken pot pie	21	75	0.58	407	105	0.18	0.4
211	Lemon chicken	39	129	1.32	243	155	15	0.5
212	Steamed fish (halibut)	9	287	0.2	82	528	28	0.43
Snacks								
213	Masala murmure (puffed rice)	94.7	207.9	6.4	0.4	16.8	128.9	1.1
214	Sundal (white chickpeas)	119.2	167.4	2.5	358.2	426.4	62.7	2.9
215	Cutlet	58.7	190.7	1.6	392.4	270.1	55	0.8
216	Peanut masala	87.1	278.3	2.1	296.1	40	8.7	3.1
217	Paneer toast	120.8	168	2.3	1866.8	145.8	31.8	0.5
218	Egg sandwich	30.2	86.2	0.7	490.3	144.1	6.8	0.1
219	Grilled chicken sandwich	17.1	94.0	1.9	966	171	21.4	0.8
220	Mixture	73.7	186.9	2.3	765.6	428.3	90.2	1.7
221	Potato chips	26.8	104.5	1.2	313.1	632.4	77.6	1.4
222	Banana chips	35.2	95.5	15.2	2893.9	497.4	31	0.2
223	Potato bajji	20	121.2	1.8	147.3	385.9	67.4	1.2
224	Bajji	30.7	69	2.2	681.2	236.9	37.4	0.5
225	Mysore bonda	102.1	270.3	3	26.5	554.3	119.5	2.3
226	Potato bonda	41.6	150.9	3.3	772.6	287	70.3	1
227	Pakoda	71.5	233.8	3.7	689.2	521	94.6	1.3
228	Maddur vada (SI)	56.1	137.2	2.3	745.7	228.3	64.7	0.9
229	Urad vada (SI)	73.8	171.1	1.9	876.3	352	76.1	1.4
230	Kachori	60.4	159.5	2.3	596.5	354.9	67.3	1
231	Thair vada (curd vada)	134.6	128.6	0.9	317.5	215.4	25.6	0.5
232	Karasev	52.9	270.1	4.3	910.1	519	112.6	1.5
233	Murukku	49.2	188.7	1.5	351.5	153.4	98.6	1.6
234	Veg puff	38.6	99.8	1.7	2,318.5	174.9	45.5	0.8
235	Sweet cookies	12.5	61.7	1.4	204.7	65	28.3	0.3
236	Biscuits (salted)	106.4	174.4	3.4	927.7	156.5	65.2	0.7
237	Biscuits (sweet/creamed)	87.8	112.8	2.1	129.5	94.8	39.3	0.4

Continued

Continued

S No	Food items	Calcium (mg)	Phos-phorus (mg)	Iron (mg)	Sodium (mg)	Potassium (mg)	Magne-sium (mg)	Zinc (mg)
238	Bhelpuri	52.4	205.4	4.4	1778.3	325.3	76.3	1.6
239	Dhokla	91.9	176.8	2.5	1118.6	404.2	74.6	1.5
240	Pavbhaji	80.8	124.4	1.5	482.1	230.1	31.4	0.6
241	Healthy green kabab	45.6	92.4	1.4	486.6	339.9	69.5	0.7
242	Corn chat	29.9	41.1	0.7	179	122.4	20.2	0.3
243	Popcorn	10	250	2.78	884	225	0.88	2.64
244	Hot dog	24	99	2.36	684	146	0.09	2.02
245	Croissant (butter)	37	105	2.03	467	118	0.33	0.75
246	Croissant (cheese)	53	130	2.15	361	132	0.34	0.94
247	Doughnut, (plain)	25	261	3	450	113	0.29	0.68
248	Egg roll	40	85	1.4	468	165	18	0.62
249	Cheese burger	167	140	2.35	626	200	0.23	1.91
250	Popcorn chicken	32	299	1.42	1140	288	0.23	0.98
251	Fried chicken, drumstick	29	211	0.97	625	250	0.14	1.96
252	Nachos with cheese	241	244	1.13	722	152	0.2	1.58
253	Taco (with beef and cheese)	89	178	1.19	397	209	0.25	1.75
254	Thai lettuce roll	45.2	61.4	1.2	123.6	241.5	18.7	0.48
255	Dim sum (wanton)	22	75.6	2.9	4.9	128.3	17.6	0.49
256	Green gram sprouts, steamed	12	28	0.6	246	101	14	0.5
257	Wo tou (steamed corn bun)	249	169	25	658	147	25	0.6
258	Garlic bread	27	87	3.05	544	103	23	0.9
259	Spinach corn and cheese sandwich	61	54.9	0.36	91.4	54.8	12	0.2
260	Mixed vegetable sandwich	71.1	96.9	1.3	367	98.2	30.5	0.4
Sweets								
261	Cake/sweet pastry	63.2	113.2	1.5	94.9	78.6	18.9	0.5
262	Payasam, kheer	105.6	91.6	0.6	62.1	150.4	21.1	0.5
263	Bread pudding	100.8	105.5	0.6	59.1	151.7	28.8	0.7
264	Ice cream	128	105	0.1	80	199	14	0.7
265	Mysore pak (rich sweet dish prepared in butter)	15.7	89	1.4	18.6	237.3	46.3	0.8

Continued

Continued

S No	Food items	Calcium (mg)	Phosphorus (mg)	Iron (mg)	Sodium (mg)	Potassium (mg)	Magnesium (mg)	Zinc (mg)
266	Peda	311.6	202.5	0.5	28.4	149.2	49.8	0.4
267	Badusha (Balushahi)	39.3	68.9	1.4	27.7	72.3	26.8	0.3
268	Kesari bhath	7.3	24.5	0.4	4.9	28	12.9	0.3
269	Kaju katli	24.3	191.7	2.5	7.3	241.2	148.5	2.6
270	Shrikhand	103.5	65.2	0.3	24.4	110.4	11.3	0.4
271	Chocolate	215	0	1.2	92	0	0	0
272	Besan ladoo	42.3	140.6	2.4	32.4	260.9	57.9	0.8
273	Boondi ladoo	14.3	74.5	1.3	11.7	115.2	36.8	0.5
274	Gajar (carrot) halwa	200.4	301.8	1	97	134.9	19.8	0.4
275	Coconut burfi	135.4	191.7	0.9	53.1	377.1	4.1	0.9
276	Jalebi	10.5	39.7	0.8	3.6	43.3	16.8	0.2
277	Kalakand	383	310.1	0.7	152.5	0	15.3	0.3
278	Rasgulla	158.6	109.7	0.1	0.8	3.1	2.6	0
279	Nariyal doodh mithai (coconut milk sweet)	41.3	234.7	2.4	5.4	425.5	24.1	2
280	Caramel custard (flan)	83	96	0.38	53	118	0.01	0.5
281	Egg custard, baked	107	113	0.35	61	148	0.01	0.5
282	Chocolate mousse	96	117	0.55	38	143	0.06	0.6
283	Apple pie	7	28	1.12	211	79	0.19	0.2
284	Brownie	42	146	2.15	255	139	0.18	0.9
Chutney and raita								
285	Green tomato chutney	56.8	58.9	2.5	436.1	159.8	29.3	0.2
286	Red capsicum chutney	60	74.6	1.1	475.9	170.5	13.9	0.6
287	Cabbage chutney	56.2	115.7	1.6	447.9	235.8	33.6	0.9
288	Green peas chutney	23.8	70.3	0.9	611.1	57.8	25.2	0.1
289	Ridge gourd chutney	47.6	41.2	0.8	315.5	105.6	37.2	0.6
290	Gherkin chutney	67	46.1	2	685.5	61.3	28.6	0.1
291	Tomato chutney	147.7	76.4	3.4	2,224.9	369.6	1.9	1
292	Mint chutney	84.1	56.8	2.4	417	151.7	30	0.4
293	Coconut chutney	4.8	51.2	0.6	232.5	86.6	13.3	0.3
294	Groundnut chutney	97.1	207.1	2.3	1,102.4	456.8	94.1	1.9
295	Chili chutney	21.9	92.9	2.7	1,853.9	287.8	207.4	1.4
296	Tamarind chutney	51.3	92.7	3.8	508.2	315.4	60.5	0.6
297	Mango chutney	19.4	92.9	1	664.9	170.2	33.1	0.5
298	Brinjal chutney	67	77.4	2.1	1,968.3	311.8	58.1	0.7

Continued

Continued

S No	Food items	Calcium (mg)	Phos-phorus (mg)	Iron (mg)	Sodium (mg)	Potassium (mg)	Magne-sium (mg)	Zinc (mg)
299	Urad dal chutney	67.7	150.1	1.5	586.9	312.8	56.6	1.2
300	Chutney powder	190.9	364.5	4.3	893.3	760.4	160.1	3.5
301	Onion raita	117.1	80.6	0.4	345.4	130	10.1	0.2
302	Vegetable raita	77.2	89.7	0.7	118.1	118	11.2	0.3
Salad								
303	Salad with green gram	42.2	119.3	1.5	513.9	318	40.6	0.9
304	Salad with macaroni	18.7	57.1	0.8	327.2	134.5	17.8	0.4
305	Crunchy salad	52.5	121.6	5.4	760.9	122.8	21.2	0.3
306	Vegetable salad	53	162.9	0.8	16.7	133.3	16.7	0.4
307	Caesar salad	86	79	0.6	83	216	9	-
308	Moong dal and green mango salad	42.2	119	1.4	513	317.3	40.5	0.8
309	Sprouts salad	13	54	0.9	6	149	21	0.4
310	Asparagus salad	23	54	0.9	14	224	14	0.6
311	Greek salad	24	-	0.6	12	220	-	-
312	Tossed salad	13	39	0.6	26	172	11	0.2
Soup								
313	Creamy broccoli soup	54.6	58.4	0.5	16.8	109.9	13.9	0.3
314	Carrot and coriander soup	130.7	649.1	1.7	280.1	180.3	27.4	0.6
315	Garlic vegetable soup	86.9	116.4	0.6	344.9	125.1	11.4	0.2
316	Noodle soup, chicken	11	36	0.35	306	117	0.06	0.17
317	Wonton soup, Chinese	5	18	0.21	406	32	0.03	0.12
318	Drumstick soup	93.8	78.8	0.5	235	156.2	12.1	0.2
319	Button mushroom soup	189.4	141.3	0.6	842.5	218.8	16.2	0.5
320	Vegetable manchow soup	19.5	45.5	0.7	228.2	48.7	12.2	0.2
321	Spinach soup	108.1	80.8	0.5	230	146.9	11	0.1
322	Chicken herb soup	16.8	54.5	0.7	235.4	20	7	0
323	Tomato soup	27.3	10.4	0.4	286.4	58.9	2.5	0.2
324	Tomato soup with cream	68	33.8	1.6	314.1	183.3	10.7	0.7
325	Tomato mint soup	26.8	15	0.3	23.3	52.3	5.6	0.1
326	Vegetable soup	34.2	96.6	0.6	32.6	131.6	16.6	0.3
327	Miso soup	35	75	1.5	970	250	33	1.1
328	Tom yum soup	23	30	0.7	359	165	3	1.3

Continued

Nutritive Value of Common Indian Cooked Foods

Continued

S No	Food items	Calcium (mg)	Phosphorus (mg)	Iron (mg)	Sodium (mg)	Potassium (mg)	Magnesium (mg)	Zinc (mg)
Beverages								
329	Tea with sugar	69.7	56.1	0.2	43.1	150.8	11.6	0.3
330	Coffee with sugar	112.4	85.1	0.2	67.8	149.9	14.3	0.4
331	Plain milk with sugar	120.5	90	0.2	73	140.1	13.4	0.4
332	Horlicks	137.7	102	0.3	93.2	168.5	15.5	0.4
333	Curd	119.6	89.7	0.2	72.6	139.4	13.4	0.4
334	Buttermilk	33.2	20.5	0.2	54.4	32.4	4.6	0.1
335	Fresh fruit juice	69.7	51.5	1.2	236.4	839.3	27.4	0.1
336	Soft drinks	3	12	0	4	1	1	0
337	Beer	5	12	0	5	25	6	0
338	Wine	8	14	0.4	8	89	10	0.1
339	Spirits (whisky/gin/rum, etc.)	0	4	0	1	2	0	0
340	Local arrack/toddy	0	0	0	0	0	0	0
341	Raw green mango squash (aam ka panna)	6.8	7.3	0.1	286.7	28.8	6.3	0
Miscellaneous								
342	Butter/cream	23.5	22.8	0.2	11	26	2	0.1
343	Ghee	0	0	0.2	2	3	0	0
344	Jam	20	11	0.5	32	77	4	0.1
345	Sugar	12	1	0.2	1	2	0	0
346	Honey	5	16	0.7	4	52	2	0.2
347	Jaggery	80	40	2.6	79	285	117	0.1
348	Cheese	790	520	2.1	1,345.2	241.9	28.5	2.6
349	Ketchup, tomato sauce	14	32	0.8	605	371	19	0.3
350	Mango pickle	29.1	28.5	0.6	3,414	71.6	18.1	0.2
351	Papad (papadum)	173.6	504.7	6.2	2,369.7	1281.4	166.9	3.7
352	Maple syrup	102	2	0.11	12	212	2.9	1.5

SI, South Indian; NI, North Indian.

Suggested Readings

1. Agricultural Research Service, United States Department of Agriculture (USDA). (2014). National Nutrient Data Base for Standard Reference: Release 25. [online] Available from: ndb.nal.usda.gov/ndb/foods/list. [Accessed September, 2014].
2. Annapurna - 2003 deluxe. Version 1.0, Product by Annapurna Associates.
3. Bharathi AV, Kurpad AV, Thomas T, Yusuf S, Saraswathi G, Vaz M. Development of food frequency questionnaires and a nutrient database for the Prospective Urban and Rural Epidemiological (PURE) pilot study in South India: methodological issues. Asia Pac J Clin Nutr. 2008;17(1):178-85.

APPENDIX 2

Carbohydrate Counting

A. List of Food Items that Provide 15 g of Carbohydrate

S No	Food items	Amount (g)	Serving
Cereals			
1	Idli	64	1½ number
2	Vegetable upma	54	⅓ cup
3	Upma	57	⅓ cup
4	Vermicelli Upma	58	⅓ cup
5	Poha (flattened rice)	42	⅓ cup
6	String hoppers (or idiyappam)	31	⅓ cup
7	Poori	33	1 number
8	Dalia (broken/cracked wheat)	43	¼ cup
9	Puttu	32	¼ cup
10	Adai	49	1 number
11	Wheat dosa	52	1 number
12	Onion dosa	44	½ number
13	Onion wheat dosa	52	1 number
14	Plain dosa	43	1 number
15	Masala dosa	49	⅓ number
16	Pesarattu (green gram dosa)	59	½ number
17	Avalakki (beaten rice)	39	⅓ cup
18	Ragi (chapatti)	32	⅓ number
19	Channa (gram) chapatti	35	½ number
20	Jowar (sorghum) chapatti	31	¾ number
21	Bajra (Millet) chapatti	31	½ number

Continued

Continued

S No	Food items	Amount (g)	Serving
22	Rice chapatti	29	¼ number
23	Tandoor chapatti	37	1¾ number
24	Chapatti (Phulka)	37	1¾ number
25	Stuffed paratha	33	⅓ number
26	Mix-vegetable methi (fenugreek) paratha	39	¾ number
27	Methi (fenugreek) chapatti	42	1½ number
28	Tomato chapatti	31	¾ number
29	Plain chapatti	31	1 number
30	Puliyogare (tamarind rice)	47	⅓ cup
31	Peas pulao	44	⅓ cup
32	Mushroom cauliflower pulao	69	½ cup
33	Pongal (rice dish)	68	¾ cup
34	Curd rice	93	½ cup
35	Chinese fried rice	56	⅓ cup
36	Tomato rice	64	½ cup
37	Masala bhath	50	⅓ cup
38	Sprouted green gram garlic rice	91	½ cup
39	Lemon rice	46	⅓ cup
40	Methi (fenugreek) pulao	63	½ cup
41	Vegetable biryani	60	⅓ cup
42	Vegetable pulao	65	⅓ cup
43	Plain rice	68	½ cup
44	Coconut rice	63	½ cup
45	Sweet pongal	39	⅓ cup
46	Chicken biryani	77	½ cup
47	Mutton biryani	97	½ cup
48	Bisibele bhath (hot lentil rice with tamarind)	114	½ cup
49	Khichdi with vegetables	72	⅓ cup
50	Bread	29	1½ slice
51	Brown bread	31	1½ slice
52	Plain ragi ball	62	¼ number
53	Ragi with rice ball	64	¼ number
54	Ragi porridge	147	½ cup
55	Vada	61	1¾ number
56	Corn flakes	51	½ cup
57	Pizza/burger	35	½ number

Continued

Continued

S No	Food items	Amount (g)	Serving
58	Vegetable noodles	59	½ cup
59	Macaroni and cheese	87	½ cup
60	Bagel	28	1 number
61	French toast	60	1 number
62	Pancake (4 inch diameter)	53	1½ number
63	Waffle (7 inch diameter)	46	½ number
64	Tortilla	30	¼ cup
65	Soba noodles, plain boiled (Japanese)	70	½ cup
66	Sômen, plain boiled (noodles, Japanese)	54	⅓ cup
67	Noodles, chowmein	181	1 cup
68	Rice noodles (cooked)	60	⅓ cup
69	Tofu pad Thai	128	¾ cup
70	Vegetable soba noodles	130	¾ cup
71	Burrito (with beans and cheese)	48	⅓ number
72	Spaghetti and meatballs	138	½ cup
73	Spaghetti in tomato and cheese sauce	71	½ cup
74	Ravioli (cheese filled)	110	½ cup
75	Lasagna, cheese	108	½ cup
76	Tortilla and black bean casserole	69	½ slice
77	Pasta in tomato sauce (plain)	105	½ cup
78	Vegetables congee	72	⅓ cup
Lentils/Curries			
79	Plain sambhar	175	1¼ cup
80	Tur lentil sambhar with vegetables	161	1¼ cup
81	Whole gram curry	127	¾ cup
82	Green leafy vegetable curry	242	2 cup
83	Paneer gravy	198	1½ cup
84	Rasam	373	3 cup
85	Kadhi (curd sambar) (NI)	415	3½ cups
86	Mosaru huli (curd sambar) (SI)	317	3 cup
87	Bengal gram curry	76	½ cup
88	Black gram dhal curry	76	½ cup
Vegetable dishes			
89	Baked vegetable	105	7½ tbsp
90	Cauliflower aloo sabji (potato vegetable)	100	5½ tbsp
91	Vegetable saagu	161	5½ tbsp

Continued

Continued

S No	Food items	Amount (g)	Serving
92	Corn palak (spinach)	129	5½ tbsp
93	Paneer matar (pea) masala	95	8 tbsp
94	Mushroom with baby corn	70	5 tbsp
95	Potato (SI)	72	3⅓ tbsp
96	Potato (NI)	65	3⅓ tbsp
97	Carrot (SI)	121	10 tbsp
98	Carrot (NI)	103	6½ tbsp
99	Fresh peas	68	3½ tbsp
100	Pumpkin	96	3¾ tbsp
101	Pointed gourd (parwal) (SI)	121	8 tbsp
102	Stuffed pointed gourd (parwal) (NI)	167	7¼ tbsp
103	Colocasia (SI)	112	8⅓ tbsp
104	Colocasia (NI)	93	5 tbsp
105	Yam palya (SI)	93	6 tbsp
106	Yam palya (NI)	59	2¾ tbsp
107	Jack fruit tender	146	6¾ tbsp
108	Raw banana palya	154	8½ tbsp
109	Bittergourd	80	3⅓ tbsp
110	Lotus stem	54	2⅓ tbsp
111	Avial (SI)	119	½ cup
112	Sweet corn, boiled	71	½ cup
113	Mashed potatoes	85	⅓ cup
114	Hash brown (potato)	47	⅓ cup
Fruits			
115	Gooseberry (amla)	12	1 number
116	Apple	112	1 number
117	Banana	44	½ number
118	Custard apple	43	½ number
119	Dates (dry)	4	¼ number
120	Grapes	174	1 number
121	Guava, country	134	1¼ number
122	Jackfruit	19	¾ number
123	Jamun (jambu)	9	1 number
124	Kiwi	124	1 number
125	Sweet lime (mosambi)	177	1½ number
126	Litchis	7	1 number

Continued

Continued

S No	Food items	Amount (g)	Serving
127	Mango	89	1 number
128	Muskmelon	600	4¼ pc
129	Orange	138	1½ number
130	Palmyra	14	¾ number
131	Papaya	167	2 number
132	Passion fruit	121	1¼ number
133	Peach	121	1½ number
134	Pears	78	1¼ number
135	Pineapple	72	1½ number
136	Plums	34	1½ number
137	Pomegranate	149	1 number
138	Sapota	40	¾ number
139	Strawberry	153	4½ number
140	Sugarcane	8	¼ number
141	Water melon	345	4½ pieces
142	Ziziphus	16	1 number
143	Fruit custard	103	½ number
144	Persimmons (kaki, raw)	81	½ number
145	Persimmons (kaki, dried)	20	½ number
Salad			
146	Salad with green gram	94	½ cup
147	Salad with macaroni	86	½ cup
148	Crunchy salad	66	1 cup
149	Vegetable salad	194	1 cup
150	Moong dal and green mango salad	95	¾ cup
Soup			
151	Creamy broccoli soup	52	¼ cup
152	Carrot and coriander soup	94	½ cup
153	Noodle soup, chicken	375	1½ cup
154	Wonton soup, Chinese	286	1¼ cup
155	Garlic vegetable soup	175	1 cup
156	Button mushroom soup	8	¼ cup
157	Vegetable manchow soup	197	1 cup
158	Spinach soup	204	1 cup
159	Vegetable soup	138	1 cup
160	Miso soup	97	⅓ cup

Continued

Carbohydrate Counting | 195

Continued

S No	Food items	Amount (g)	Serving
Beverages			
161	Tea with sugar	167	1⅓ glass
162	Coffee with sugar	169	1½ glass
163	Plain milk with sugar	176	1½ glass
164	Horlicks	143	1¼ glass
165	Curd	343	1¾ glass
166	Fresh fruit juice	58	½ glass
167	Soft drinks	144	¾ glass
Snacks			
168	Masala murmure (puffed rice)	23	1 cup
169	Sundal (white chickpeas)	52	⅓ cup
170	Cutlet	53	1¾ number
171	Peanut masala	67	½ cup
172	Paneer toast	29	½ number
173	Mixture	58	½ cup
174	Potato chips	26	½ cup
175	Banana chips	42	¾ cup
176	Potato Bajji	52	2½ number
177	Mysore bonda	39	1⅓ number
178	Potato bonda	42	1⅓ number
179	Pakoda	35	¾ number
180	Maddur vada	35	1¾ number
181	Urd vada	57	2½ number
182	Kachori	35	½ number
183	Thair vada (curd vada)	131	2 number
184	Karasev	26	½ cup
185	Murukku	22	½ number
186	Vegetable puff	39	½ number
187	Sweet cookies	24	1¼ number
188	Biscuits (salted)	17	1½ number
189	Biscuits (sweet/creamed)	18	1½ number
190	Bhel poori	31	⅓ cup
191	Dhokla	44	1¾ number
192	Pav bhaji	128	2¼ number
193	Popcorn	26	2¼ cup
194	Hot dog	82	¾ number

Continued

Continued

S No	Food items	Amount (g)	Serving
195	Croissant (butter), small	33	¾ number
196	Croissant (cheese), small	32	¾ number
197	Doughnut (plain), medium sized	33	¾ number
198	Doughnut (sugared/glazed), medium sized	30	¾ number
199	Cheese burger, McDonalds	54	½ number
200	Nachos with cheese	47	¼ cup
201	Taco (with beef and cheese)	76	¾ number
202	Thai lettuce roll	176	2 number
203	Dim sum (steamed wonton/bao)	31	1 number
204	Wo tou (steamed corn bun)	34	1 number
205	Garlic bread	36	¾ slice
206	Spinach (palak) corn and cheese sandwich	50	½ number
207	Mixed vegetable sandwich	48	½ number
Sweets			
208	Cake/sweet pastry	30	½ number
209	Payasam, kheer	62	⅓ cup
210	Bread pudding	57	¼ cup
211	Ice cream	64	1¾ scoop
212	Mysore pak	36	½ number
213	Peda	32	¾ number
214	Badusha	15	⅓ number
215	Kesari bhath	53	1½ Cup
216	Sweet pongal	57	¼ Cup
217	Kaju katli	43	2¼ number
218	Shrikhand	47	¼ Cup
219	Chocolate	26	¾ number
220	Besan ladoo	27	½ number
221	Boondi ladoo	22	¼ number
222	Carrot halwa	24	¾ tbsp
223	Coconut burfi	30	½ number
224	Jalebi	20	½ number
225	Kalakhand	27	½ number
226	Rasgulla	117	2⅓ number
227	Narayal doodh mithai (coconut milk sweets)	25	½ number
228	Caramel custard (flan)	66	¼ cup
229	Egg custard, baked	136	½ cup

Continued

Continued

S No	Food items	Amount (g)	Serving
230	Chocolate mousse	93	¼ cup
231	Apple pie	40	¼ slice
232	Brownie	23	½ number
Miscellaneous			
233	Jam	22	4½ tsp
234	Sugar	15	3¾ tsp
235	Honey	19	3¾ tsp
236	Jaggery	16	2⅓ tsp
237	Maple syrup	22	1 tbsp

SI, South Indian; NI, North Indian.

B. Low Carbohydrate Foods: These Foods Can Be Consumed in Moderate Amounts

Vegetables	
• Green leafy vegetable • Lady's finger • Radish • Cabbage • Beans • Cauliflower • Brinjal • Mushroom • Capsicum • Drumstick	• Bottle gourd • Ridge gourd • Chow chow marrow • Asparagus • Broccoli • Brussels sprouts • Celery • China cabbage (bok Choy) • Bamboo shoot • Wax gourd (Tung Qwa)

Note: Nonvegetarian food, nuts and some milk products are low in carbohydrates, but are very high in fat which is not good for diabetic or overweight patients.

APPENDIX 3

Seven Day Menu with Recipes and Nutritive Value

A. Recipes and Nutritive Values

Green Gram (Moong) Dal and Green Mango Salad

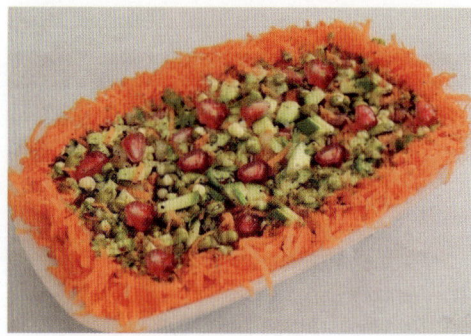

The above image indicates two servings: Weight of one serving is 80 g.

Ingredients
- Green gram (moong) sprouts: 1 cup
- Pomegranate fruit: 2 tablespoon (tbsp)
- Green mango (cut into tiny pieces): ½ cup
- Chopped coriander leaves: 2 tbsp
- Finely chopped cucumber: 2 tbsp
- Grated carrot: 2 tbsp
- Lemon juice: as required
- Salt: as required
- Black pepper powder: as required.

Method
- Mix lemon juice, salt, and pepper for the dressing
- Mix green gram sprouts, cut green mango, pomegranate, cucumber, carrot, and coriander leaves in a bowl and add dressing to it before serving.

Vegetable Cutlet (Shallow Fried)

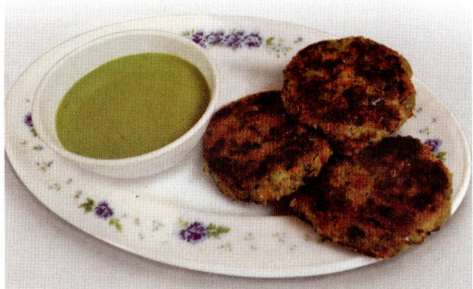

The above image indicates one and half serving: Weight of one serving is 110 g.

Ingredients

- Medium sized potato: 1
- Carrot (finely chopped): 2 tbsp
- Beans (finely chopped): 2 tbsp
- Green peas: 1 tbsp
- Corn: 1 tbsp
- Green chilli, finely chopped: 1
- Ginger, chopped: ¼ tsp
- Green coriander leaves, chopped: ½ tbsp
- Dry mango powder: ¼ tsp
- Ground black pepper: ¼ tsp
- Chilli flakes: 1½ tsp
- Oregano: ¼ tsp
- Bread crumbs: ¼ cup
- Corn flour: 1 tsp
- Salt to taste
- Oil to shallow fry.

Method

- Boil the potatoes until they are tender. Once cooked, mash the potatoes and set aside
- Boil carrot, beans, peas and corn, and drain out all the water
- Mix all the ingredients together, adjust salt and pepper to your taste (retain some amount of bread crumbs for coating at the end)
- Make flat round patties and roll them in breadcrumbs and set aside
- Heat the oil on medium heat in a frying pan and shallow fry the cutlets until golden-brown on both sides
- Serve hot.

Lady's Finger-Curd Curry (Dahi Bhindi)

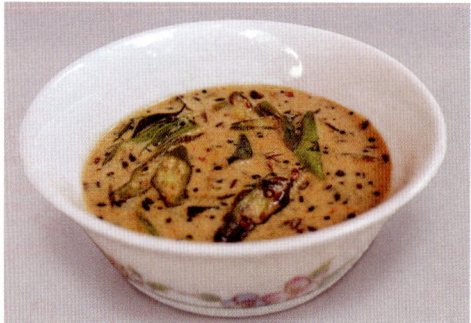

The above image indicates one serving: Weight of one serving is 70 g.

Ingredients

- Lady's finger (cut into 2 inch pieces): ¾ cup
- Low fat curds: 1 cup
- Coriander powder: 2 tsp
- Red chilli powder: 2 tsp
- Gram flour: ½ tsp
- Cumin seeds: 1 tsp
- Mustard: 1 tsp
- Fennel seeds: 1 tsp
- Asafoetida: a pinch
- Curry leaves: 5–7
- Oil: 1 tsp
- Salt to taste.

Method

- Stir fry ladie's finger till they are cooked
- Combine curds with coriander powder, red chilli powder, gram flour, salt and two tablespoons of water
- Heat oil in a non-stick pan and add the cumin seeds, mustard seeds, fennel seeds, asafoetida and curry leaves
- When seeds crackle, add curd mixture and lady's finger and bring it to boil. Simmer for 3–4 minutes
- Serve hot.

Corn Chat

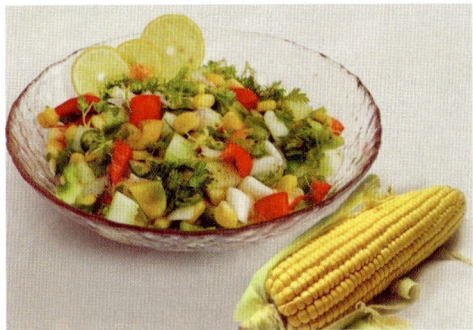

The above image indicates two servings: Weight of one serving is 75 g.

Ingredients

- American sweet corn: ½ number
- Onion: 1 medium sized
- Tomato: 1 medium sized
- Red capsicum: ¼ number
- Yellow capsicum: ¼ number
- Green capsicum: ¼ number
- Cucumber: ½ number
- Green chilli: 1 number
- White pepper powder: a pinch
- Lemon juice: 1 tbsp
- Chat masala (chat powder): ½ tsp
- Salt to taste
- Green coriander leaves (chopped) for garnish.

Method

- Remove the corn kernels from the cob and steam
- Prepare the chat dressing by mixing lemon juice, salt and chat masala (chat powder) well in a bowl. Add a pinch of white pepper
- Add finely diced cucumber, onions, deseeded and diced tomatoes, finely chopped green chilli, and capsicum to the steamed corn and toss well. Add the chat dressing over the corn mixture
- Add chopped coriander and serve.

Crunchy Salad

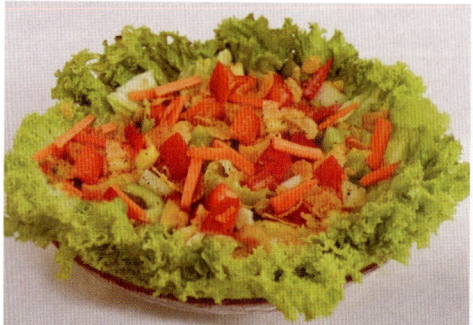

The above image indicates two servings: Weight of one serving is 65 g.

Ingredients

- Green capsicum: ¾ number
- Tomato: 1½ number
- Cucumber: ½ number
- Onion: 1 number
- Pineapple: 4 slices
- Iceberg lettuce: 4 leaves
- Corn flakes: ½ cup
- Olive oil: 2 teaspoon (tsp)
- Apple cider vinegar: 1 tsp
- Salt to taste
- Chat masala (chat powder): ¼ tsp
- Roasted cumin powder: ¼ tsp (optional)
- Lemon juice: as required

Method

- Chop the capsicum, tomato, cucumber, onion, pineapple into cubes and mix in a bowl
- Soak the iceberg lettuce in ice cold water for 10 minutes and tear the leaves into pieces
- Add corn flakes into the bowl
- Add salt, cumin powder, chat powder, lemon juice, apple cider vinegar, and olive oil, and mix well
- Serve.

Healthy Green Kebab

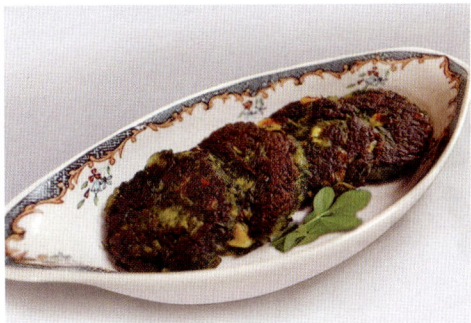

The above image indicates two servings: Weight of one serving is 90 g.

Ingredients

- Boiled potato: 200 g
- Boiled green peas: 40 g
- Boiled spinach: 40 g
- Boiled fenugreek leaves: 15 g
- Chopped green coriander leaves: 2 tsp
- Chopped green chilli: ¾ tsp
- Chopped ginger: ½ tsp
- Chat powder: ½ tsp
- Dry mango powder: ½ tsp
- Bread crumbs: 2 tbsp
- Oil: 1 tbsp
- Salt to taste.

Method

- Boil potatoes, green peas, and mash until soft
- Squeeze out excess water from the boiled spinach and methi (fenugreek) leaves—chop finely
- Finely chop green chillies, green coriander, and ginger
- Mix all the above ingredients along with chat powder, dry mango powder, and salt. Add bread crumbs for binding
- Divide the mixture into five equal parts. Shape them into a ball and then press it in between your palm to flatten it
- Shallow fry on both sides
- Serve hot.

Tortilla and Black Bean Casserole

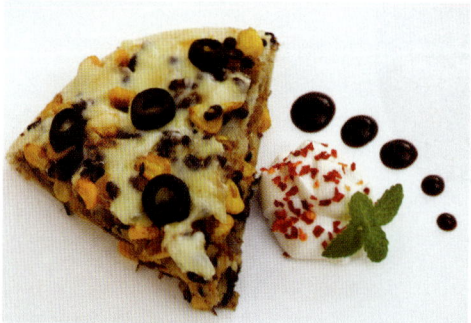

The above image indicates one serving: Weight of one serving is 150 g.

Ingredients

- For tortillas:
    - Wheat flour: 1 cup
    - Butter: 1 tbsp
    - Baking powder: ¾ tsp
    - Salt: to taste
- For casserole topping:
    - Onion: 5 medium sized, chopped
    - Green chilli: 2 number
    - Black pepper powder: ¼ tsp
    - Garlic, finely chopped: 3 number
    - Cumin powder: 1 tsp
    - Olive oil: 1 tbsp
    - Black beans: 2 cups, soaked overnight
    - Vegetable stock: 1 cup
    - Sweet corn kernels: 1 cup
    - Low fat cheddar cheese, grated: ½ cup
    - Salt to taste.

To Make Vegetable Stock

Chop one cup of mixed vegetables (carrots, beans, cauliflower, cabbage, potato) and boil it in three cups of water until the liquid is reduced to half. Drain the water from the vegetables and you have your stock ready.

Method

Tortilla
- In a bowl mix flour, salt, and baking powder. Add butter to it and mix it well between the palm of your hands until the ingredients are evenly mixed. Add about one-third cup of warm water and knead the dough well until it is soft and is not sticky. Divide the dough into four round balls and roll it to the diameter that is 1 inch smaller than the tin you are using to bake the casserole.

Casserole
- Add oil to a pan and sauté one-third of the chopped onions, chopped green chilli, black pepper, and cumin powder till onions are soft. Add garlic and cook for a minute
- Drain the water from the beans and add it to the above mixture along with the vegetable stock. Boil it and cook until the liquid is reduced to about one-third of its original volume. Add the remaining chopped onions, sweet corn, and salt. Sauté well until cooked. Remove the pan from the heat and divide the contents into four parts
- Grease the baking tin with a few drops of oil. Place one tortilla on the base and cover it with one-fourth of the topping mixture and sprinkle one-fourth of the grated cheese over it. Repeat this until you have four layers of tortilla and topping
- Now place the tin in a preheated oven at 180°C for about 15–20 minutes or until heated through. Remove sides of the pan and slice the casserole into wedges and serve hot.

Note: The above recipe makes four servings.

Caesar Salad

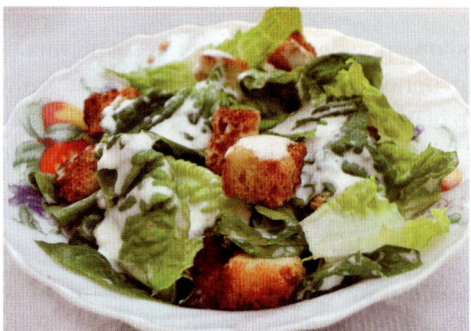

The above image indicates one serving: Weight of one serving is 210 g.

Ingredients

- Grated Parmesan cheese: ½ tbsp
- Low fat mayonnaise: ½ tbsp
- Milk: ½ tbsp
- Lemon juice: ½ tbsp
- Garlic salt/powder: ¼ tsp
- Romaine lettuce: 5 leaves
- Salad croutons: as desired
- Salt to taste.

To Make Salad Croutons

Mix one tsp olive oil with a pinch of salt and ½ tbsp dried garlic powder. Take two bread slices, trim the edges off, and cut into small cubes. Mix the bread cubes with olive oil mixture and bake it at 180°C for 10–15 minutes.

Method

- Make the salad dressing by whisking the mayonnaise, cheese, milk, lemon juice, garlic, and salt in a small bowl
- Cut the lettuce into small pieces and place it in a large bowl
- Drizzle with dressing and toss well to coat the lettuce
- Serve with salad croutons.

Spaghetti with Tomato and Cheese Sauce

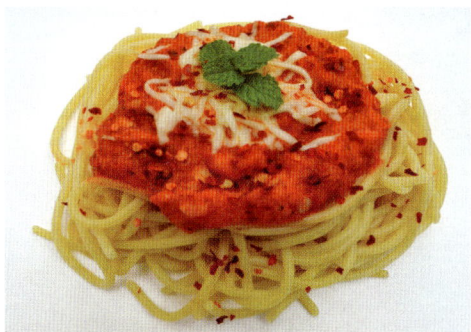

The above image indicates one serving: Weight of one serving is 250 g.

Ingredients

- Spaghetti: 100 g
- Garlic, peeled and sliced: 1 cloves
- Low fat feta cheese: 10 g
- Tomatoes, boiled and pureed: 3 number
- Fresh basil leaves (Tulsi): 5
- Chilli flakes: 1 tsp
- Oregano: ½ tsp
- Salt to taste
- Olive oil: 1 tbsp.

Method

- Heat olive oil in a pan and when the oil sizzles, add garlic and sauté for a minute
- Add the pureed tomatoes and salt, and mix well
- Cut the feta cheese into small cubes and add it to the sauce
- Allow the sauce to cook for about 15 minutes or until it reduces to about half its original volume
- Now, chop the basil leaves (tulsi) into small pieces and add to the sauce. Allow it to cook in the sauce for 2 minutes
- Add oregano and chilli flakes and sauté for about a minute
- Cook the spaghetti in hot water with a teaspoon of oil
- Once the spaghetti is cooked, drain the water, rinse the spaghetti in cool running water, and keep aside
- Finally mix the cooked spaghetti with the sauce and toss everything gently until the sauce is evenly coated on the spaghetti
- Serve hot.

Tossed Salad

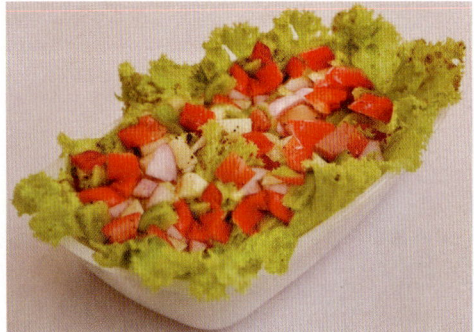

The above image indicates two servings: Weight of one serving is 75 g.

Ingredients

- Iceberg lettuce: ½ number
- Green capsicum: ¾ number
- Cucumber: ½ number
- Tomato: 1 number
- Onion: 1 number

Dressing

- Olive oil: 2 tbsp
- Balsamic vinegar: ½ tbsp
- Lemon juice: 1 tbsp
- Salt to taste
- Black pepper powder: as desired.

Method

- Wash all the vegetables thoroughly
- Cut the capsicum and onion into cubes
- Deseed the tomatoes and cucumber; cut them the size of the capsicum pieces
- Tear the lettuce into small pieces and keep them in ice cold water for sometime
- Mix vinegar, lemon juice, olive oil and to it, add pepper and salt. Mix it well
- Mix all the ingredients and season it with the oil-vinegar mixture just before serving.

Thai Lettuce Roll

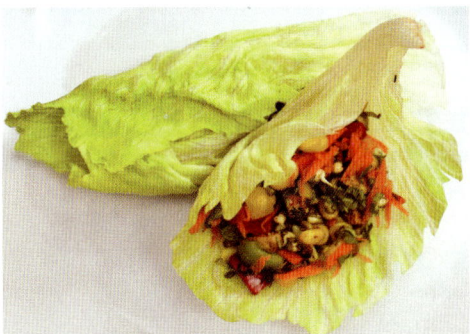

The above image indicates two servings: Weight of one serving is 100 g.

Ingredients

- Fresh iceberg lettuce: 2 leaves
- Ginger, grated: ½ tsp
- Garlic, finely chopped: 2 cloves
- Green chilli: 2 number
- Red and yellow capsicum, diced: 3 tbsp
- Onions, sliced: 1 number
- Cottage cheese, cut into thin strips: 4 tbsp
- Carrot, julienned: ½ number
- American sweet corn: 3 tbsp
- Shredded cabbage: 4 tbsp
- Celery: ½ stalk
- Green gram (moong) sprouts: ½ cup
- Lime juice: 1 tbsp
- Soy sauce: 1 tsp
- Chilli sauce: 1 tsp
- Oil for stir-frying: 1 tbsp.

Method

- Heat oil in a wok and add garlic, ginger. Add green chilli, onions, and celery. Stir-fry for 1 minute
- Add cottage cheese, carrot, sweet corn, cabbage and capsicum. While you stir-fry, add lime juice, soy sauce, and chilli sauce and sauté for a minute
- Add the green gram (moong) sprouts and stir-fry briefly to mix. Remove from heat and add salt to taste. Your filling is ready
- Separate the leaves of the lettuce and place 1–2 heaped tablespoons of filling in the center of each lettuce leaf
- Roll it and serve.

Tofu Pad Sew

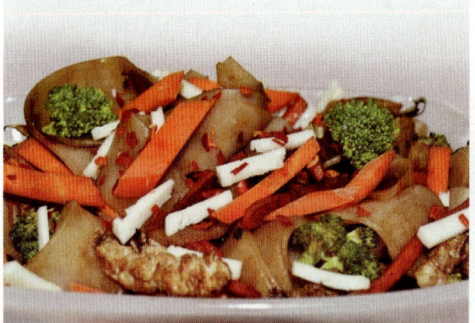

The above image indicates one serving: Weight of one serving is 150 g.

Ingredients

- Dried, flat rice noodles (pad sew): 100 g
- Fresh lime juice: 1 tbsp
- Soy sauce: 1 tbsp
- Tabasco sauce: 1 tsp
- Green chilli: 1 number
- Sugar: ¼ tsp
- Oil: 1 tbsp
- Egg whites, lightly beaten: 1 number
- Firm tofu, drained, thinly sliced and patted dry: ¼ cup
- Cabbage, shredded: ¼ cup
- Broccoli, chopped: ¼ cup
- Carrots, peeled and shredded: 1 medium sized
- Garlic, minced: 2 cloves
- Spring onions, white and green parts separated and thinly sliced: 4 number
- Salt to taste
- Fresh cilantro leaves: 3 tbsp.

Method

- Boil the noodles for 4–5 minutes and drain the water immediate and rinse it with cold water
- In a small bowl, whisk together lime juice, soy sauce, tobasco sauce, and sugar
- Coat a pan with half teaspoons of oil on a medium flame and add egg white and swirl the pan to coat the bottom and cook until just set, about 1 minute. Transfer it to a plate and cut it into thin strips

- Add four teaspoons oil to a wok and heat. Add tofu and cook until golden brown on both sides. Remove from heat and keep aside
- Now cook carrots, broccoli, cabbage, garlic, spring onion whites, and green chilli in a pan with one teaspoons oil and add lime juice mixture to it. Add noodles and cook, stirring frequently for a minute. Add egg and tofu and gently toss to combine. Season to taste with salt
- Divide among four plates and top with cilantro and spring onion greens and serve hot.

Dim Sum

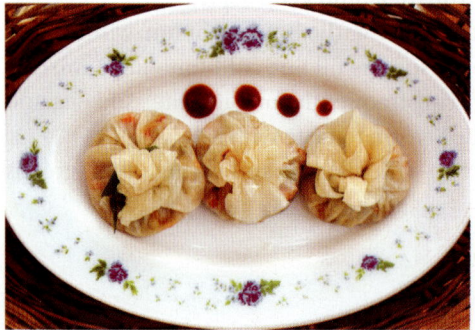

The above image indicates one serving: Weight of one serving is 105 g.

Ingredients

- Dough:
  - Refined wheat flour: ½ cup
  - Salt to taste.
- Filling:
  - Finely chopped mixed vegetables (cabbage, carrot, beans): 4 tbsp
  - Oil: 1 tsp
  - Onion, finely chopped: 2 tbsp
  - Garlic, chopped: ¼ tsp
  - Salt to taste
  - Vinegar: ¼ tsp
  - Black pepper: ¼ tsp.

Method

- Mix the refined wheat flour and salt and knead to a stiff dough, with water
- Heat oil and add the onion and garlic. Sauté till a little soft and add the vegetables
- Continue to sauté till the vegetables are slightly cooked
- Take it off the heat and mix in the salt, vinegar, and black pepper
- Roll the dough thin (translucent) and cut into 4–5 inch circular sheets
- Take a sheet and place some filling in the center. Bring the edges together and press to seal
- Steam for about 10 minutes and serve.

Vegetable Soba Noodles

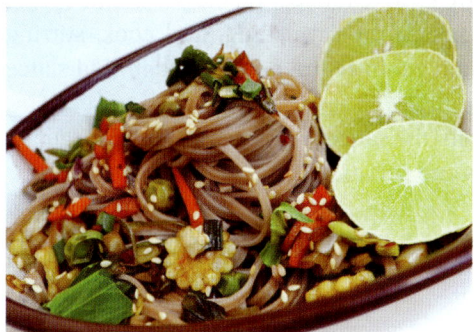

The above image indicates one serving: Weight of one serving is 235 g.

Ingredients

- For sauce:
    - Water: 1/3 cup
    - Soy sauce: 2 tbsp
    - Tabasco sauce: 2 tsp
    - Brown sugar: 1 tsp
    - Chilli flakes: 1 tsp
- For noodles:
    - Sesame seeds: 1 tbsp
    - Oil: 1 tbsp
    - Ginger, finely chopped: 1 tsp
    - Garlic, finely chopped: 1 tsp
    - Baby corn, sliced: ¼ cup
    - Cabbage, thinly sliced: ¼ cup
    - Spring onions, thinly sliced: 3 number
    - Soba (buckwheat noodles): 70 g
    - Green peas: ¼ cup.

Method

- Mix the water, soy sauce, tabasco, sugar, and chilli flakes well and keep it aside
- Roast sesame seeds in a dry pan over low or medium heat until pale golden and keep it aside in a small bowl
- Cook soba noodles in a pot of boiling salted water until noodles are just tender. Drain the water, rinse in running cold water and keep aside

- Heat oil in a wok over medium-high heat and sauté ginger and garlic for half a minute. To this add baby corn, cabbage, green peas, and spring onions leaving aside one teaspoon for garnishing, and cook, stirring occasionally, until baby corn and cabbage are a little tender. Add sauce and simmer for 2 minutes
- Mix the cooked soba noodles with the sauce and vegetable mixture gently and garnish with spring onions and serve.

B. Seven Day Sample Menu

	Day 1 Monday (South Indian)	Day 2 Tuesday (North Indian)	Day 3 Wednesday (Indian)	Day 4 Thursday (Continental)	Day 5 Friday (Continental)	Day 6 Saturday (Pan Asian)	Day 7 Sunday (Pan Asian)
Early morning	Coffee/green tea	Coffee/green tea	Coffee/green tea	Coffee/green tea	Coffee/green tea	Coffee/green tea	Coffee/green tea
Breakfast	Vegetable upma	Tomato chapatti	Idli	Brown bread toast	Oats/cornflakes/muesli	Congee with vegetables	Rice
	Green tomato chutney	Skimmed curds	Sambhar and mint chutney	Egg white scrambled	Skimmed milk	Boiled egg white	Miso soup
	Fruit	Fruit	Fruit	Fruit	Raisins and walnuts		Fruit
Mid-morning	Roasted peanuts	Masala murmure (puffed rice)	Steamed green gram sprouts	Boiled corn	Fruit salad	Thai lettuce roll	Egg roll
Lunch	Plain rice	Tandoori chapatti	Chapatti	Pasta in tomato sauce	Mashed potato	Vegetable fried rice	Chicken noodle soup
	Sambhar with vegetables	Brinjal curry	Black gram curry	Garlic bread	Grilled chicken sandwich	Lemon chicken	Steamed wonton/ Dim sum
	Round gourd curry/thondaikai curry	Ladie's finger-curd curry	Plain rice	Caesar salad	Steamed vegetables	Asparagus salad	Vegetable salad
	Green gram dal and green mango salad	Sprouts salad	Ladie's finger curry				
	Skimmed buttermilk	Fruit	Crunchy salad				
	Fruit		Fruit				
Tea	Tea	Tea	Tea	Tea	Tea	Tea	Tea
	Vegetable cutlet (shallow fried)	Corn chat	Healthy green kebab	Spinach corn sandwich	Mixed vegetable sandwich	Wo Tou (steamed corn bun)	Tofu Bao (steamed bun)

Continued

Continued

	Day 1 Monday (South Indian)	Day 2 Tuesday (North Indian)	Day 3 Wednesday (Indian)	Day 4 Thursday (Continental)	Day 5 Friday (Continental)	Day 6 Saturday (Pan Asian)	Day 7 Sunday (Pan Asian)
Dinner	Vegetable soup	Tomato soup	Spinach soup	Broccoli soup	Chicken herb soup	Vegetable manchow soup	Tom yum soup
	Sorghum (jowar) chapatti	Fenugreek leaves (methi) paratha	Fenugreek (methi) leaves	Tortilla and black bean casserole	Spaghetti in tomato and cheese sauce	Tofu Pad Thai	Vegetable soba noodles
	Whole gram curry	Kadhi	Bengal gram dal curry	Greek salad	Tossed salad		Steamed fish
	Brinjal curry	Bitter gourd curry	Cauliflower curry			Fruit	
	Skimmed curd	Fruit	Skimmed curd				
Nonvegetarian							
Recipes	Green gram dal and green mango salad	Lady's finger-curd curry	Crunchy salad	Tortilla and black bean casserole	Spaghetti in tomato and cheese sauce	Thai lettuce roll	Dim sum
	Vegetable cutlet (shallow fried)	Corn chat	Healthy green kebab	Caesar salad	Tossed salad	Tofu Pad Thai	Vegetable soba noodles

Note:
- Use minimum oil while cooking paratha, curry, and fried rice.
- Restrict fruits high in glycemic index like banana, mango, pineapple, custard apple, sapodilla (chikoo) and jackfruit.
- Add minimum amount of butter while baking garlic bread.
- Use a small portion of low fat feta cheese to make Greek salad.
- Use whole wheat flour to make tortillas.
- Serve steamed or boiled vegetables with Congee.
- Use a cabbage filling for steamed wontons.

APPENDIX 4

Sample Exchange List

A. Images of Standard Measurements

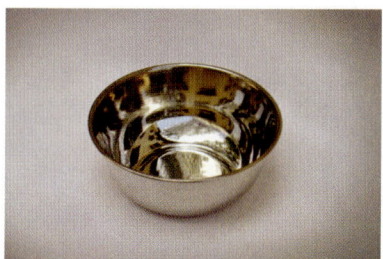

Cup (1 cup = 150 g)

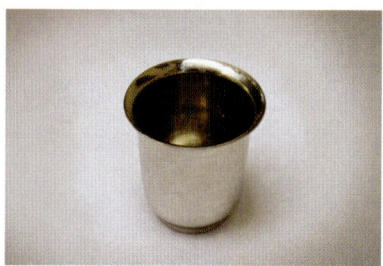

Glass (1 glass = 120 mL)

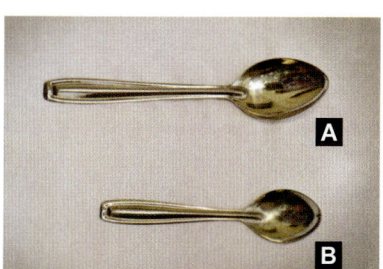

A, Tablespoon (1 tablespoon = 15 g);
B, Teaspoon (1 teaspoon = 5 g)

B. Sample Exchange List for Continental Menu

		1,200 kcal		1,400 kcal		1,600 kcal		1,800 kcal		2,000 kcal	
		Serving	Amount	Serving	Amount	Serving	Amount	Serving	Amount	Serving	Amount
Early morning	Coffee/green tea	1 glass	120 mL	1 glass	120 mL	1 glass	120 mL	1 glass	120 mL	1 glass	120 mL
Breakfast	Brown bread toast	2 number	48 g	2 number	48 g	3 number	72 g	3 number	72 g	4 number	96 g
	Egg white, scrambled	1 number	35 g	1 number	35 g	2 number	70 g	2 number	70 g	2 number	70 g
	Fruit	1 number	100 g	1 number	100 g	1 number	100 g	1 number	100 g	1 number	100 g
Mid-morning	Boiled corn	½ cup	75 g	½ cup	75 g	½ cup	75 g	1 cup	150 g	1 cup	150 g
Lunch	Pasta in tomato sauce	½ cup	125 g	½ cup	125 g	¾ cup	187 g	1 cup	250 g	1 cup	250 g
	Garlic bread	1 slice	43 g	1 slice	43 g	1 slice	43 g	1 slice	43 g	2 slices	86 g
	Caesar salad	½ cup	106 g	½ cup	106 g	¾ cup	160 g	1 cup	213 g	1 cup	213 g
Tea	Tea	½ glass	60 mL	1 glass	120 mL	1 glass	120 mL	1 glass	120 mL	1 glass	120 mL
	Spinach corn sandwich	½ number	46 g	1 number	92 g	1 number	92 g	1 number	92 g	1 number	92 g
Dinner	Broccoli soup	½ cup	125 g	¾ cup	187 g	1 cup	250 g	1 cup	250 g	1 cup	250 g
	Tortilla and black bean casserole	1 slice	150 g	1 slice	150 g	1 slice	150 g	1 slice	150 g	1 slice	150 g
	Greek salad	½ cup	53 g	¾ cup	80 g	¾ cup	80 g	1 cup	106 g	1 cup	106 g

C. Sample Exchange List for Pan Asian Menu

		1,200 kcal		1,400 kcal		1,600 kcal		1,800 kcal		2,000 kcal	
		Serving	Amount	Serving	Amount	Serving	Amount	Serving	Amount	Serving	Amount
Early morning	Coffee/tea	1 glass	120 mL	1 glass	120 mL	1 glass	120 mL	1 glass	120 mL	1 glass	120 mL
Breakfast	Congee with vegetables	¾ cup	130 g	1 cup	170 g	1¼ cup	212 g	1½ cup	255 g	2 cups	340 g
	Boiled egg white	1 number	33 g	1 number	33 g	1 number	33 g	2 number	66 g	2 number	66 g
	Thai lettuce roll	2 number	200 g	2 number	200 g	2 number	200 g	2 number	200 g	2 number	200 g
Mid-morning	Vegetable fried rice	1 cup	170 g	1 cup	170 g	1¼ cup	212 g	1½ cup	255 g	1¾ cup	298 g
Lunch	Lemon chicken	2 pieces	50 g	3 pieces	75 g	3 pieces	75 g	3 pieces	75 g	4 pieces	100 g
	Asparagus salad	½ cup	90 g	¾ cup	135 g	¾ cup	135 g	1 cup	180 g	1 cup	180 g
Tea	Tea	1 glass	120 mL	1 glass	120 mL	1 glass	120 mL	1 glass	120 mL	1 glass	120 mL
	Wo Tou (steamed corn bun)	2 number	70 g	3 number	105 g	3 number	105 g	3 number	105 g	3 number	105 g
Dinner	Vegetable manchow soup	½ cup	103 g	1 cup	207 g	1 cup	207 g	1 cup	207 g	1 cup	207 g
	Tofu Pad Thai	¾ cup	113 g	1 cup	150 g	1 cup	150 g	1½ cup	225 g	1½ cup	225 g
	Fruit	1 number	100 g	1 number	100 g	1 number	100 g	1 number	100 g	1 number	100 g

D. Sample Exchange List for Indian Menu

		1,200 kcal		1,400 kcal		1,600 kcal		1,800 kcal		2,000 kcal	
		Serving	Amount	Serving	Amount	Serving	Amount	Serving	Amount	Serving	Amount
Early morning	Coffee/green tea	1 glass	120 mL	1 glass	120 mL	1 glass	120 mL	1 glass	120 mL	1 glass	120 mL
Breakfast	Idli	2 number	90 g	2	90 g	3 number	135 g	4 number	180 g	5 number	225 g
	Sambhar	1/2 cup	70 g	1/2 cup	70 g	1/2 cup	70 g	3/4 cup	105 g	1 cup	140 g
	Mint chutney	2 tbsp	30 g	2 tbsp	30 g	2 tbsp	30 g	3 tbsp	45 g	3 tbsp	45 g
	Fruit	1 number	100 g	1	100 g	1 number	100 g	1 number	100 g	1 number	100 g
Mid-morning	Steamed green gram sprouts	1/4 cup	40 g	1/2 cup	80 g	1/2 cup	80 g	1/2 cup	80 g	1/2 cup	80 g
Lunch	Chapatti	1 number	22 g	1 number	22 g	1½ number	33 g	2 number	44 g	2½ number	55 g
	Black gram dal curry	1/2 cup	70 g	1/2 cup	70 g	3/4 cup	105 g	3/4 cup	105 g	3/4 cup	105 g
	Plain rice	1/2 cup	75 g	1/2 cup	75 g	1/2 cup	75 g	1/2 cup	75 g	1/2 cup	75 g
	Lady's finger curry	6 tbsp	120 g	6 tbsp	120 g	8 tbsp	160 g	9 tbsp	180 g	10 tbsp	200 g
	Crunchy salad	1 cup	65 g	1 cup	65 g	1 cup	65 g	1 cup	65 g	1 cup	65 g
	Fruit	1 number	100 g	1 number	100 g	1 number	100 g	1 number	100 g	1 number	100 g
Tea	Tea	1/2 glass	60 mL	1 glass	120 mL	1 glass	120 mL	1 glass	120 mL	1 glass	120 mL
	Healthy green kebab	1 number	43 g	1 number	43 g	1 number	43 g	2 number	86 g	2 number	86 g
Dinner	Spinach soup	1/2 cup	75 g	1/2 cup	75 g	1/2 cup	75 g	1/2 cup	75 g	3/4 cup	115 g
	Methi (fenugreek) leaves paratha	1 number	28 g	1½ number	42 g	2 number	56 g	2 number	56 g	2	56 g
	Bengal gram dal curry	1/2 cup	70 g	1/2 cup	70 g	1/2 cup	70 g	1/2 cup	70 g	1/2 cup	70 g
	Cauliflower curry	3 tbsp	100 g	3 tbsp	100 g	4 tbsp	130 g	4 tbsp	130 g	5 tbsp	160 g
	Skimmed curd	3/4 glass	75 g	1 glass	100 g	1 glass	100 g	1 glass	100 g	1 glass	100 g

tbsp, tablespoon; tsp, teaspoon.

E. Example of Sample Exchange with Images

	Early morning	Breakfast	Mid-morning	Lunch	Evening snack	Dinner
1,200 kcal	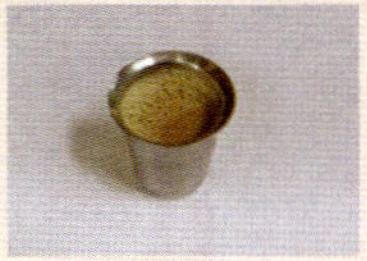 1 glass coffee	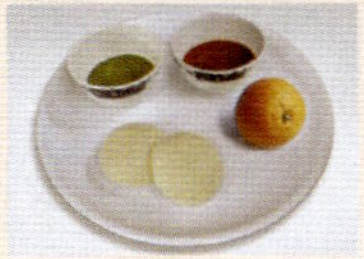 2 Idli, ½ cup sambhar, 2 tbsp chutney, 1 fruit	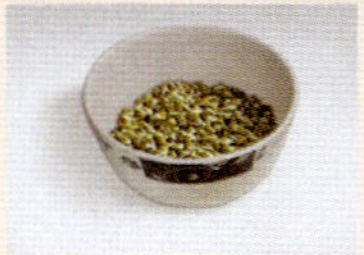 ¼ cup steamed green gram sprouts	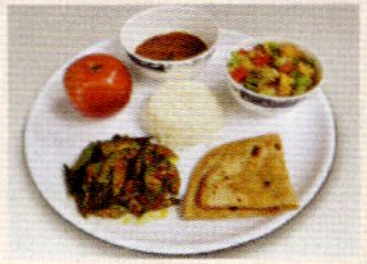 1 chapatti, ½ cup black gram dal, ½ cup rice, 6 tbsp ladies' finger curry, 1 cup salad, 1 fruit	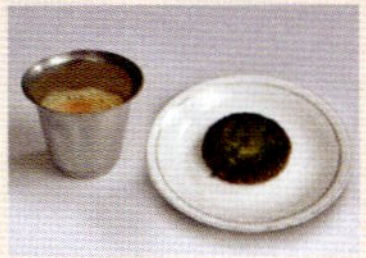 ½ glass tea, 1 healthy green kebab	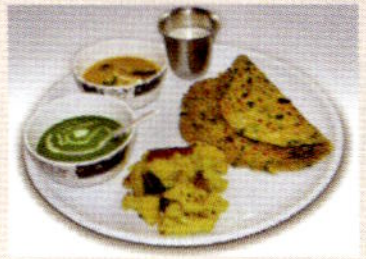 ½ cup spinach soup, 1 fenugreek paratha, ½ cup Bengal gram dal, 3 tbsp cauliflower curry, ¾ glass skimmed curd
1,600 kcal	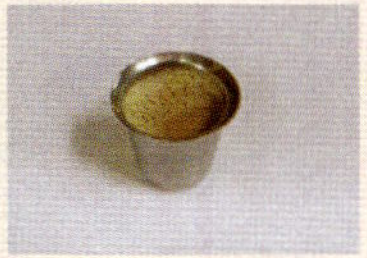 1 glass coffee	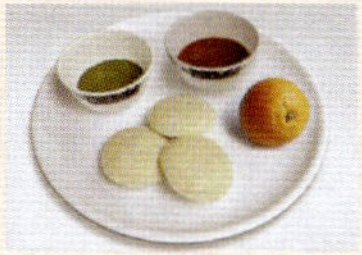 3 Idli, ½ cup sambhar, 2 tbsp chutney, 1 fruit	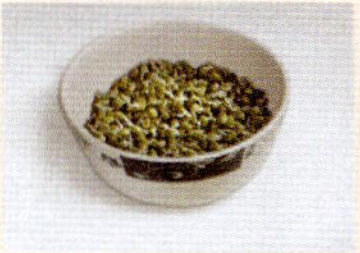 ½ cup steamed green gram sprouts	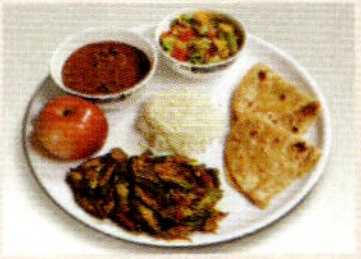 1½ chapatti, ¾ cup black gram dal, ½ cup rice, 8 tbsp ladies' finger curry, 1 cup salad, 1 fruit	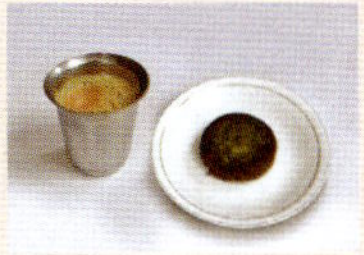 1 glass tea, 1 healthy green kebab	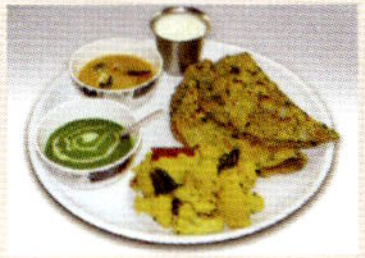 ½ cup spinach soup, 2 fenugreek paratha, ½ cup Bengal gram dal, 4 tbsp cauliflower curry, 1 glass skimmed curd
2,000 kcal	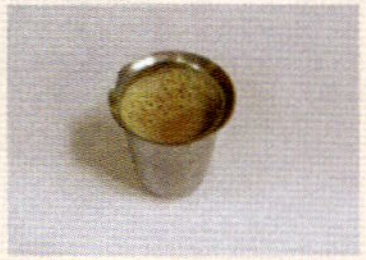 1 glass coffee	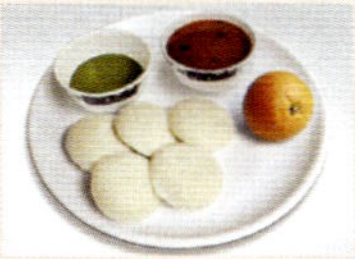 5 Idli, 1 cup sambhar, 3 tbsp chutney, 1 fruit	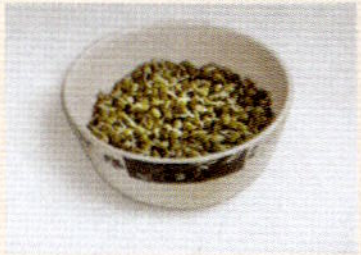 ½ cup steamed green gram sprouts	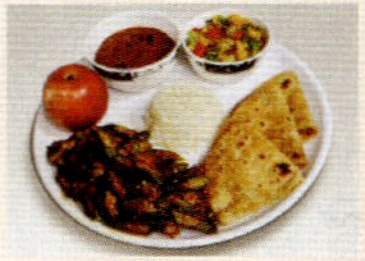 2½ chapatti, ¾ cup black gram dal, ½ cup rice, 10 tbsp ladies' finger curry, 1 cup salad, 1 fruit	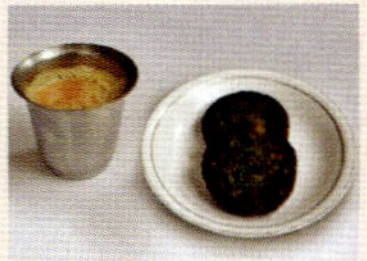 1 glass tea, 2 healthy green kebab	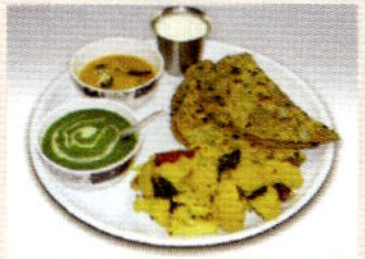 ¾ cup spinach soup, 2 fenugreek paratha, ½ cup Bengal gram dal, 5 tbsp cauliflower curry, 1 glass skimmed curd

APPENDIX 5

Energy Cost of Common Activities

Category	Activity	PAR
Conditioning exercise	Mild stretching, stretching, hatha yoga	2.5
	Calisthenics (e.g., push-ups, sit-ups, pull-ups, jumping jacks), heavy vigorous effort	8
	Weight lifting, free weight, power lifting or body building, vigorous effort	6
	Weight lifting, free, general, light or moderate effort	3
	Health club exercise, general	5.5
	Stair-treadmill ergometer, general	9
Running	Jogging, general	7
Dancing	Aerobics, general	6.5
	Ballroom, slow dancing, samba, tango, cha cha	3
	Ballroom, fast (disco, folk, square), line dancing, Irish step dancing, polka, contra, country	4.5
Home activities	Washing clothes (sitting, indoor)	2.6
	Carpet sweeping, sweeping floors	3.3
	Cleaning, heavy or major (e.g., wash car, wash windows, clean garage), vigorous effort	3
	Wash dishes: standing or in general (not broken into stand/walk components)	2.3
	Mopping, vacuuming	3.5
	Putting away groceries (e.g., carrying groceries, shopping without a grocery cart), carrying packages, cooking or food preparation: walking, serving food, setting table, implied walking or standing	2.5
	Kneading dough	3.4
	Making tortillas/chapattis, scraping coconut	2.4

Continued

Continued

Category	Activity	PAR
	Sitting-knitting, sewing, wrapping presents, peeling vegetables	1.5
	Implied standing: laundry, fold or hand clothes, put clothes in washer or dryer, packing suitcase, making bed	2
	Implied walking: putting away clothes, gathering clothes to pack, putting away laundry, ironing	2.3
	Moving furniture, household items, carrying boxes	6
	Scrubbing floors, on hands and knees, scrubbing bathroom, bathtub	3.8
	Sweeping garage, sidewalk or outside of house	4
	Sitting-playing with child(ren)-light, only active periods	2.5
	Standing-playing with child(ren)-light, only active periods	2.8
	Walk/run-playing with child(ren)-moderate, only active periods	4
	Walk/run-playing with child(ren)-vigorous, only active periods	5
	Child care, standing-dressing, bathing, grooming, feeding occasional lifting of child—light effort, carrying small children, window cleaning	3
	Elder care, disabled adult, only active periods	4
	Breastfeeding	1.1
	Cleaning grains, deshelling groundnuts	1.2
	Walk, run, playing with animals, moderate, only active periods	4
	Watering plants, feeding animals	2.5
Home repair	Carpentry, general, workshop, wiring, plumbing	3
	Laying or removing carpet, painting	4.5
	Eating and drinking	1.4
	Roofing	6
Inactivity, quite	Lying, sitting quietly and watching television, listening to music, lying in bed awake, watching a movie in theater, reclining-writing, reading, talking or talking on phone, meditating	1
	Sleeping	0.9
	Standing quietly (standing in a line)	1.2
Fishing	Fishing, general	3
Gardening	Gardening, general	4
Music	Drums	4
	Flute (sitting), horn	2
	Piano or organ, trumpet, violin, conducting	2.5
	Guitar, classical, folk (sitting)	2
	Guitar, rock and roll band (standing)	3
	Marching band, drum major (walking)	3.5

Continued

Continued

Category	Activity	PAR
Occupation	Bakery, general	3.2
	Building road (including hauling debris, driving heavy machinery), using heavy power tools such as pneumatic tools (jackhammers, drills, etc.), coal mining, general	6
	Carpentry, general, electric work, plumbing	3.5
	Carrying heavy loads, such as bricks, moving boxes, carrying moderate load upstairs, forestry, general	8
	Construction, outside, remodeling	5.5
	Custodial work: cleaning sink, toilet, dusting, vacuuming, light effort, chambermaid, making bed (nursing)	2.5
	Custodial work: general cleaning, mopping, moderate effort	3.5
	Farming, general	4.3
	Fire fighter, general	12
	Machine tooling, general	3.6
	Masonry, concrete	7
	Moving, pushing heavy objects, 34 kg or more (desks, moving van work)	7.5
	Operating heavy duty equipment/automated, not driving, tailoring, general, shoe repair, general, police, directing traffic (standing)	2.5
	Printing (standing)	2.3
	Steel mill, general	7.4
	Truck driving, loading and unloading truck (standing)	6.5
	Typing, electric, manual or computer	1.5
	Walking on job, <3.2 km/hour (in office or laboratory area) very slow	2
	Walking on job, 4.8 km/hour, in office, moderate speed, not carrying anything	3.3
	Walking on job, 5.6 km/hour, in office, brisk speed, not carrying anything	3.8
	Walking, pushing a wheelchair, teach physical education, exercise, sports classes (non-sport play)	4
	Digging	5.6
Occupation: Military training	Drill	4.5
	March (slow)	3.2
	March 2–4 m/hour (3.2–6.4 km/h) with 27 kg load	4.9
Self-care	Bathing (sitting), eating (sitting)	1.5
	Grooming (washing, shaving, brushing teeth, washing hands, putting on make-up), sitting or standing, dressing, undressing, talking and eating or eating only (standing)	2
	Hairstyling	2.5

Continued

Continued

Category	Activity	PAR
Sports	Billiards	2.5
	Bowling, Frisbee playing, general	3
	Archery (non-hunting)	3.5
	Coaching: football, soccer, basketball, baseball, swimming, etc. Gymnastics, general, horseback riding, general, juggling, kickball, table tennis, ping pong, volleyball, track and field (short, discuss, hammer throw)	4
	Badminton, social singles and doubles, general, golf, general	4.5
	Cricket (batting, bowling), children's games (hopscotch, four-square, dodge ball, playground apparatus, marbles, jacks), skateboarding, tennis, doubles	5
	Boxing, punching bag, drag racing, pushing or driving a car, track and field (high jump, long jump, triple jump, javelin, pole vault)	6
	Badminton, competitive, skating, roller, soccer, casual, general, tennis, general, swimming laps, freestyle, slow, moderate or light effort	7
	Basketball (game), hockey (field), polo	8
	Football, competitive	9
	Judo, karate, kick boxing, rope jumping, moderate, general, track and field (steeplechase, hurdles), swimming laps, freestyle, fast, vigorous effort	10
	Boxing, in ring, general, handball, general, squash	12
Transportation	Bicycling, general	8
	Bicycling, cycling on a dirt road	7
	Automobile or light truck (not a semi) driving	2
	Riding in a car, bus or truck	1
	Motor scooter, motorcycle	2.5
	Driving heavy truck, tractor, bus	3
	Walking around/strolling	2.1
	Walking slowly	2.8
	Walking quickly	3.8
	Walking uphill	7.1
	Walking downhill	3.5
	Climbing stairs	5
	Pulling a rickshaw (one person/no load)	5.3
	Pulling a rickshaw (two person)	7.2

PAR, physical activity ratio.

Suggested Readings

1. Ainsworth BE, Haskell WL, Whitt MC, Irwin ML, Swartz AM, Strath SJ, et al. Compendium of physical activities: an update of activity codes and MET intensities. Med Sci Sports Exerc. 2000;32(9): S498-504.
2. Joint FAO/WHO/UNU. (2004). Human energy requirements. Report of a Joint FAO/WHO/UNU Expert Consultation, Rome, 17–24 Oct 2001. FAO Food and Nutrition Technical Report Series 1 [online] Available from: www.fao.org/3/contents/64705f04-87cc-556d-8292-ee763b53a102/y5686e00.htm. [Accessed August, 2014].
3. Rao S, Gokhale M, Kanade A. Energy costs of daily activities for women in rural India. Public Health Nutr. 2008;11(2):142-50.
4. Sujatha T, Shatrugna V, Venkataramana Y, Begum N. Energy expenditure on household, childcare and occupational activities of women from urban poor households. Br J Nutr. 2000;83(5):497-503.

APPENDIX 6

Case Studies

Case 1: Childhood Obesity

A 12-year-old visits the nutrition clinic with her parents. Her weight is 76.6 kg, and she is 159.8 cm tall. Her parents are concerned about her weight. Her eating habits and nutritional status are given below:
- Body mass index (BMI): 29.9 kg/m^2
- Dietary assessment
    - Eats large quantities of rice three times a day
    - Does not snack much, but prefers to eat three large meals
    - Water intake is low
    - Eats her meals in front of the television (TV)
    - Does not like to eat vegetables
- Other habits
    - She is sedentary and prefers to watch TV most of the time
    - Feels shy to involve in any form of games in the evening
    - Sleeps for 5–6 hours everyday

Dietary history also reveals that about 4–5 L of oil is used per month for a four-member family in cooking.

Questions

1. How will you classify her BMI?
2. What dietary changes would you suggest for her?
3. What are the behavioral modifications that she can begin to make?
4. How important are her parent's role in the treatment plan?

Answers

1. The child is classified as obese, based on BMI for her age.
2. The dietary changes that can be suggested for her include:

- Consume small frequent meals rather than large meals
- Increase water intake
- The child needs to be encouraged to increase her vegetable intake. Suggestions can be provided to the mother to serve it in an attractive way, i.e., chapatti roll with vegetable filling, stuffed parathas and grilled sandwich with leftover vegetables.

3. The behavioral modifications that she can begin to make are
   - Eating meals together with the entire family
   - Avoiding watching TV during meal times and to restrict TV viewing
   - To sleep for a minimum of 7–8 hours/day
   - The parents should be advised to encourage the child in some form of sports or recreational activity.

4. Parents are integral to the child's dietary plan and need to be involved in the entire process, therefore:
   - Imparting *nutrition education* to the parents is of primary importance.
   - Educating the mother on healthy methods of cooking will ensure a decrease in the fat content of the meals and increase in fiber content.
   - Parents should ensure that the availability of junk foods and fried snacks are minimal in the household to decrease its frequency of consumption.
   - The parents need to be reminded that they are the role models for the child and thus bringing about a change in the eating habits of the entire family will encourage the child to adhere to dietary guidelines more efficiently.

> **Important**
>
> Any change in the diet and lifestyle should be slowly incorporated to the childs daily routine in order to attain sustainable changes.

Case 2: Adult Obesity

Neeru is a 31-year-old lady. Her weight has been gradually increasing in the last 3 months by 6 kg. Currently she weighs 67 kg and is 147 cm tall. She has a strong family history of obesity with both of her parents being obese. She is an Assistant Manager at a firm and leads a sedentary lifestyle. She reports having no time for any physical activity and manages to get barely 4 hours of sleep. Since she has to reach her office by 7.30 am, she is not able to make time for breakfast and her lunch is often from the office cafeteria. Dinner is her main meal and she eats it around 11.00 pm. She reveals that she has tried numerous weight loss regimes for short-term with no success. Her goal is now to lose 6 kg weight in a month and wants a very low-calorie diet to attain her goal.

Questions

1. Calculate and classify her BMI.
2. What are the required changes in her dietary pattern?
3. What are the lifestyle modifications that you can suggest to her?
4. Do you think her weight loss targets are reasonable, achievable and sustainable?

Answers

1. $$\text{BMI} = \frac{\text{Weight (kg)}}{\text{Height (m}^2)}$$

   $$\frac{67}{1.47 \times 1.47} = 31.0 \text{ kg/m}^2$$

   She is classified as grade 1 obese.
2. It is essential to make her realize the importance of breakfast and explain that skipping breakfast with subsequent overeating during the day could be one of the reasons contributing towards her weight gain. If time is a constraint, then healthy ready to eat or easy to prepare foods like wheat flakes, muesli or oatmeal with fruits, brown bread sandwich can be eaten. Since she eats her lunch regularly at the cafeteria, it is important to educate her to choose healthy foods low in calorie, high in fiber. She should be advised to eat an early, light dinner. Advice on managing the portion size of her meals, with emphasis on small frequent meals should also be provided.
3. The lifestyle changes she can make are:
    - To start doing some form of exercise (walking, running, or jogging) for 60 minutes a day. Additionally, some form of resistance exercise should be prescribed thrice a week. Exercise could aid her in losing weight and preserving muscle mass
    - Undertaking simple measures to decrease sedentary time such as taking stairs instead of the elevator, avoiding usage of vehicle to nearby destinations, gardening, playing with kids
    - Get adequate sleep of about 7–8 hours in the night. Lower sleep duration has shown to be associated with increased body weight and waist circumference.

4. Her goals for weight loss are not realistic and sustainable. She has to be educated on achievable weight loss targets and the importance of weight management after the initial weight loss. Setting unrealistic goals that are not achievable can demotivate an individual on a weight loss regime and make them fall off the band wagon.

> **Important**
>
> Incorporating regular physical activity into the lifestyle is essential for achieving and sustaining weight loss.

Case 3: Gestational Diabetes

A 28-year-old lady in her second trimester of pregnancy is admitted to the hospital with symptoms of gestational diabetes mellitus (GDM). Her oral glucose tolerance test (OGTT) revealed her blood glucose to be 150/130/115 mg/dL, and she currently weighs 68 kg. She has a maternal history of type 2 diabetes. She eats three meals and two light snacks daily. She works from home, which is primarily on her laptop, and is sedentary for the rest of the day except for some light exercise classes every alternate day.

Questions

1. What are the assessments that need to be conducted on this patient to arrive at the energy requirements?
2. Describe the key points that should be considered while planning her diet.
3. She expresses concern about continuing her exercise, what would you suggest her?
4. What are the additional energy and protein requirement for the patient?

Answers

1. The assessment include:
    - Weight history: Weight gain in previous pregnancies (if any), significant weight fluctuations (gain or loss) during present pregnancy, weight fluctuations prior to pregnancy are all recorded
    - Prepregnancy weight: To determine if there is adequate or excess weight gain
    - Physical activity assessment: To assess the physical activity level of the patient

- Dietary assessment: 24-hour recall of a weekday and weekend to capture details on the meal patterns, food preferences and snacking habits.
2. Medical nutrition therapy (MNT) for a patient with GDM should focus on both the maternal and fetal health, providing necessary nutrients for fetal development, maintaining blood sugar levels, preventing ketosis and achieving appropriate weight gain. It is important to:
    - Include late night and early morning snacks to prevent ketosis
    - Provide adequate energy and protein intake to support fetal growth
    - Ensure that micronutrients intake is adequate to support pregnancy.
3. The patient needs to be advised to consult with the treating doctor regarding continuing the exercise. If continuing, care should be taken such that:
    - Strenuous exercise should be avoided
    - A small serving of carbohydrates can be consumed when necessary, before and after exercise to prevent hypoglycemia.
4. The additional requirements are:[1]
    - Energy: 230–280 kcal/day
    - Protein: 5.5 g/day.

Important

Medical nutrition therapy should focus on both maternal and fetal health and to prevent/delay the onset of diabetes, obesity and cardiovascular problems.

Case 4: Type 1 Diabetes

A 14-year-old Indian boy walks into the nutrition clinic with his parents complaining of hypoglycemic episodes during his swimming classes for which he has enrolled recently. He swims for about 1 hour daily with small breaks in between. He was diagnosed with type 1 diabetes at the age of 12 year and has since then been on insulin. This is his first visit to a nutritionist/dietician. His assessment shows:
- Anthropometric data:
    - Height: 153 cm
    - Weight: 46.1 kg
- Biochemical data:
    - Random blood sugar (RBS): 78 mg/dL

- Glycosylated hemoglobin (HbA1c): 6.9%
- Creatinine: 0.6 mg/dL
- Sodium: 143 mEq/L
- Potassium: 4.7 mEq/L
- Serum cholesterol: 200 mg/dL
- Low-density lipoprotein (LDL): 180 mg/dL
- High-density lipoprotein (HDL): 40 mg/dL
- Triglycerides: 410 mg/dL
- Dietary data:
    - Breakfast: 8.00 am; a glass of milk and two slices of bread
    - Lunch at school: 12.30 pm; 1½ cup of vegetable pulao
    - Evening: 4.30 pm; 3–4 biscuits and a glass of milk
    - Dinner: 8.30 pm; 2 chapatti with ½ cup of sambhar

Questions

1. Calculate the energy, protein, and fat requirements of the child.
2. What would you suggest for his hypoglycemic episodes?
3. What dietary modification would you suggest after assessing the biochemical data?
4. What are the key points that you would advise him on?

Answers

1. Following the Indian Council of Medical Research (ICMR), 2010 guidelines:[1]
    - The energy, protein, and fat requirements for a 14-year-old boy are:
        - Energy = 58 kcal/kg/day
        - Protein = 1.14 g/kg/day
        - Fat = 25% of the total energy intake
    - Therefore, the energy requirement would be 46 × 58 = 2,668 kcal/day.
    - Protein requirement would be 46 × 1.14 = 52.4 g.
    - Fat = 25% of the total energy intake = 2668/100 × 25 = 667 kcal
    - 667/9 = 74 g (since 1 g of fat gives 9 kcal)
        - Energy = 2,668 kcal
        - Protein = 52.4 g
        - Fat = 74 g.
2. The suggestion for avoiding hypoglycemic episodes include:
    - The child should be advised to consume about 55–60 g (that is 1–1.5 g/kg) of quick acting carbohydrates like fruit or a sandwich half an hour before he starts his practice. Additionally, replenishing the body with electrolytes and glucose if necessary during practice is important

- Readily digestible form of carbohydrate (like fruit juice, white bread, milk, fruits, and yogurt) should be available for consumption, immediately postpractice to prevent hypoglycemia.
3. Biochemical data assessment shows high triglyceride values, borderline serum cholesterol and low HDL values. Hence, his diet should be modified to decrease the triglycerides, cholesterol and increase HDL cholesterol in the body.
    - The carbohydrate intake from refined carbohydrates such as white bread, rice, pasta should be restricted and replaced by complex carbohydrates like whole wheat, broken wheat and red millet (ragi)
    - Sweets (cakes, pastries, chocolates, candies, Indian sweets, ice creams) should be restricted and consumed only during special occasions
    - Foods rich in omega-3 fatty acids like fish (salmon, mackerel, and sardine), flaxseeds, walnuts, soy products should be included in the diet, as it helps in lowering the triglycerides and increasing the HDL
    - Foods high in saturated fats like red meat, fried foods, butter and cheese should be restricted
    - Bakery items contain trans-fat and should be restricted
    - Include fiber-rich foods such as whole grains, whole cereals, legumes, fruits and vegetables.
4. To ensure maintenance of blood sugar levels and prevention of hypoglycemia, the involvement of the parents of the child in the nutrition care plan is essential. Nutrition education should be provided to understand the disease condition; identify and manage hypoglycemia; adjust insulin doses to match the carbohydrate intake.
    - Advice on the following need to be given:
        o Distribution of carbohydrates consistently throughout the day and inclusion of complex carbohydrates like whole grains [brown rice, wheat, ragi (red millet), whole grain cereals], vegetables, legumes and whole grains
        o Consumption of small frequent meals rather than three large meals
        o Restricting intake of foods rich in fat
        o Monitoring of blood glucose levels and consuming adequate fluids before any physical activity/exercise to prevent hypoglycemia and dehydration
- Regular follow-up sessions to be planned.

Important

Nutrition education for the child should be an ongoing process with the parents/family being involved in the education and treatment plan.

Case 5: Type 2 Diabetes

Ravindra Pandey, aged 64 years, was admitted to the hospital with complains of chest pain, swelling of both feet and fatigability. He was diagnosed with diabetes mellitus 7 years back. Since 2 years, his blood sugars and blood pressure have not been under control. He is retired and is involved with some voluntary service 2–3 times/week. His meal habits are regular (three meals with evening coffee or tea), and he generally eats at home. He drinks alcohol occasionally, but does not smoke. He has gained around 5 kg weight since retirement. His nutritional assessment results are:
- Weight: 87 kg
- Height: 168 cm
- Blood pressure: 180/120 mmHg
- Urine output: 600 mL/day
- He has been advised a diet with fluid restriction of 1.2 L.

Laboratory results
- Fasting blood sugar: 152 mg/dL
- Glycosylated hemoglobin (HbA1c): 7.1%
- Creatinine: 1.4 mg/dL
- Sodium: 137 mEq/L
- Potassium: 5.8 mEq/L
- Blood urea nitrogen: 65 mg/dL.

Questions

1. What are the nutrients that are restricted for this patient?
2. Since the patient has been advised fluid restriction, list down the foods that are considered as fluids and what can be done to reduce his thirst?
3. Do you think regular self-monitoring of blood glucose (SMBG) will help this patient?

Answers

1. The nutrients that are restricted include protein, sodium, potassium, and phosphorous.
    - The dietary plan should be designed to provide enough protein for the body without causing excessive amounts of urea and creatinine. Proteins of high biological value such as eggs, fish, poultry, milk, and legumes should be recommended
    - Since the patient has hyperkalemia (high levels of potassium in blood), potassium should be restricted. Foods rich in potassium include tinned and homemade soups, bananas, avocados, spinach, greens, mushrooms, dried peas, beans, baked beans, potatoes, pumpkin,

chocolate, cocoa, tomato pastes and purees, fruits, vegetable juices, tender coconut water, dried fruit, nuts, seeds, and high-fiber breakfast cereals
- Sodium has to be restricted since the patient is having elevated blood pressure. The intake of sodium should be restricted to 2,400 mg/day. Foods high in salt and sodium include: canned foods, some frozen foods, processed foods such as cheese, fast foods such as pizza, salty snacks such as chips, salted nuts, sauces chutneys, pickles, and any product where baking soda or baking powder is included
- Phosphorus is a mineral found in many foods and is excreted through kidneys. Dietary sources of phosphorus are bran of rice and oats, wheat germ, soyabean, processed meats, flaxseeds, sesame seeds, milk and its products like curds, ice cream, cheese, nuts like groundnuts, almonds, cashews, and beverages containing phosphates or phosphoric acid.

2. Foods that are considered as fluids are soups, milk, coffee, tea, ice creams, fruit juices, buttermilk, lassi, soft drinks, alcohol, etc. To keep thirst under control the following may be helpful to the patient:
   - Gargling with ice-cold water
   - Sucking an ice cube
   - Sipping small amounts throughout the day
   - Using smaller cups/glasses while drinking fluids.
3. Yes, SMBG will help this patient as it is an important component of diabetic therapy. Regular monitoring of blood sugars will help:
   - The doctors in deciding the treatment regime
   - In recognizing hypoglycemia and hyperglycemia
   - In better glycemic control
   - The patient to adjust dietary and physical activity plan according to the blood glucose levels on a regular basis.

Important

Treatment should focus not only to control blood sugars, but also to prevent any complications and comorbidities.

Reference

1. National Institute of Nutrition. (2009). Nutrient Requirements and Recommended Dietary Allowances for Indians: A Report of the Expert Group of the Indian Council of Medical Research. [online] Available from: icmr.nic.in/final/RDA-2010.pdf. [Accessed August, 2014].

Index

Page numbers followed by *f* refer to figure and *t* refer to table.

A

Air displacement plethysmography 24
   validity of 25
Alcohol intake 43, 112
American Diabetic Association 120
Anemia 130
Anthropometry 13
Artificial sweeteners 96

B

Barker hypothesis 44
Basal
   energy expenditure 3*f*
   metabolic rate 2, 3, 8, 68
Bioelectrical impedance analysis 27, 28
Blood
   cholesterol 132*t*
   pressure 17
Body
   composition 4, 20
   fat estimation 16
   mass index 14, 21, 36, 92, 117, 140
      classification of 14*t*
   size 4
   weight 23
Bone mass 23
Boyle's law 25

C

Calculating daily energy requirements 59
Caralluma fimbriata 139
Carbohydrate 109
   intake 94, 120
Cardiovascular disease 107, 111, 121, 128, 131
Carotid artery intima-media thickness 98
Cognitive behavioral therapy 80
Complementary and alternative medicine 136, 137
Cushing's syndrome 17

D

Diabetes 17, 40, 121, 136
   mellitus 52
   prevention program 41
Diabetic
   ketoacidosis 125
   nephropathy 126
   neuropathy 131
Dietary
   assessment methods 19*t*
   calcium 65
   data 17
   fat 111
      types of 132*t*
   fiber 41, 64, 109, 110
Direct calorimetry 5
Disease control and prevention 15
Doubly labelled water 5, 6
Dual energy X-ray absorptiometry 22, 27
   validity of 27
Dyslipidemia 107

E

Energy
  Expenditure
    components of 3
    measurements of 5
  medicine 141
  requirement 1, 2, 127
  therapies 137

F

Fasting blood glucose 17
Fat
  free mass 4, 21, 23
  intake 42, 98
Fluid intake 130
Food and
  agricultural association 8
  drug association 110
Formulating meal plan 100

G

Gestational
  diabetes mellitus 116-118
  weight gain 10
Glomerular filtration rate 127
Glycemic
  control 132
  index 37, 42, 62, 95, 97t, 99, 110, 120

H

Heart rate monitoring 5, 6
High
  density lipoprotein 17, 69, 128, 132
  protein diets 61
Hydrodensitometry 23, 24
  validity of 24
Hydrometry 26
  validity of 26
Hyperglycemia 125
Hyperlipidemia 17
Hypertension 17, 107, 132, 133
Hypoglycemia 126
Hypothyroidism 17

I

Indian Council of Medical
  Research 7, 8

International obesity task force
  standards 15
Intrauterine growth
  retardation 44
Isotope dilution method 26

L

Lagenaria siceraria 143
Loss of skeletal muscle lipoprotein
  lipase 69
Low
  calorie diets 59
  carbohydrate diet 61, 108
  density lipoprotein 37, 132, 142
  fat diet 61, 107
  glycemic index diets 62

M

Maintenance of weight loss 63
Medical nutrition therapy 51, 92, 106,
  117, 125
Metabolic syndrome 17
Micronutrients 43, 111
Mind-body medicine 137, 140
Momordica charantia
  abreviata 143

N

Nephropathy 107
Neutron activation analysis 22
Non-nutritive sweeteners 96
Non-starch polysaccharide 36, 41
Nutrients 36
Nutrition in complications of
  diabetes 125
Nutritional management 54, 93, 127,
  131

O

Obesity 40, 80, 84, 107, 121, 136
  abdominal 40
  and diabetes, nutritional management
    of 51
  nutritional management of 51
Osteopathic manipulative
  medicine 141
  treatment 141

P

Phosphate restriction 130
Plethysmography 25*f*
Polycystic ovarian syndrome 17
Polyunsaturated fatty acid 61, 98
Postprandial blood glucose 17
Potassium
    content of foods 129*t*
    restriction 128
Premature coronary heart disease 131
Protein 110
    intake 37, 96
    requirement 127

R

Resting metabolic rate 3, 58, 69

S

Serum triglycerides 17
Skinfold measurements 29
Sodium restriction 128
Strategies for diabetes prevention 41
Substituted monounsaturated fats 94
Sucrose 110

T

Tapas acupuncture technique 142
Thermic effect of food 3
Thyroid stimulating hormone 17

Total body
    bone mineral 27
    mineral/body weight 23
    water/body weight 21
Total energy expenditure 2
    measurements of 1
Total testosterone 17
Traditional Chinese medicine 137, 142
Type 1 diabetes mellitus 91, 93*t*, 99
Type 2 diabetes 107, 107*t*
    mellitus 91, 106, 125, 138

U

United Nations University 8
Urinary albumin excretion 128

V

Very low-calorie liquid diet 60, 107, 108
Vitamin 111
    and micronutrients 98

W

Waist
    circumference 15, 15*t*, 40
    hip ratio 16, 40
Weight
    gain 40, 119
    management 107
Wier's equation 5